NATURE'S MEDICINE

Plants That Heal

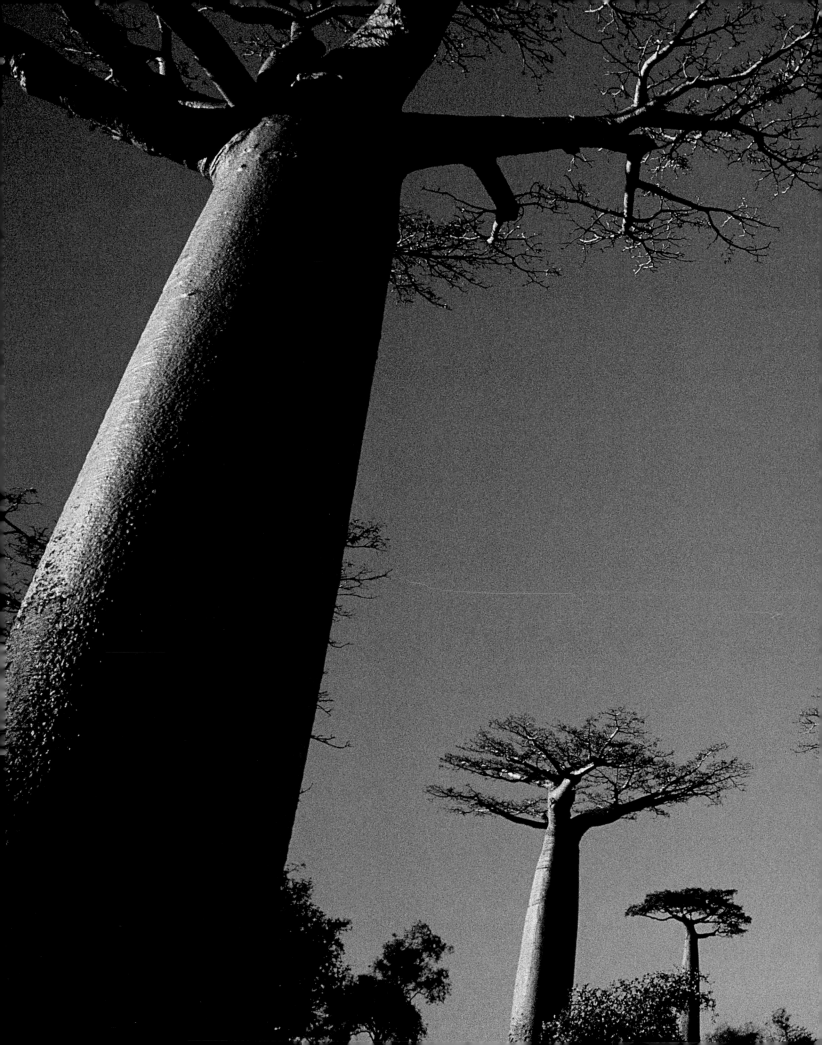

NATURE'S MEDICINE
Plants That Heal

BY JOEL L. SWERDLOW, PH.D.

PHOTOGRAPHS BY LYNN JOHNSON

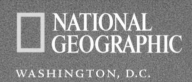

WASHINGTON, D.C.

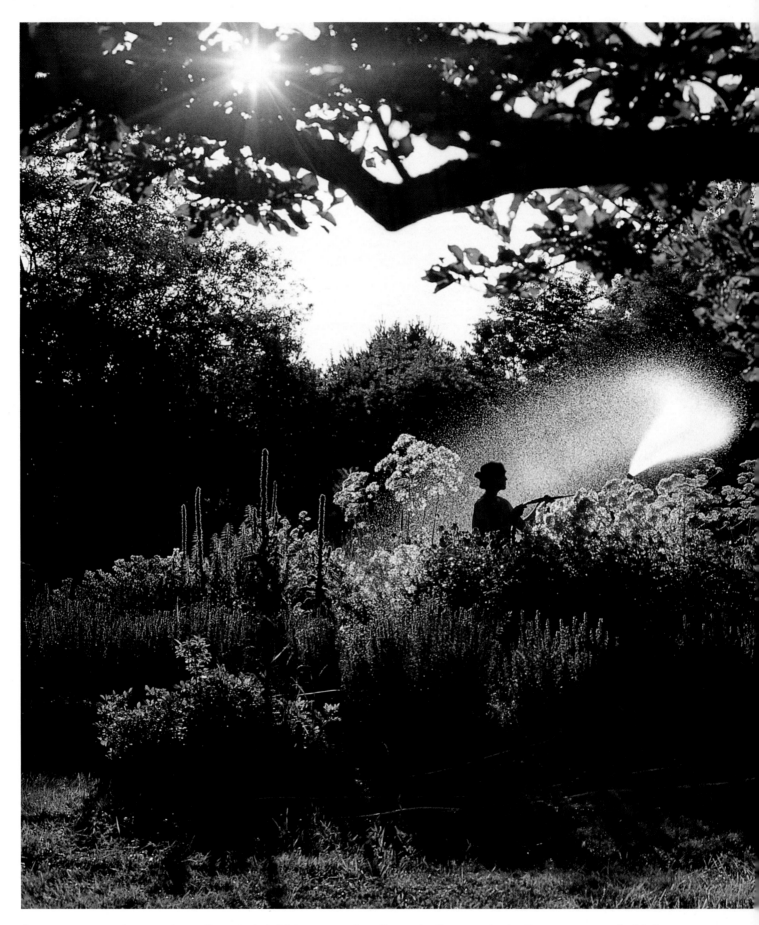

A woman waters plants at Avena Botanicals in Maine, a supplier of organically grown herbs. PRECEDING PAGES: In Madagascar a man

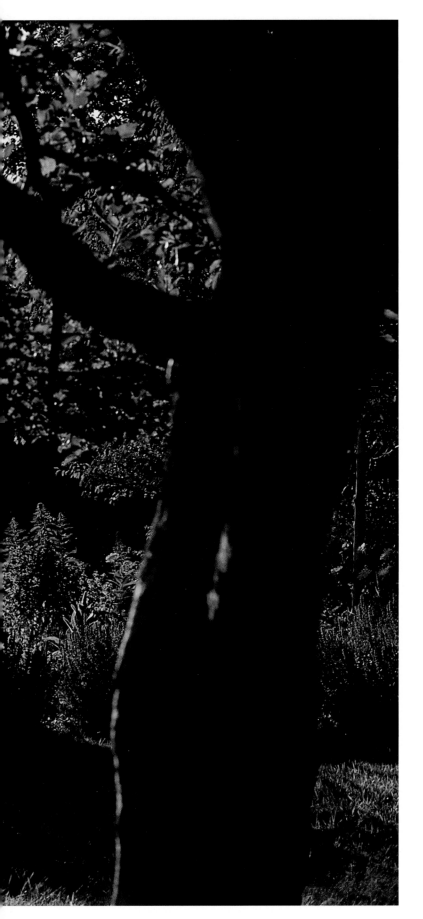

DEDICATED WITH LOVE TO MARJORIE L. SHARE

CONTENTS

harvests bark from a baobab tree; the people use it to treat back pain.

A Plant That Cures

My brother, Paul, was a doctor at one of America's leading medical centers. On April 4, 1984, he collapsed while making rounds. The diagnosis was acute myelogenous leukemia. Although Paul knew that modern medicine had little to offer, he faced his new reality with grace and a determination to live.

During long days in the hospital with Paul I witnessed leukemia treatment firsthand. It was, to say the least, rough. One of the things I learned was that a plant, the Madagascar rosy periwinkle, had yielded chemicals that cure most cases of acute lymphocytic leukemia, also known as childhood leukemia, an uncontrolled growth of primitive lymphatic cells. Surely, I thought, a plant somewhere must cure Paul's leukemia, which involved the bone marrow. But to this day modern science has found no such plant.

On February 28, 1985, Paul died. The image of other plants like the rosy periwinkle stayed with me. Madagascar has more than 10,000 known plant species, perhaps 70 or 80 percent of which are indigenous. Yet no plant indigenous only to Madagascar other than the rosy periwinkle has contributed to any drug approved by the U.S. Food and Drug Administration (FDA).

When I tried to find out why, research quickly revealed that the question far transcended Madagascar. Although 25 to 50 percent of prescription drugs in the industrialized world come from plants, no new drug has come out of the Amazon forests beyond those based on plants brought to Europe by the conquistadores and their successors more than 300 years ago.

No modern pharmaceutical drug, with one possible exception, is based on Native Americans' use of plants; only one comes from Ayurveda, India's ancient medical system; and only two drugs come out of China's massive plant pharmacopoeia. And in the past 40 years the FDA has approved fewer than a dozen plant-based drugs.

A decade after my brother's death I traveled to Madagascar for the NATIONAL GEOGRAPHIC article that grew into this book. I hoped to find, amid its wildlife and its traditional healers, an understanding of how we might better take advantage of what plants offer.

I rented a four-wheel-drive vehicle and drove across the island, accompanied by Nat Quansah, an ethnobotanist who is an expert in Madagascar's medicinal plants. In Antananarivo, Madagascar's capital, Philippe Rasoanaivo, a Western-trained pharmacological researcher, told me about a rural healer who had a reputation for collecting plants that could work wonders with cancer.

The healer lived far to the south, but Philippe had gone to see him. The journey had taken two days, much of it traveling by bullock cart in areas with no roads. The area was so isolated that the healer spoke only a local dialect of Malagasy.

The healer provided leaves from a plant that he described to Philippe as good for *omamiadana*, which roughly translates to "killing little by little"—cancer. Once back at his laboratory, Philippe sent the leaves to a pharmaceutical company in Switzerland. Months later the company wrote back with its test results: The leaves were extremely effective against cancer. Swiss researchers were excited, and so Philippe went back to see the healer in southern Madagascar. The healer, fearful that his secrets would be stolen, refused to give him any more leaves. So Philippe, accompanied by a Malagasy botanist, picked some on his own.

Philippe was confident because he had watched the healer carefully and had saved a few of the original leaves. The Swiss pharmaceutical company found, however, that this second batch of leaves showed no anticancer activity. Some variable that was detected only by the healer had effected the plant's chemical output.

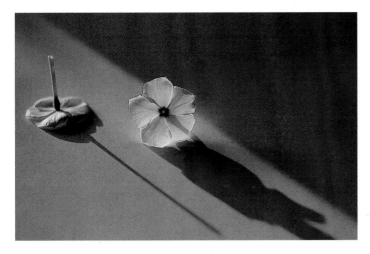

Drugs from the Madagascar rosy periwinkle cure childhood leukemia and some other cancers. The herb's power raises a question: Why do we get so few medicines from plants?

This story was my first lesson on why so few pharmaceutical drugs—prescription medicines approved by government regulators—have come from plants. No pharmaceutical company is likely to invest research monies in a plant it may not be able to obtain and whose chemical content may not be medically effective. Madagascar, however, awakened me to a much broader perspective—one that takes better advantage of all that plants have to offer.

My awakening began as I sat on the dirt floor in the thatch-roofed home of an elderly woman who was the healer in a remote village.

On straw mats surrounding her were sticks, leaves, grasses, bark, wood chips, oils, seeds, and nuts. People in her village, like nearly two-thirds of the world's 6.1 billion people, cannot afford Western pharmaceutical drugs and must rely on plant-based traditional medicine.

As I watched the healer use plants to treat everything from colds to cancerous tumors, I began to realize that my focus on government-approved pharmaceutical drugs was far too narrow.

For years, my wife, Marjorie Share, and others had been telling me how Western medicine—which only uses drugs with one active ingredient—had forgotten and overlooked powerful plant chemicals that affect a huge range of human ailments. Some of these chemicals, they claimed, even stimulate the human immune system, something modern medicine has not yet managed to accomplish. These people seemed to work hard to find accurate and useful information, reading books, seeking studies, and telling each other about physicians and other healers who knew about herbs.

I began to wonder: How much of what I had heard back at home and of what I was seeing in this far corner of the world was wishful thinking, and how much had some foundation in fact—whether or not scientifically proven?

Then I experienced what some people call the "Aha! moment."

In a hospital ward in eastern Madagascar, young children lay dying of malaria. For many, treatment with chloroquine, the most effective modern antimalarial drug, was useless because the parasite that causes malaria had developed resistance to it. But local traditional healers had identified several plants that allowed the chloroquine to work. The plants somehow seemed to overcome the parasite's ability to keep the medicine from permeating its outer cell wall.

How had the traditional healers known the plants would do this? They certainly had not learned it over centuries of trial and error, because chloroquine had been on the island for at most a few decades.

Where, furthermore, does such plant power originate, why do plants have it, and why should any plant produce chemicals—whether used as a pharmaceutical drug or a botanical remedy—that cure a human disease? Why, in the words of William Shakespeare, do herbs possess such "powerful grace?"

I returned home from Madagascar realizing how much I had yet to learn.

That is why I wrote this book.

I hope it provides some answers, raises new questions, and offers a framework for understanding a fast-changing topic that increasingly generates news headlines and sales revenues. Together, Americans and Europeans now spend billions of dollars annually on botanical remedies, a total that rises dramatically each year.

The time to focus on medicinal plants is now. Amid some incorrect assumptions—such as the widely held belief that "we are now getting most of our pharmaceutical drugs from plants"—growing scientific knowledge, public pressure, and economic forces are making extraordinary advances in how we use medicinal plants.

To shape a future that utilizes the full potential of medicines from plants, we must first understand where we are and how we got here.

Chemicals From Plants

The story of plant chemicals started about 1.5 billion years ago, when algae first evolved in the ocean. About 435 to 500 million years ago the first known land plants began to appear in wet mud at the edge of bodies of fresh water. Once on land, plants enjoyed access to more sunlight, carbon dioxide, and minerals, which they transformed into stored sugars and oxygen.

As millions of years passed, plants grew in size and differentiated. Their evolution escalated about 375 million years ago, when many began to rely on two types of spores, male and female, for reproduction. The next major step was the appearance of gymnosperms, seed-producing plants such as present-day pine trees. Further sophistication came with angiosperms, or flowering plants, which enclose their seeds in an ovary, usually encased inside a flower. This development occurred about 150 million years ago, relatively recently in evolutionary terms. The appearance of angiosperms seems to have been sudden; they quickly dominated other plants and became one of the most widespread life-forms. After studying fossil evidence, Charles Darwin supposedly called flowering plants an "abominable mystery." It is one students of evolution still have not deciphered.

Until the 1990s scientists thought that most of the chemicals produced by flowering and other plants were useless waste products of the plants' basic metabolism. They called these chemicals secondary metabolites to distinguish them from primary metabolites such as sugars and amino acids that are essential for functions such as absorbing water. But we now know that secondary metabolites perform a huge array of functions.

Many chemicals in flowering plants, in fact, became more sophisticated than those of animals, which can rely on sensory organs. Instead of eyes, for example, flowering plants developed proteins in light-sensitive compounds that collect clumps of light energy. Such chemical sensory devices extend throughout a plant's contact with the outside world. Plant roots detect nitrates and ammonium salts in the soil, elements vital to their growth, and move toward them. To help with reproduction, other chemicals attract animals that serve as pollinators. Unable to run away, and faced with microbes, insects, and animals that wanted to eat them, plants also developed an arsenal of bioactive substances—compounds that affect living cells—with which to wage chemical warfare.

This sophisticated arsenal often includes chemical communications. Sensing the arrival of a disease-causing virus, some plants release chemicals that begin to protect their leaves and travel through the air to alert nearby plants of the approaching virus. Neighboring plants receive this message and start to generate their own defensive chemicals. In another example, a plant may sense from a caterpillar's saliva that its leaves are being eaten. If the caterpillar is a species that is particularly destructive, the plant issues substances that summon a wasp. The wasp lays eggs in the caterpillar, which kill it when they hatch.

This bioactivity makes many plant chemicals harmful to humans. Evidence indicates that early hominids—mammals who walked on two legs and had opposable thumbs—appeared about five to six million years ago. Hominids, who ate numerous plants, needed enzymes to counteract plant toxins. They developed genes that produce such enzymes, which helps explain some of the fundamental genetic variations among humans today.

Bioactivity also suggests why a plant like the rosy periwinkle combats acute lymphocytic leukemia. The periwinkle produces chemicals to kill its enemies. That these chemicals impede a particular kind of cancer seems to be a coincidence—but then, Aristotle warned that "nature does nothing without a purpose."

To obtain medicines from complex and frequently dangerous plant chemicals required experimentation. "The first fellow that picked an herb to cure himself had a bit of pluck," James Joyce noted in *Ulysses*. All forms of hominids probably experimented with plants. Archaeologists have found pollen from at least eight species of flowers in the dirt of a Neandertal burial cave in Iraq that dates back 60,000 years. All eight species are still found in Iraq, and seven are traditionally used to treat wounds, dysentery, asthma, inflammation, toothache, and other ailments.

The eight Iraqi flowers do not grow together naturally; they had to be collected into a bouquet. Were they left because they were beautiful, or did whoever left them know about the flowers' medicinal value? Was one of the bodies buried in the cave a healer?

———

By 30,000 years ago Neandertals and other hominids had given way to *Homo sapiens*, or modern humans. As hunter-gatherer nomads, humans used plants for food, medicine, clothing, shelter, and weapons. About 11,000 years ago, during what is called the agricultural revolution, humans began to cultivate certain plants, particularly those that produce grain.

Of all these uses of plants, only the medicinal evoked a deep spiritual response from humans, for whom the medicine man was almost always a spiritual leader. Plants, according to ancient beliefs, are the mediators between humans and the Creator, and often can grant eternal life. In the *Epic of Gilgamesh*, a Sumerian prose poem dating from before 2000 B.C., a god tells the hero, who has just arrived at the mouth of the rivers at the ends of the Earth, "Gilgamesh, you came here exhausted and worn out. What can I give you so you can return to your land? I will disclose to you a thing that is hidden.…There is a plant…whose thorns will prick your hand like a rose. If your hands reach that plant you will become a young man again."

Gilgamesh decides to test the plant, but he and his ferryman stop to eat some food. The story continues: "Gilgamesh went down and was bathing in the water. A snake smelled the fragrance of the plant, silently came up and carried off the plant."

Gilgamesh was the best known story in the Middle East at the time of the events recorded in the Bible. Its influence is evident in descriptions of the Garden of Eden, where the snake reappears, boasting about a fruit that grows on the "tree of knowledge of good and evil." Eat it and you become immortal, the snake promises. The fruit of another tree, the "tree of life," says the snake, makes you "live forever." These two trees, in turn, appear in the Koran, the holy book of Islam, which has its own Garden of Eden story.

Chinese myths that date back thousands of years likewise describe Penglai, Fangzhang, and Yingzhou, islands with palaces of gold and silver, pure white birds and animals, and magic herbs that provide immortality. More recently, a Han epic from the 4th to 5th centuries A.D. mentions the "herb of deathlessness." This herb, according to legend, "seems to have the form of sprouts of water-grass, [with leaves] three to four feet long. If this plant is laid upon a man who has been dead for [as much as] three days, he will come to life again at once. If it is eaten, it will give longevity and immortality."

———

The medicinal relationship between plants and humans was, of course, far more than spiritual. Collecting medicinal plants and trying to learn about them are among mankind's oldest professions. Desire for medicinal plants, furthermore, has been fundamental to commercial trade. As soon as people anywhere established contact with other societies, one of their first activities was to exchange medicinal plants and knowledge about them.

Known written records about medicinal plants date back at least 5,000 years to the Sumerians, who lived in Mesopotamia; the Babylonians, another Mesopotamian civilization, which dates to the second millennium B.C.; and the Egyptians, whose Nile River-based culture began to flourish around 3000 B.C.

Two other ancient civilizations, in India and China, are still thriving after thousands of years and continue to mystify modern science. They offer lessons that could be invaluable as Westerners try to obtain more pharmaceutical drugs from plants and attempt to better understand herbal medicine.

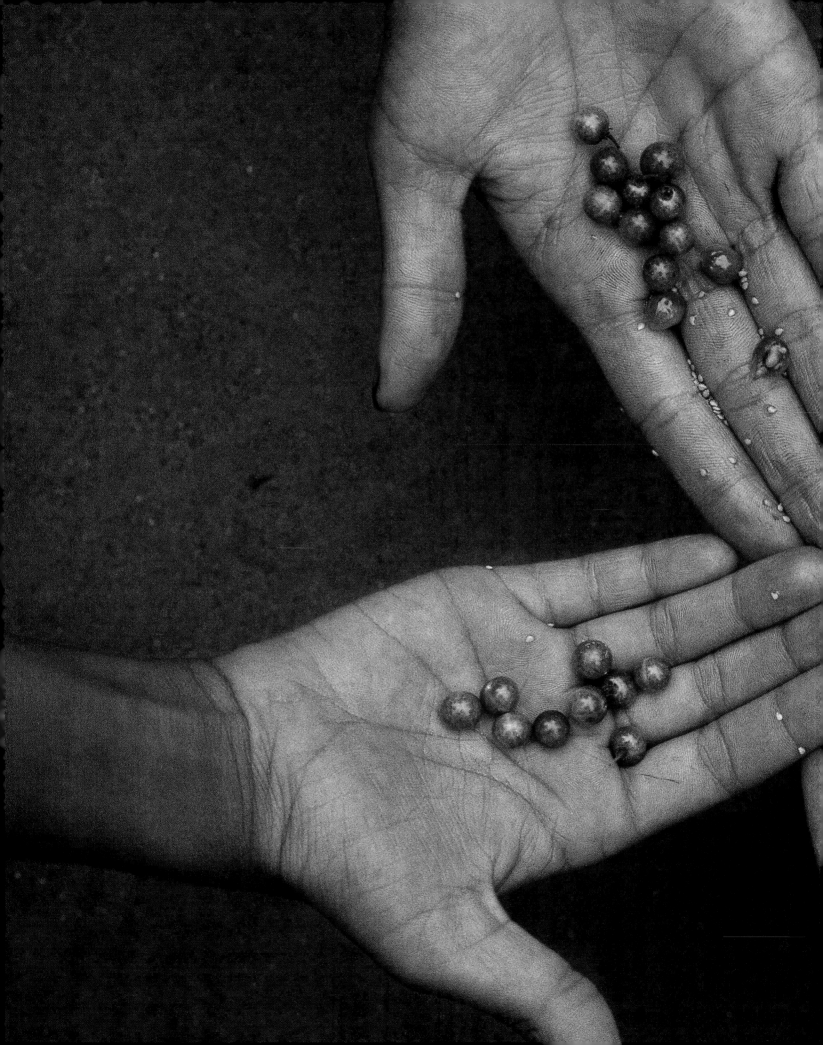

ANCIENT CIVILIZATIONS
TO THE
BIRTH
OF MODERN
SCIENCE

CHAPTER ONE

Herbal Medicine of India and China

In late 1998 *JAMA*, the *Journal of the American Medical Association*, published a study examining how the herb mugwort, when allowed to smolder on the little toe of pregnant women (and removed before it became too hot), affected fetuses in the dangerous breech position. Researchers tested the ancient Chinese practice of burning mugwort on a designated acupuncture point to cause the fetuses to move into a safer headfirst orientation.

"It is bizarre," said Dr. George Lundberg, then *JAMA* editor, in describing the results of the study. Seventy-five percent of fetuses carried by women who experienced the burning mugwort moved to a headfirst position. Of the fetuses carried by women in a control group that did not receive the mugwort treatment, a significantly lower number—48 percent—moved to a headfirst position.

The pharmacy of a hospital of traditional medicine, one of many in China, stores blossoms, seeds, and bark. Employees combine the ingredients of each tray and boil them to make cough medicine.

PRECEDING PAGES: Five young girls in Coimbatore, in southern India, hold seeds they will brew into a cough treatment. The girls grow dozens of plants in small kitchen gardens that provide herbal remedies for family use. Such remedies, some of which have surprised modern science with their effectiveness, date back thousands of years.

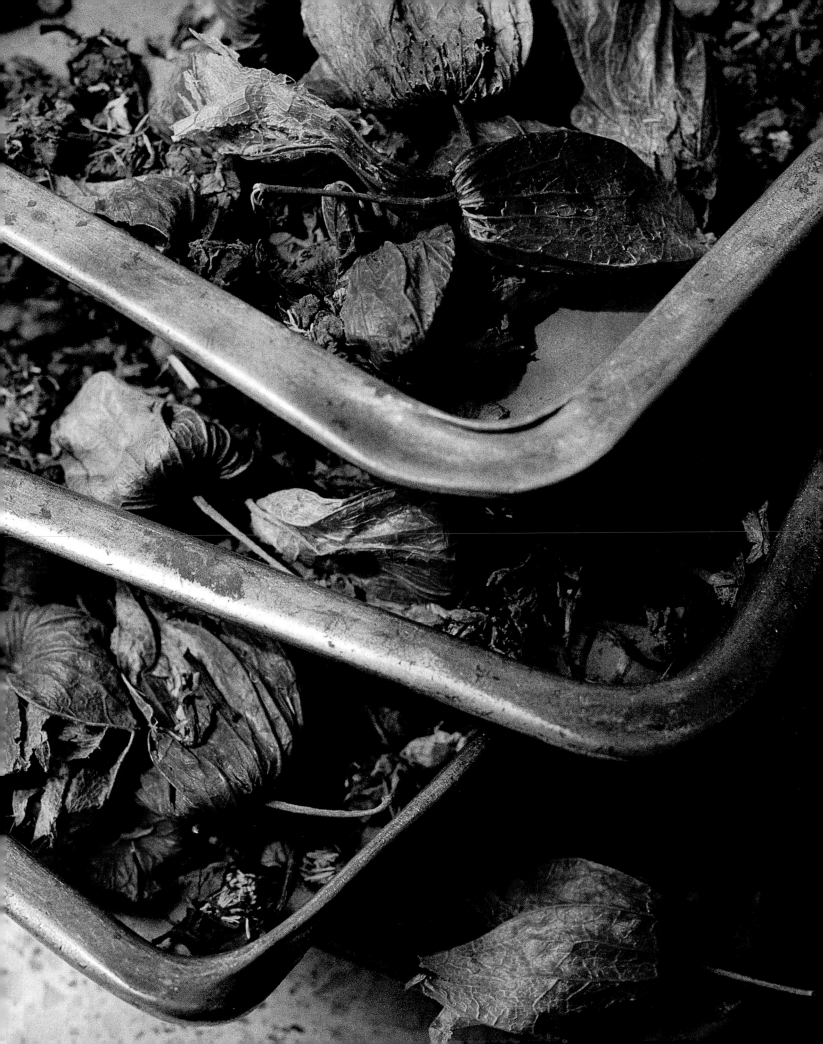

VARIOUS STORIES, describing events that occurred thousands of years before recorded human history, explain the origins of Ayurvedic medicine, the ancient Indian system of maintaining health and fighting disease. In these stories knowledge was transferred from a god to a virtuous sage. Often this sage then, himself, became a god, using his medicinal knowledge as a vehicle.

In one version, Brahma, the creator-god aspect of the Hindu trinity of Brahma, Vishnu, and Siva, passed this "wisdom of long life" to other gods, including Indra, god of storms and battles. Brahma heard the appeals from a group of enlightened sages who were meditating in an effort to find ways to end human suffering and, impressed by their sincerity, revealed the secrets of medicines.

According to tradition, these secrets were passed on in the form of hymns, prayers, incantations, chants, and ritual formulas that included information about how to use plants. The first known written versions of these stories, recorded in Sanskrit, are called the Vedic texts and consist of the *Rig Veda*, *Sama Veda*, *Yajur Veda*, and *Atharva Veda*.

Archaeological evidence dates the origin of these Vedic texts to the second millennium B.C., when nomadic Aryan tribes from north of the Black Sea entered southern Asia through the mountain passes of present-day Afghanistan. These stories, archaeologists say, remained oral for centuries before being written down in stages beginning around 1200 B.C. The *Rig Veda* discusses healing in a spiritual context. The father of mankind, named Manu, offers the source of all healing medicines—*soma*—to the gods. The medicines, described as "so pure, so strengthening, so comforting," include plants.

In a scene that captures the heart of the Vedic attitude toward plants, a doctor prepares to treat someone who is seriously ill. After meditating on 107 healing herbs, the doctor blesses them and then blesses the patient. The doctor praises him "in whom the plants gather like kings in the assembly" and expresses his hope that "the plants have driven out whatever wound was in the body" and that "flying down from the sky, the plants spoke: that man shall not be harmed…."

Addressing a plant he is about to use, the doctor says, "You are supreme, a remedy for need and a blessing for the heart." Then the doctor speaks to all plants, asking them to come to the aid of their compatriot about to be enrolled in medicinal duty: "You growing plants who hear this, and those who have gone far away, all coming together, unite your power in this plant."

The plants answer, "Whomever the Brahmin priest treats, we will carry him across…." That the plants address the doctor as "Brahmin priest" highlights the close relationship between spirituality and healing in Vedic tradition.

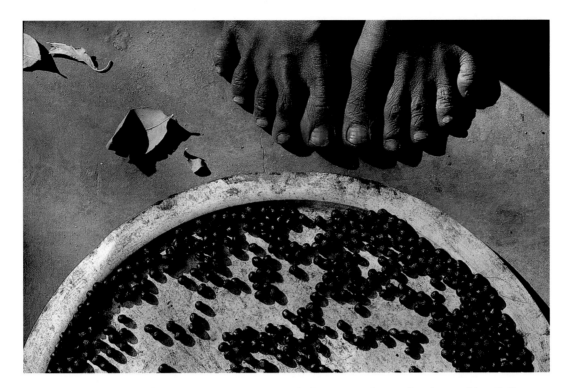

A tray of tarlike *kayakalpa vati* pills sits at a worker's feet at an Ayurvedic clinic in New Delhi. Workers cook ingredients over an open fire, then fashion each tablet by rotating the sticky substance between their palms. Dried in the sun, then packaged, the pills are used as a rejuvenating potion for a variety of illnesses.

Detailed references to plant-based medicines are not found in the Vedic texts, hymns, and other ritual texts. However, writing about specific plant prescriptions dates from at least the seventh century B.C. The practice seems to have been adopted and compiled by Buddhist monks around the fourth century B.C., not long after the Buddha himself wandered through northeast India.

———

THE WORD *AYURVEDA*, a combination of the Sanskrit words for "life" and "knowledge," may have been coined in the fourth century B.C. to associate these plant remedies and recipes with the *Rig Veda* and other basic Vedic texts. Ayurvedic remedies and recipes are quite specific. The bark from the dita tree, a tall evergreen cultivated throughout India, is used to treat malaria, chronic diarrhea, fevers, and skin diseases. The fruit of the bael tree relieves diarrhea, dysentery, and intestinal problems; its roots treat melancholia and heart palpitations; and its leaves can be used as a poultice to reduce inflammation. Two types of pigweed—red-flowered and white-flowered—are used to treat anemia, heart disease, cough, intestinal colic, and snakebite. Red-flowered pigweed also treats insomnia, rheumatism, and chronic alcoholism.

The first known Sanskrit medical treatises with detailed analyses of treatment date approximately from between 200 B.C. and A.D. 200. The *Caraka Samhita* describes uses for 500 medicinal plants, and the *Sushrata Samhita* shows how to use 760.

These plants form the core of Ayurvedic medicine, *(Continued on page 20)*

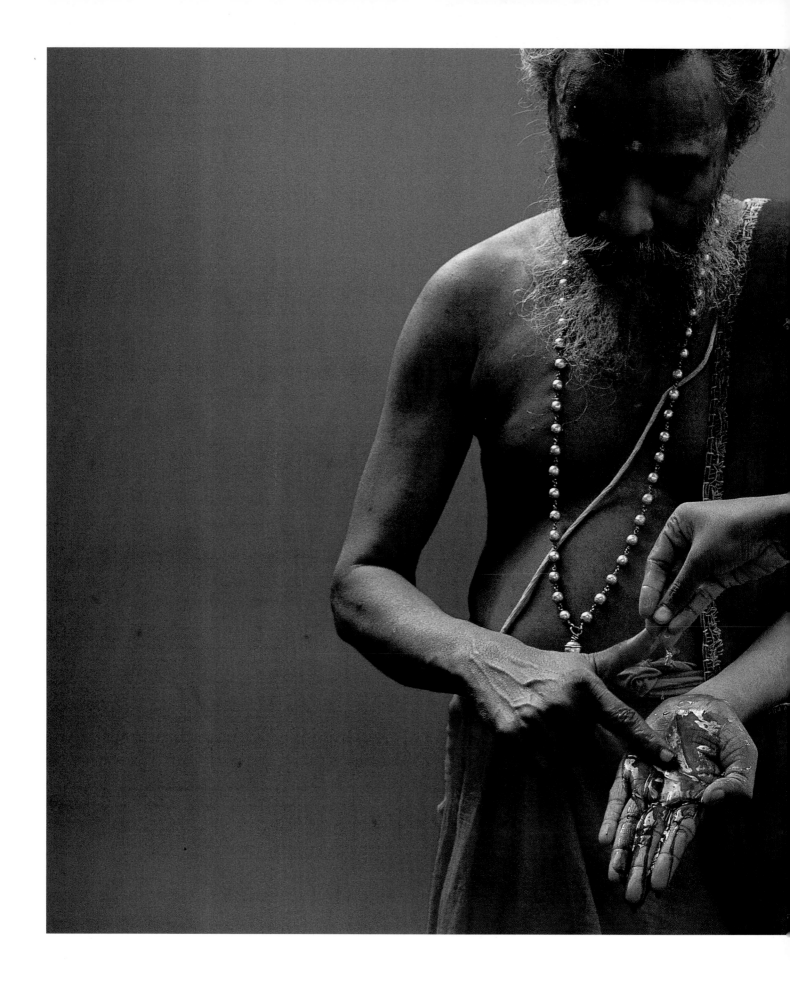

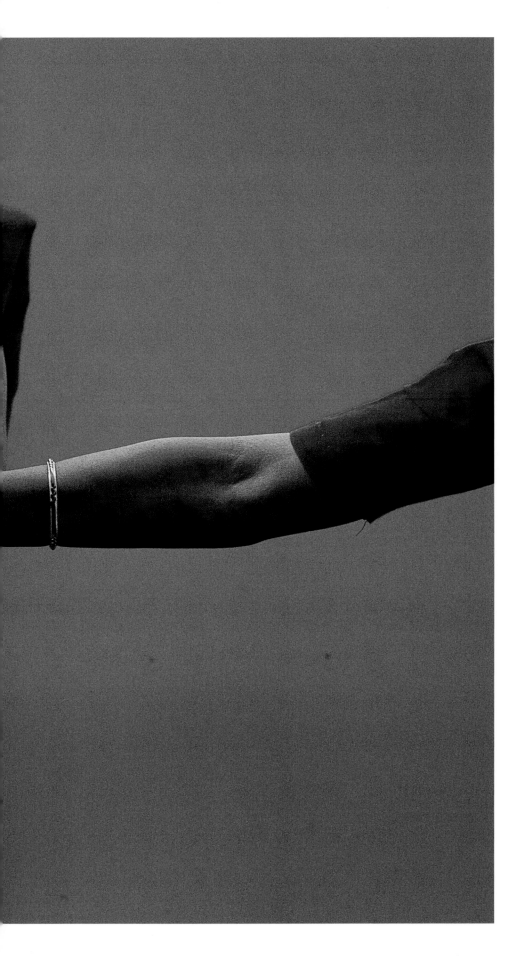

Swami Brahmananda, a Siddha healer in Bangalore, India, tests a combination of minerals and herbs that have been mixed together and heated. Siddha, an ancient medical system of the Tamil culture in southern India, uses herbs to reduce the toxic effect of metals such as iron and gold in remedies. Preparing a Siddha remedy can take up to 30 days, following rules written centuries ago on the pages of a book made of palm leaves. In Siddha belief, as in northern India's Ayurvedic medicine, healers are holy men.

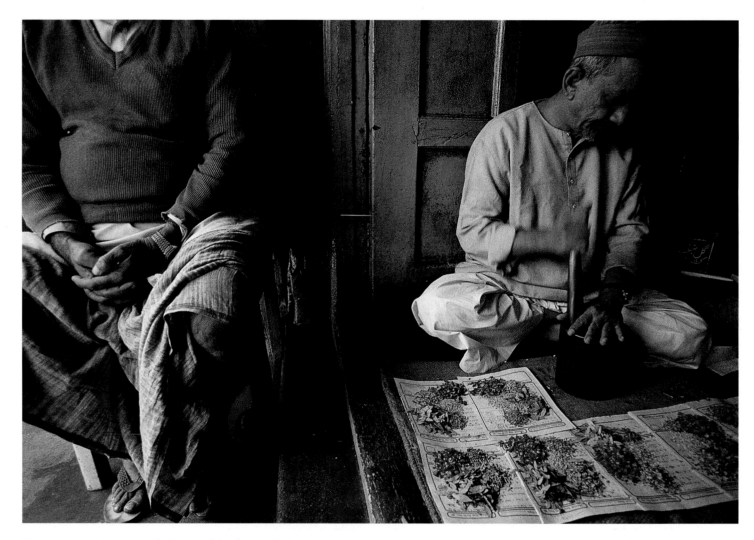

For 30 years Muzzamur Rahman of Lucknow, India, has prepared medicines according to the centuries-old traditions he learned from his father in this same shop. Rahman combines a variety of plant and animal parts, as well as minerals, in each formula. A patient waits while he makes a week's worth of packets to treat a common cold; each will be boiled and drunk as a tea.

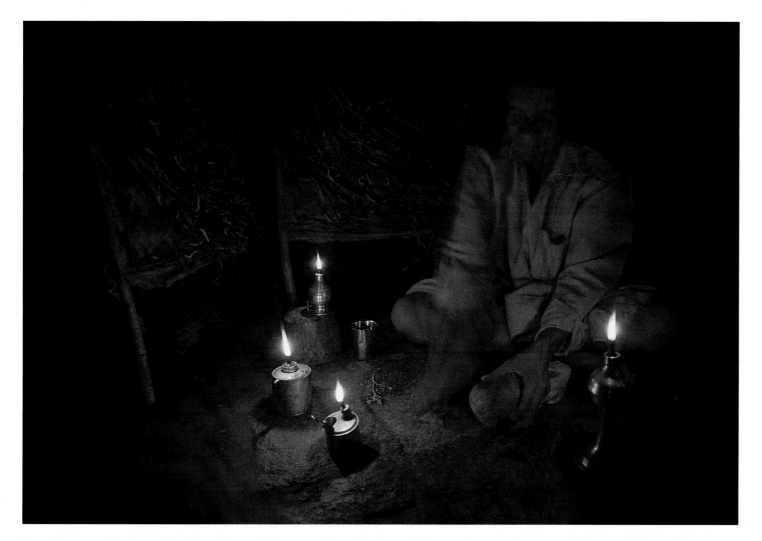

In a village outside Bangalore, in southern India, a traditional healer grinds one of seven plants he combines to help snakebite victims. Elements of the plants may chemically interact with components of the venom and may trigger responses such as increased blood pressure or muscle contractions that could help a person survive a snakebite. In such poor rural areas cost or distance from a medical facility often precludes the use of a modern antivenom. Like all healers, this one accepts occasional gifts, usually food, but receives no cash payment for his services. Mulberry leaves and silkworms, his main source of income, line panels behind him.

which also uses animal parts such as bones and gallstones, and minerals such as sulfur, arsenic, lead, copper sulfate, and gold. Extensive and complex procedures are used to elicit nontoxic and therapeutic material from these substances.

Influenced by Arab medicine—which, for example, introduced opium to India as a treatment for dysentery—the golden age of Ayurvedic medicine continued until approximately A.D. 1000. During that time Indian scientists accurately described the circulation of blood in the human body. Surgeons removed tumors and performed cesarean sections and plastic surgery, practices not common in Europe until the advent of what we now call the scientific revolution in the 16th to 18th centuries.

Indian scientists realized that microbes exist and that they can be found in the human body, but did not associate them with disease. Instead, their approach was essentially preventive, stressing that the key to health is to live in balance with all of nature. To achieve this balance, Ayurveda—which is still widely practiced in India and worldwide—says that the body cannot be healed without healing the mind and spirit. Ayurveda emphasizes that medicine must focus on the whole person, and not simply on symptoms.

Humans, Ayurveda asserts, have one of three body types, and associated with each type are some of the five elements (earth, fire, water, air, and space) that make up the universe. These body types are *vata* (wind—air and space); *pitta* (fire and water); and *kapha* (earth and water). No matter what its type, according to Ayurveda, each body has 13 *srotas*, or channels through which substances circulate. The channels can be large, like intestines and arteries, or small, like capillaries. If the srotas are open and free-flowing, the person is healthy, while blockage—usually by improperly digested food and liquids—often produces disease. Diagnosis, usually accomplished by interviewing patients and taking their pulses, consists of determining the nature of any imbalance among the five basic elements.

After making a diagnosis, an Ayurvedic physician will probably recommend appropriate changes in sleep and eating habits. Medicines, most consisting of a dozen or more plants and other substances, are suggested. These prescriptions and their dosages can vary among patients with the same symptoms. Unlike Western medicine, Ayurvedic often has no standard treatments.

As in ancient times, prescriptions are prepared in a wide variety of ways. The plant parts might be boiled together and given as a decoction, the material that remains after much of the water has boiled away. The ingredients might be infused, steeped in water to get soluble properties without bringing about the chemical changes that could come

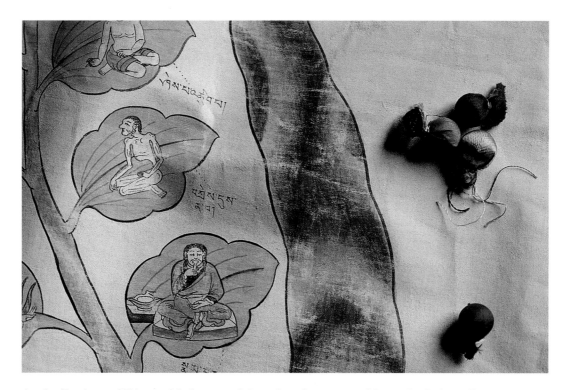

At the Traditional Tibetan Medicine and Astrology Institute in Dharmala, India, pills rest on an ancient Tibetan medical text. Pharmacists wrap each pill in the color of silk that indicates its healing properties: Red works on the heart, and blue affects the mind. Employees who make the medicine pray as they labor, believing that their devotions and positive spiritual intentions make the medicine more pure, and perhaps more powerful.

with boiling. The plant parts might be allowed to ferment. They might be given when freshly picked or after aging. The patient might take them as a warm tea, a cold drink, a liquid extract, and more commonly as ground herbs in a pill or as a powder.

THE GREATEST THREAT to Ayurvedic medicine has come from invasions. Muslims imposed their beliefs and practices on parts of India they conquered in the 11th and 12th centuries, and Great Britain ruled the subcontinent as a colony from the mid-17th to the mid-20th centuries. The British prohibited funding of Ayurvedic colleges and clinics, outlawed the publishing or sale of Ayurvedic textbooks, and depicted the belief in, or practice of, Ayurveda as a sign of barbarism.

Local Indian officials fought back as best they could. In 1921, for example, the government of Madras (on the Bay of Bengal, and home of the influential British East India Company) issued a report on Ayurvedic medicine that concluded, in part, "No Western scientist should think of criticizing Ayurveda until he has learnt the Sanskrit language and studied the subject for some years under a competent Acharya [a Hindu teacher who provides instruction in the Vedic texts]."

British physicians, outraged at any hint that Ayurveda might have something legitimate to offer, led the assault on this bulletin. The *British Medical Journal* mocked the Madras report and Ayurvedic medicine for relying on *(Continued on page 28)*

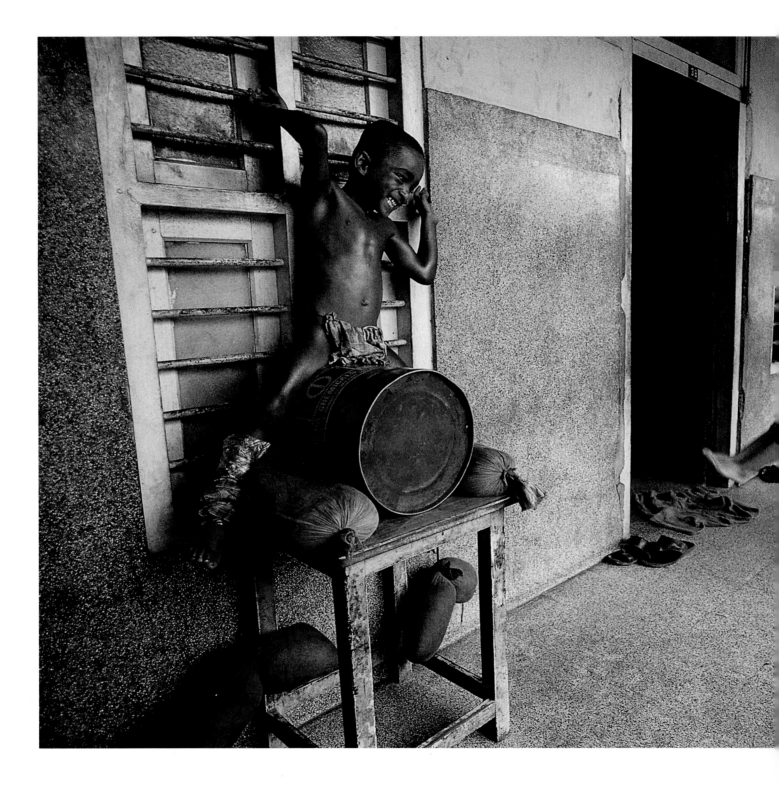

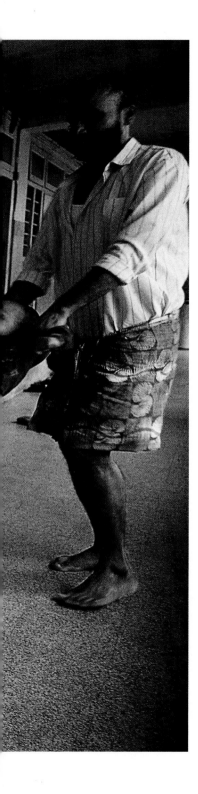

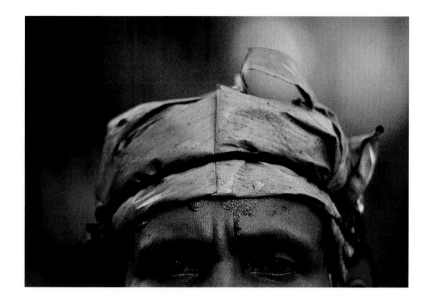

His father and brother divert the attention of seven-year-old Surendra Sindhe (left) as he undergoes traction at an orthopedic hospital in Coimbatore, India. He has cerebral palsy. Ayurvedic doctors prescribed herbal oil massages to soften his bones and hope that traction can straighten his curved legs. Modern science has yet to test such treatments even as practitioners and patients testify to amazing results. One growing impediment is that local healers fear that researchers may steal their knowledge. Concern about biopiracy is attracting more attention as governments negotiate treaties that define ownership of nature's secrets. A patient in a mental facility in Kerala State (above) undergoes an Ayurvedic treatment called *thalapotichil.* Doctors place a poultice of herbs on his head and cover it with a banana leaf to seal in moisture. Such transdermal—through the skin—delivery of medicines is becoming more common in the West.

FOLLOWING PAGES: Transdermal medication helps a 33-year-old woman in a Coimbatore, India, hospital combat arthritis. In a treatment called *kizhi,* attendants wrap rice powder in gauze, soak it in herbal oil, and aggressively massage the patient's entire body.

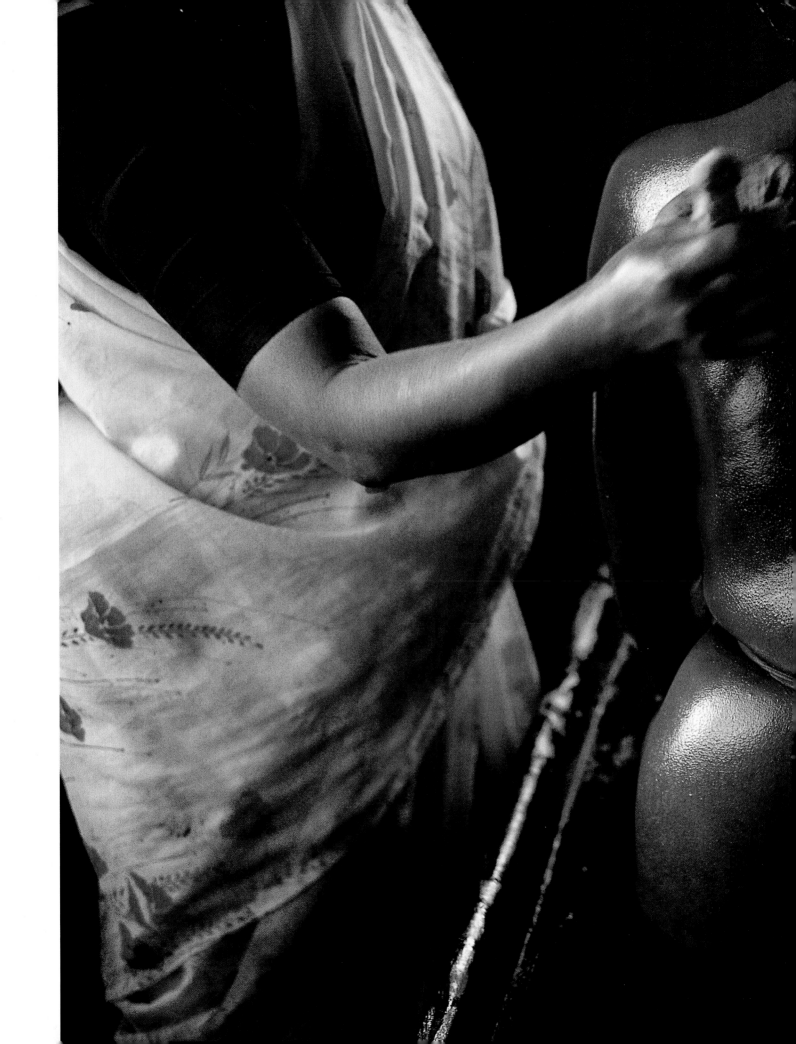

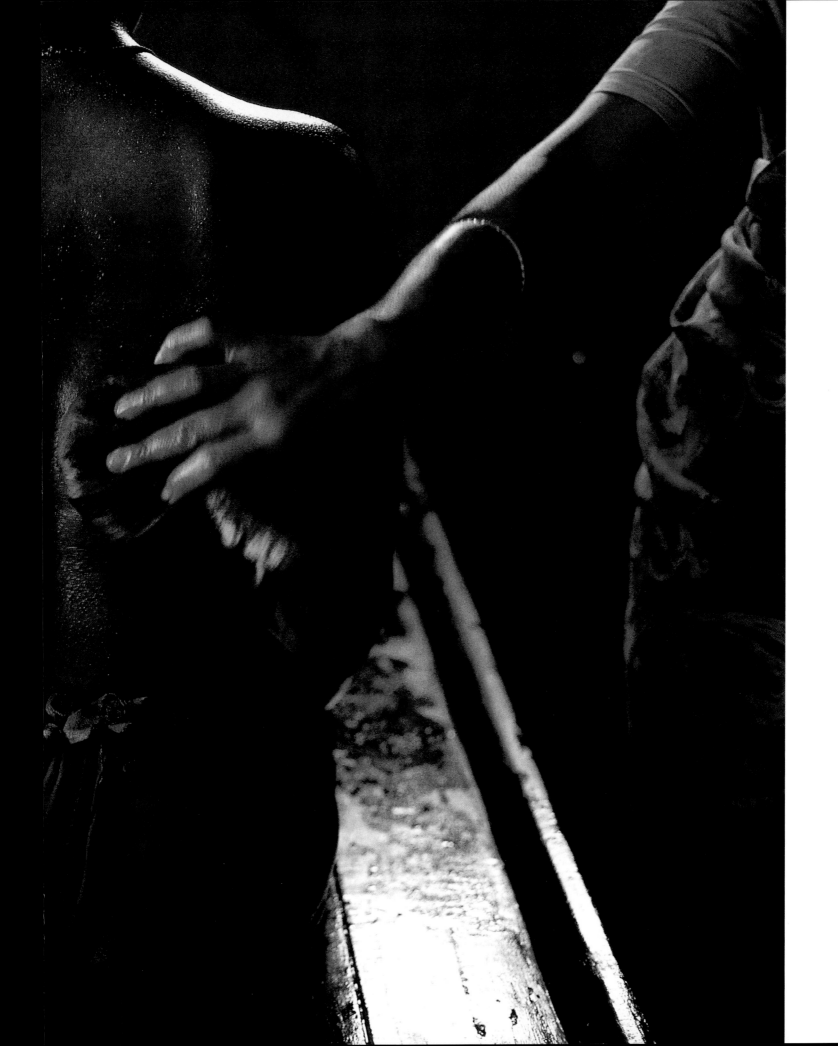

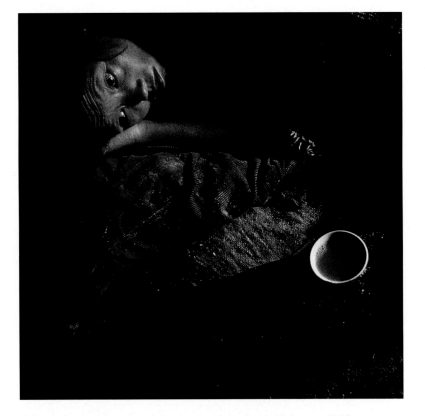

Herbal tea laced with yak butter is the only medicine available to a mother in western Tibet (above). Badly jaundiced and bleeding since the birth of a child two months before, she was too weak to travel to the nearest hospital. A healer palpates the stomach of a woman with recurring abdominal pain (right) who has come to his office on the western Tibetan Plateau. Traditional herbal medicines and Western drugs sent to the outpost by the Chinese government litter the floor, but they are often outdated, and patients frequently must resort to home remedies.

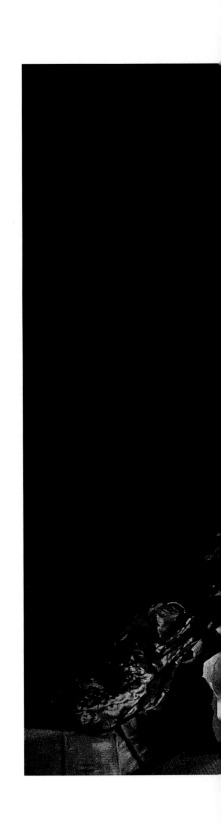

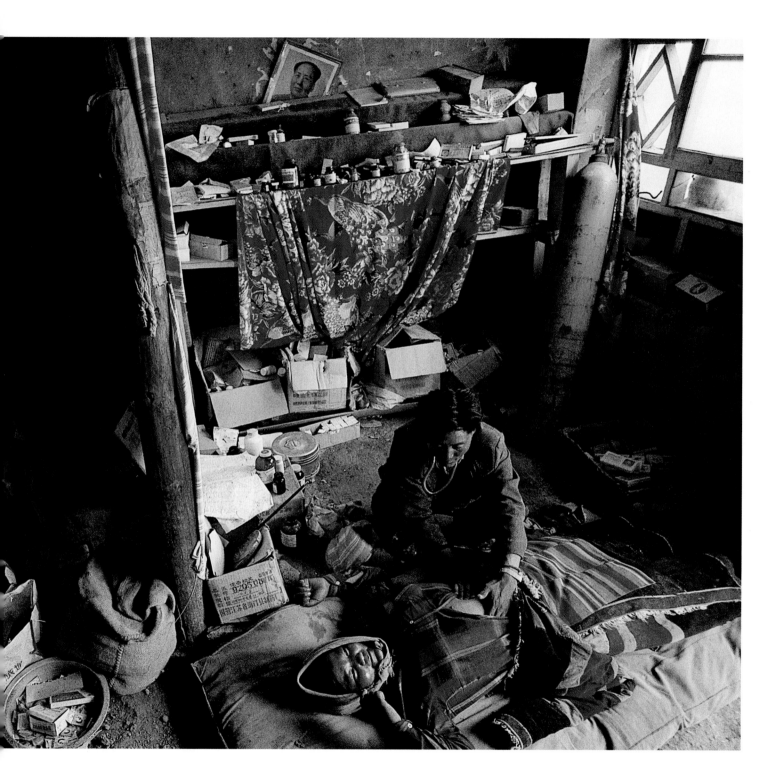

"unsupported metaphysical and theoretical dogmas." The Madras government, the *Journal* said, should be "planting modern science in the country, by the agency of scientists and teachers trained in Western methods, instead of endeavouring to stimulate the belated indigenous systems into renewed activity." In a subsequent letter published in the *Journal*, a British doctor called Ayurveda a "fantastic system of so-called medicine" whose "views on drugs are primitive." Such attitudes had a major impact. Even after India achieved independence in 1947, many of its leaders, institutions, and people wanted to become modern and sophisticated, which meant rejecting the Ayurvedic tradition. "India must break with much of her past and not allow it to dominate the present," Jawaharlal Nehru, the political leader of India's independence movement and its first prime minister wrote. "Our lives are encumbered with the deadwood of this past; all that is dead and has served its purpose has to go."

Now, thanks in part to its growing popularity in the West, Ayurvedic medicine is enjoying a revival in India.

———————

LIKE AYURVEDA, INDIAN FOLK MEDICINE, called *lok swasasthya paramparas,* or local health traditions, demonstrates considerable durability. These traditions lack the systematic beliefs that underlie Ayurveda and are mostly oral. Their practitioners have no written texts of their own, but they often use the *Caraka* and *Sushrata Samhitas.*

The traveler in contemporary India will often encounter Indian folk medicine in the form of stories like the following: A Western-trained university professor in Calcutta, a physiologist who publishes in European and American scientific journals, is approached by one of his students. The student says, "I live in a rural village, and in my village is a healer who picks plants that counteract the poison if you are bitten by a cobra. The healer says he got the recipe for the plants from his father, who got it from his father."

Many villagers in India must rely on such plant-based medicine because modern antivenom is not available to them. This antidote to snakebite, made from antibodies in horses that have been injected with venom, is expensive and may require refrigeration. The villagers do not have money to pay for such medicines. They are expensive, and they are in short supply.

The physiologist goes out into the countryside with the student and meets the healer. Unsophisticated on issues such as ownership and profit, the healer provides a plant that the doctor takes back to his laboratory. There he prepares cobra and viper venom to give to his laboratory rats. He injects the rats with a lethal dose 50—the

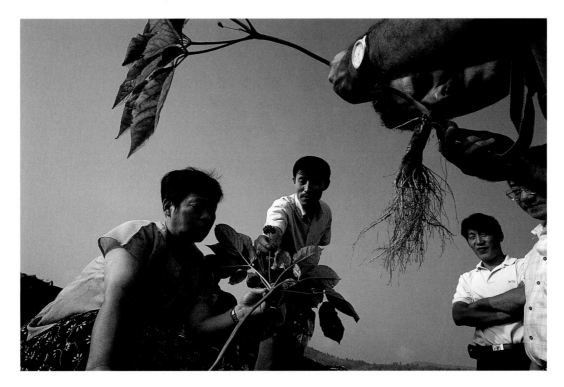

Eyeing the roots of a plant, Greg Pennyroyal of Leiner Health Products, a manufacturer of herbal preparations, joins Chinese colleagues in northeastern China to examine ginseng for possible export to the United States. Taking herbs to maintain health, basic to traditional Chinese medicine, is a concept new to many Westerners.

dosage at which 50 percent of the animals will die—and yes, 50 percent of them die. Next, he administers the same dosage to a new group of rats, along with an extract of the plant provided by the healer. None of the animals die.

The physiologist returns to the healer, who has grown suspicious. What if this stranger makes his anti-poison potions, the secret to much of his success, public. His livelihood could disappear. "I won't give you any more plants," the healer says.

The physiologist is not worried. He has asked a colleague, a botanist, to examine the first specimen provided by the rural healer. He knows just which plant to pick. He does so, and again tries his lethal dose experiment. This time, however, even with the plant antidote, all the laboratory rats die.

"What went wrong?" he asks the botanist.

"Each of those plant species has dozens or hundreds of subspecies, many of which we haven't yet identified," the botanist replies. "In addition, to obtain plant parts that would have the same chemical composition as that of the plants the healer had picked, you might have to know exactly when to pick them. In the morning or night can make a difference. Is the plant old or young? What is growing nearby?"

This story could be told hundreds, probably thousands, of ways about local treatments for the entire range of human ailments. The modern world has little knowledge of or interest in these stories. But researchers in India, using modern, scientific techniques and standards, are examining some traditional *(Continued on page 36)*

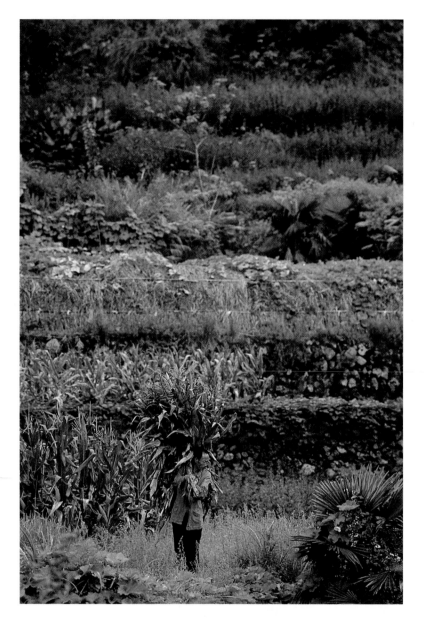

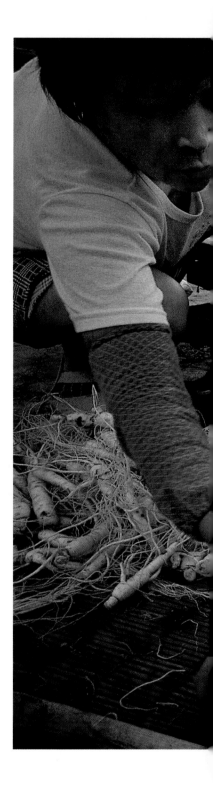

Much of the land near the eastern Chinese city of Ningbo yields medicinal crops. Beyond a farmer carrying corn from his fields, herbs line the hillside. At a processing plant, workers sort recently harvested ginseng. They will wash and scrape the root, then allow it to dry naturally. Chinese, as well as other people around the world, use ginseng as a tonic to restore energy. Studies show that it can stimulate the immune system, increase alertness, and help people deal with stress.

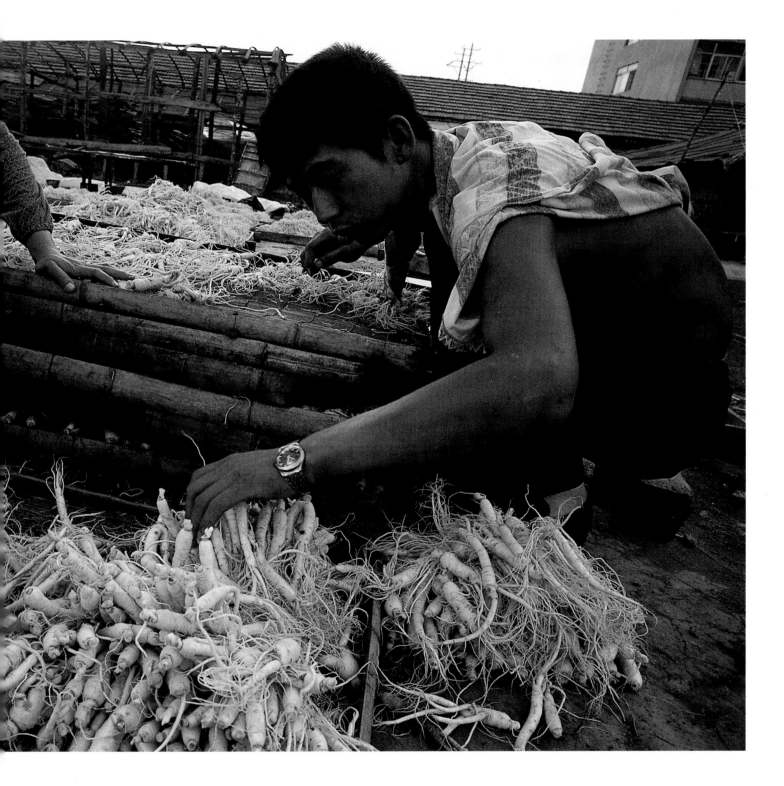

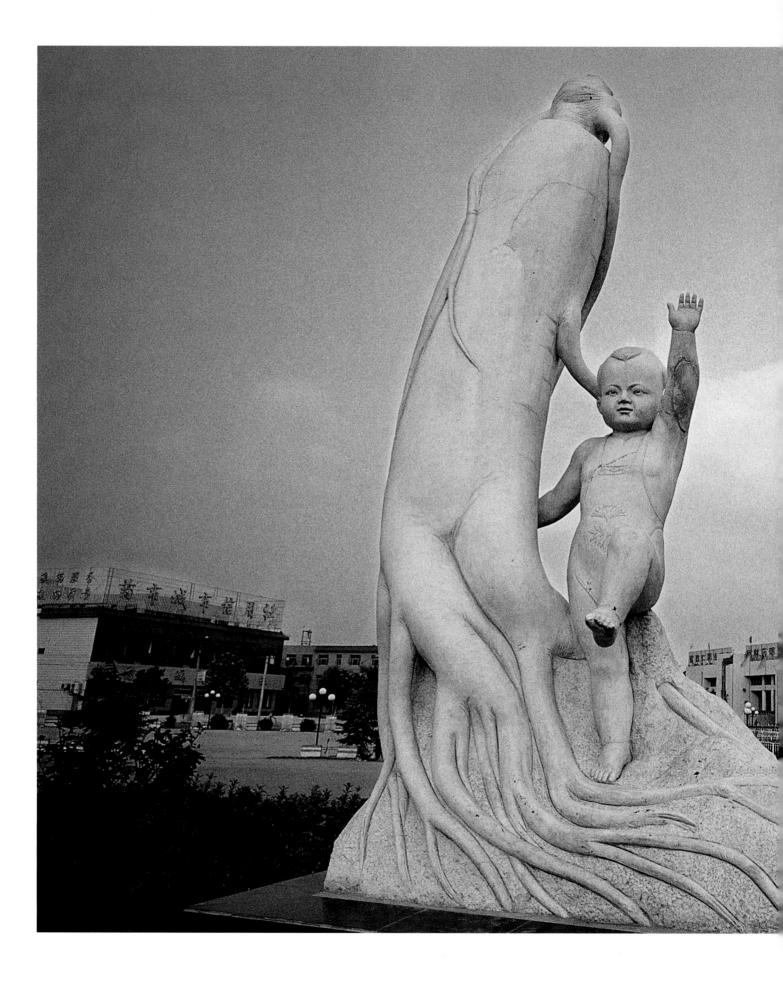

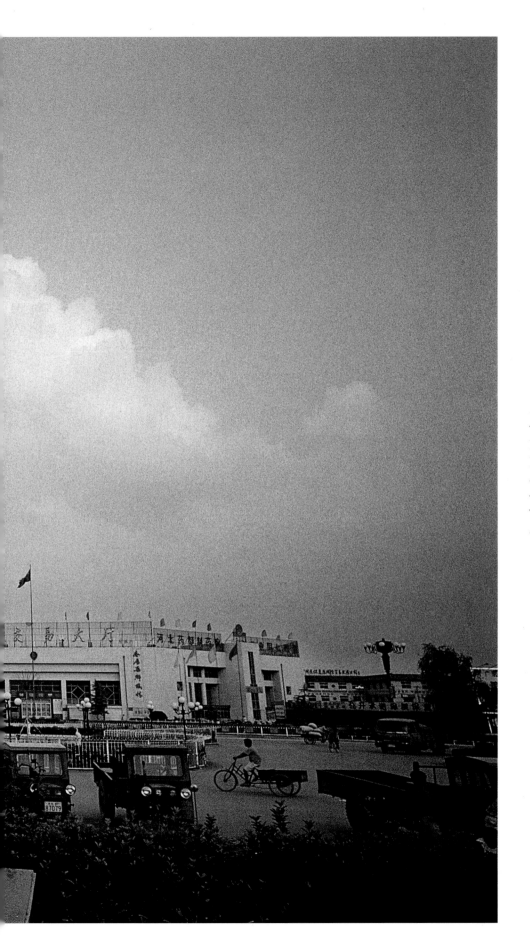

Several stories tall, a concrete tribute to the mighty ginseng presides over the herbal market in Anguo. The city, located about three hours' drive south of Beijing, boasts a 2,000-year-old tradition as the herbal center of China. Traditional Chinese especially cherish ginseng as a remedy because of its resemblance to the human form.

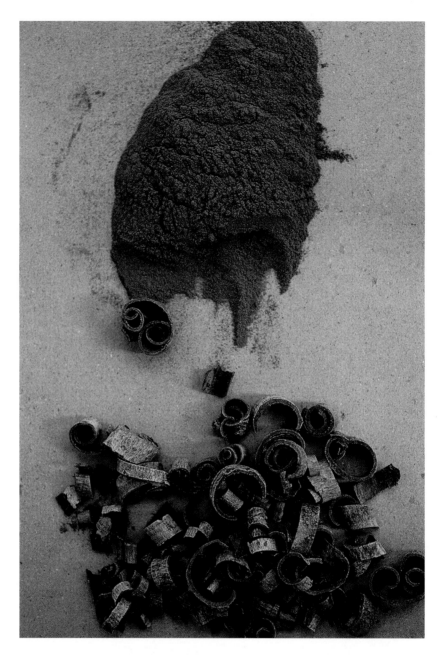

Thin shavings of *hou po,* or magnolia bark, become a reddish powder when ground (above) in a medicine shop in China. Healers use the powder to treat gastrointestinal problems such as indigestion, vomiting, and diarrhea. Merchants from across China throng the city of Anguo's state-run herbal market, one of the country's largest. Virtually any herbal, mineral, or animal material used in traditional Chinese medicine can be found in Anguo.

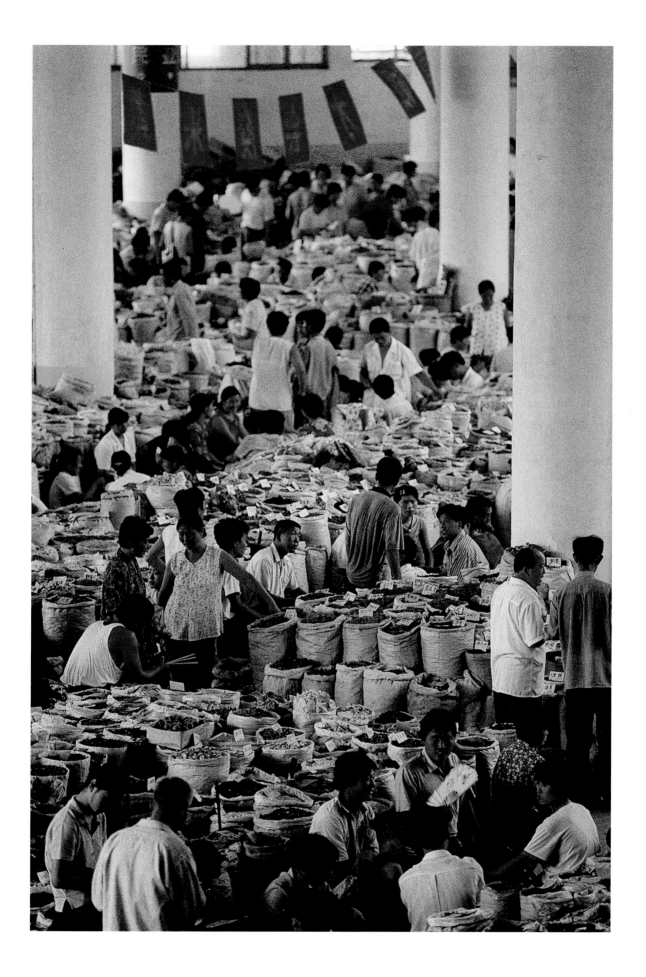

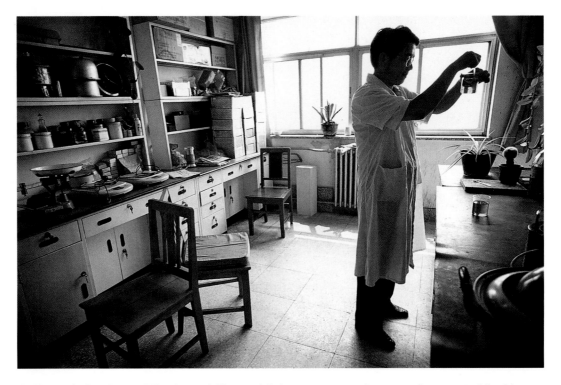

At Beijing's Academy of Traditional Chinese Medicine, a researcher tests fizzy anticold tablets that dissolve in water. Workers at the academy search for more modern delivery systems for traditional remedies. Despite their strong herbal tradition, the Chinese people are becoming too impatient to brew medicines the old-fashioned way.

treatments, as well as the Ayurvedic use of plants.

Although the ongoing research of Ayurvedic medicine is often limited by lack of money, indications are that plants used in India offer potent weapons against cancer, diabetes, and other major diseases. In one study the addition of peppers, including *Piper longum*—an herb known in Ayurveda to increase the *agni,* or metabolic fire—triples the effectiveness of the antibiotic rifampin, which is used to treat tuberculosis.

———

CHINESE MEDICINE, LIKE AYURVEDA, traces its history to unwritten legends thousands of years old. According to this oral tradition, three emperors who reigned from the 29th to the 27th centuries B.C. laid the foundations for Chinese medicine. In chronological order they were Fu Hsi, author of the yin-yang doctrine; Shen Nung, the first herbalist; and Huang Ti, who wrote the earliest known book on Chinese medicine.

These emperors taught that all creation, including humanity, is a marriage of two polar elements, the yin and the yang. Within the human body, this marriage applies to various attributes such as cold and hot, wet and dry, and body and mind. To remain healthy is to keep these attributes in harmony. The teachings posit that the body consists of *qi* or *chi* (energy—the animating force that moves along pathways called meridians); moisture (liquid that protects and nurtures tissue); and blood (which leads to muscles and organs). The teachings conclude that the body, like all of nature, consists of five elements: water, fire, earth, metal, and wood. Each is associated with an organ sys-

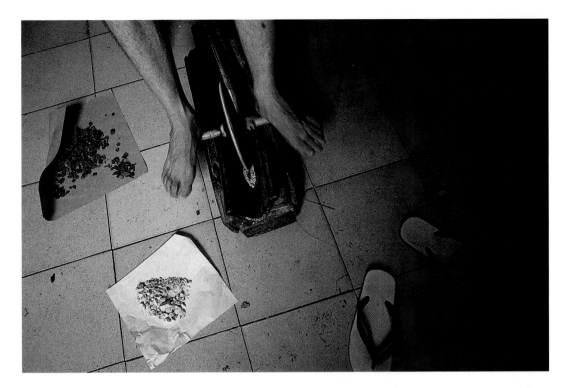

In a medicine shop that dates from 1770, one of the oldest in the northeastern Chinese city of Ningbo, a worker grinds seeds. Traditionally, if a remedy is for external use, the preparer grinds with his feet; if for internal consumption, he works the wheel with his hands.

tem—the wood element, for example, affects functions of the liver and the gall bladder.

The emphasis of Chinese medicine is on prevention. Once a patient's condition is diagnosed, treatment—which, as with Ayurveda, varies to meet the needs of each individual—can include acupuncture, massage, change in diet, and medicinal herbs.

Legend says that Shen Nung, the father of Chinese medicinal plants, gathered, tasted, and classified all the herbs himself. He then provided details on preparation and dosage.

Most likely, the knowledge of herbs and the details on how best to use them came from hundreds, even thousands, of years of trial and error. The Chinese method of delivering some drugs by soaking a cloth in herbs and resting it on the skin is an example of how useful insights evolved. This transdermal delivery, which allows drugs to reach the bloodstream without first going through the digestive system, is becoming more common in modern medicine.

THE STEADY GROWTH in the number of herbs used in Chinese medicine, as well as the complexity of the formulas, followed the pattern found in Ayurveda: use of minerals and animal parts along with plants. In Chinese medicine ingredients included stag antlers and antelope horns, bear bile, dragon's teeth (possibly the bones of prehistoric animals); insects; shells; rocks; gemstones; metals; minerals such as mercury, sulfur, arsenic, zinc sulfate, gypsum, and lead. No written record documents the experimentation that led to such recipes, and a tradition of folk medicine *(Continued on page 42)*

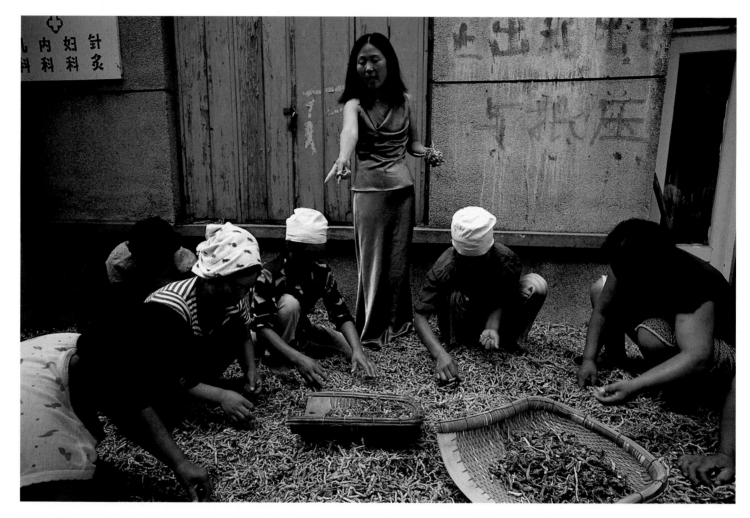

Under the vocal and strict supervision of their boss, laborers at an Anguo processing plant sort *Polygonatum,* or Solomon's seal, a member of the lily family, onto bamboo trays. The plants will be used in a longevity tonic. Like most herbs, these are classified and ranked according to size and color.

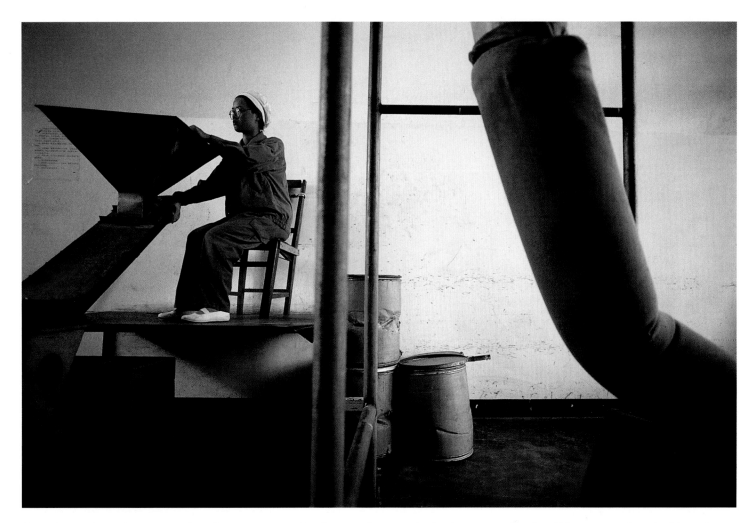

A worker in the milling room of a plant-processing facility grinds magnolia bark into powder. It will be exported to the United States. Magnolia moderates the effects of the potent bioactivity in other plants and acts as a catalyst.

FOLLOWING PAGES: In Beijing's Xi Yuan Traditional Chinese Medicine Hospital a special program for diabetics combines herbal medicine, massage, and a blend of meditation and exercise called *Qi Gong*. One *Qi Gong* master focuses a patient's energy around his heart; another meditates. The program, which encourages the mind and the body to work as one and makes the diabetic patients active participants in controlling their own health, has helped lessen their need for insulin and other drugs.

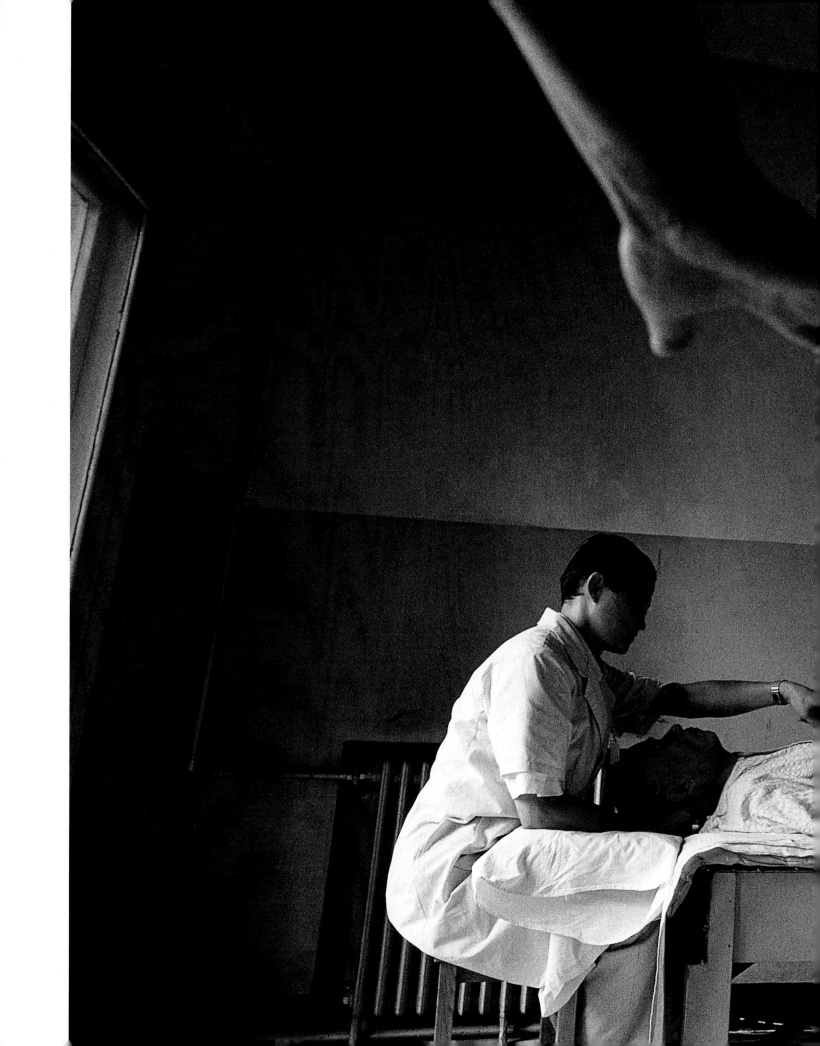

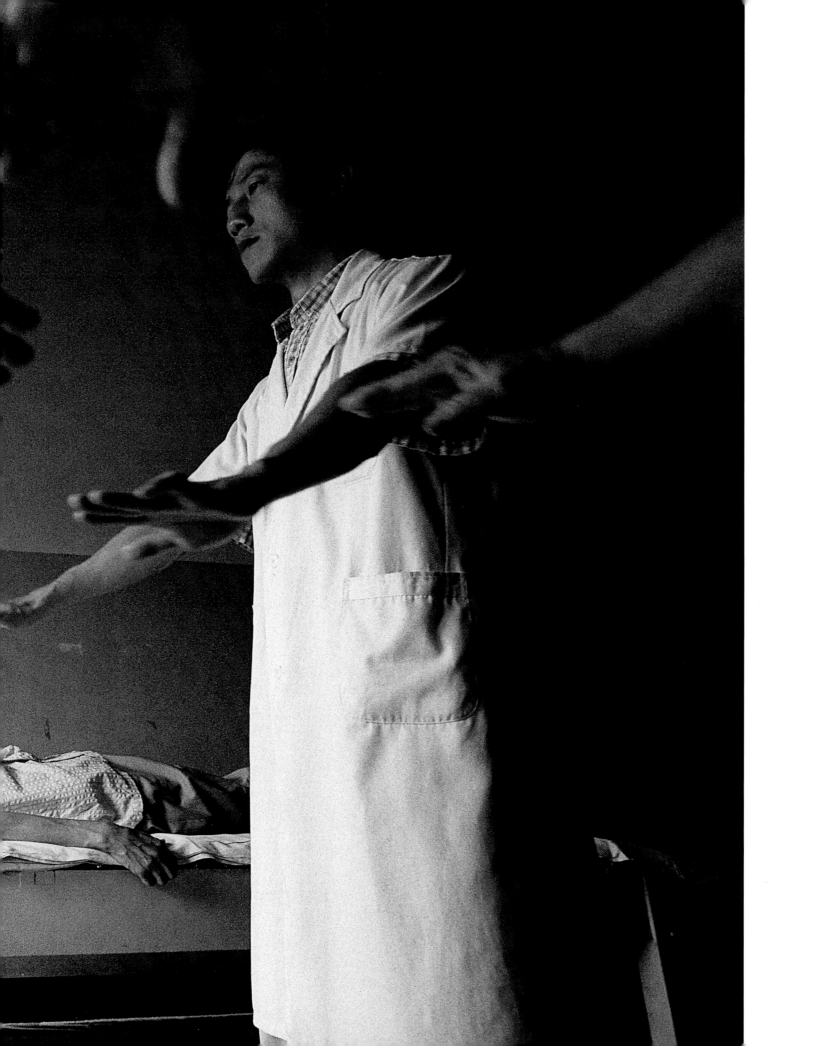

with no written material or formal structure has emerged.

Chinese pharmacopoeias, books that list medicinal preparations, first appeared during the western Han Empire (200 B.C. to A.D. 205). Although the authors of these pharmacopoeias are not known, these books appeared at around the same time that China developed a uniform written language. Perhaps by coincidence, this was also when Ayurvedic texts were first written in Sanskrit.

The relationship between Chinese and Ayurvedic medicine remains a mystery. Contact between the two cultures might have come from the spread of Buddhism or from trade. Travel between China and India via water or land certainly dates back far into antiquity.

The extent of cross-pollination between the two medical approaches is unclear, but anything purely Indian or Chinese probably existed only temporarily. While scholars argue about how much the two systems learned from each other and which is older, evidence of shared knowledge is strong. Although the Chinese seem to have been continually suspicious of "barbarian," or non-Chinese healers, their use of non-Chinese plants has a long history. At least as early as the first millennium B.C., the Chinese were receiving herbs not only from India but also from what Europeans later named the Spice Islands. Herbs from Java and the west coast of Africa also made their way to China, and medicinal herbs were prominent in diplomatic exchanges. In 667, for example, the ambassador from Rum, part of the Byzantine Empire in present-day Turkey, gave the emperor of China a pill that had, according to one source, as many as 600 ingredients.

————

A MEDICINAL PLANT that grows in the forests of Thailand and Myanmar, the chaulmoogra tree, provides some insight into the Chinese pharmacopoeia. Chaulmoogra, whose fruit is large and round, with many seeds embedded in the pulp, probably arrived in China around the 14th century. It was prepared according to a complex formula. No one knows if this formula arrived from Thailand along with the plant. One traditional method of preparing oil from chaulmoogra is to remove the husks from 3.3 pounds of seeds, excluding any that have turned yellow, and grind them into a fine powder. Seal it tightly in an earthenware jar and put the jar in boiling water, making sure that no steam escapes. Boil until a black and tarlike oil emerges. Mix one ounce of the oil and three ounces of the root and seed of the *Sophora flavescens* shrub into a paste. Combine the paste with wine and roll into pills the size of a seed from the sterculia plant. Swallow 50 of these pills with hot wine before each meal.

How did such detailed instructions evolve? Which were important and which were medically unnecessary rituals passed from generation to generation? What, for example, would happen to the chemical composition of the final pill if steam had been allowed to escape during boiling? Much of the formula does have a sound basis. Adding an extract of the root of the perennial shrub *Sophora flavescens* fights nausea, a strong side effect of taking chaulmoogra oil. The *Sophora flavescens* may have come to China from India, highlighting the international nature of this cure.

————————

IN THE EARLY 15TH CENTURY desire for increased trade, including interest in new medicinal plants, prompted China to launch ocean expeditions that easily could have precluded or eclipsed the later voyages of Christopher Columbus and other Europeans. Among the events that stimulated interest in such voyages was the publication of a book, *Hui yao fang—Pharmaceutical Prescriptions of the Muslims*.

China at the time, the beginning of the Ming dynasty, had about 60 million people, roughly one-quarter of the world's population. In 1404 a prince named Zhi Di seized power from his father and ordered construction of an oceangoing fleet. Workers soon built or refitted for ocean travel more than 1,600 vessels.

Many of these ships, called *bao chuan* (treasure boats), were 400 feet long and 160 feet wide, more than four times larger than the vessels used by Columbus later in the century. Among other innovations, the Chinese ships had watertight bulwark compartments, similar in construction to the segments of a bamboo stalk. The largest ships had nine masts and luxury cabins complete with balconies. Each ship had its own medicinal herb garden, and crew members included doctors and herbalists to collect plants in foreign countries.

A fleet consisting of hundreds of ships completed seven voyages between 1405 and 1433. These expeditions visited nearly 30 lands, ranging from islands near the north coast of Australia to the east coast of Africa. Commanding this fleet was Zheng He, a court eunuch who was a Mongol and a Muslim. Zheng He's mission was to collect information, accept tributes for the emperor, and establish trade relations. Medicinal plants, spices, and herbs, many worth their weight in silver or gold, were among the most important items of trade.

The journal of Ma Huan, a Muslim interpreter who accompanied Zheng He, describes a typical stop. It was in the town of Dhufar, which the Chinese called Tsu-Fa-Erh, on the south coast of Arabia: "When the treasure-ships of the Central Country [China] arrived there, after the reading of the imperial will and the conferment of presents was finished, the king sent chiefs everywhere to issue instructions to the

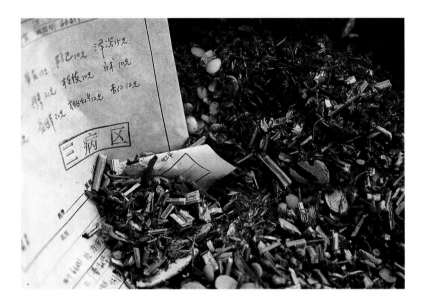

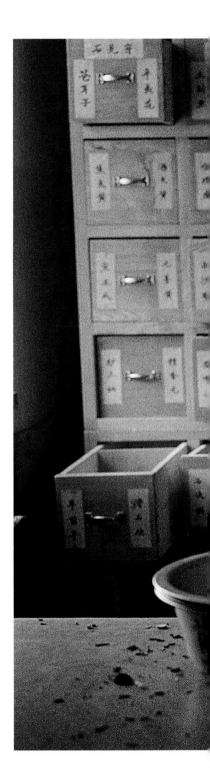

In the pharmacy of the Xi Yuan hospital in Beijing, a worker measures one of many ingredients that go into a single remedy (right). Each drawer behind her contains a type of seed, root, twig, or other part of various plants. One prescription (above) contains Chinese mother-wort, apricot kernels, cassia twigs, safflower flower, water plantain, and red-rooted sage. Such mixtures, often based on ancient formulas, contain uncounted numbers of chemicals that act upon the human body. Modern medicine has yet to develop methods to test the mecha-nisms of a remedy with so many different ingredients. Some studies do show that complicated Chinese herbal remedies provide risk-free health benefits.

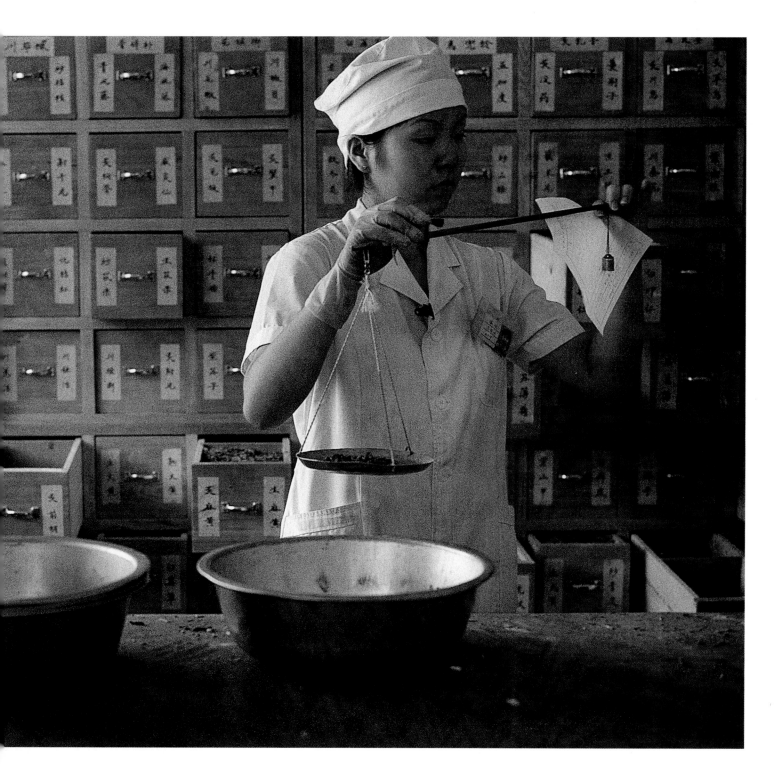

people of the country [and] they all took such things as frankincense, dragon's blood, aloes, myrrh, benzoin, liquid storax, and *mu-pieh-tzu* [all medicines derived from plants], and came to barter them for hemp-silk, porcelain ware, and other such articles."

Travelers, including Marco Polo and Arab traders, had told the Chinese about a land far to the west called Europe. To get there, Zheng He could have circumnavigated Africa, or sailed east across the Pacific, in which case he would have stumbled upon the Americas. But the Chinese had no desire to visit Europe. They knew it to be a source of wool and wine and did not particularly want or need to import either.

Zheng He pursued stories about rare drugs and powerful medical practices in present-day Sri Lanka, the Maldives, Thailand, and Africa. Among his most fruitful stops was Calicut, a city-state on the west coast of India and a center for the subcontinent's herb and spice trade. Calicut had been an important free port since the 13th century. Traders could come at any time and take on fresh water and provisions. They paid no tax if they had no sales, and a tax of one-fortieth of the amount they did sell—a tax considered very low at the time.

Ambassadors from the countries Zheng He visited often returned with him to live in the Ming capital of Nanjing and, later, Beijing. The Chinese people were forbidden to sell these foreigners coins, metals, weapons, artisans' tools, or medicinal herbs. Such herbs, along with books about health, were among top items desired by other countries.

These rules demonstrated the Chinese leaders' desire to control outflow of medicinal knowledge and herbs. But the presence of foreigners raised much larger concerns. Whether or not to maintain contact with the outside world remained a divisive issue within China's royal palace.

———————

AMID CONTINUED PALACE INTRIGUE under a series of emperors, China increasingly cut ties with other countries. The emperor canceled, renewed, and then canceled again plans for new expeditions—and all official records of Zheng He's voyages were destroyed. One emperor forbade purchase of raw copper, silk, and horses from Mongols to the north, and he ordered that no one repair or construct treasure ships.

Beginning in 1500 the government imposed a death sentence on anyone who built a ship with more than two masts. By 1551 it was a serious crime to even sail a ship with more than one mast.

Although history often moves by chance and whim, it is easy to forget that it could have taken other paths. What would the contemporary world be like, including our use of medicinal plants, if China had continued its voyages of discovery? Africa and the

Western Hemisphere could have been colonized by the Chinese instead of Europeans. Perhaps even more significantly, what we call the scientific revolution could have occurred in China.

For centuries before Zheng He's journeys, China had been using the printing press, glass, paper, gunpowder, and the compass. The country had the expertise and the accumulated capital necessary for an explosion of progress in scientific knowledge and technical capability. No one knows why this did not happen. Among the best guesses: Chinese researchers never developed widespread use of quantification in their approach to experiments, or effective ways to share information with each other. The Chinese, furthermore, were satisfied with their role as what they called the Middle Kingdom, which they believed to be located in the center of the Earth and the universe. They had little desire to discover and conquer new worlds. A final impediment to change was Chinese political unity. Orders came from the emperor, whom the Chinese people believed to be a direct link to heaven. When the emperor said that voyages of discovery would stop, they stopped. In contrast, when the king of Portugal in the late 15th century refused to finance Columbus's proposed voyage, Columbus went to the king and queen of Spain.

If the Chinese had continued their voyages of discovery, and if more modern science had emerged in China, our medicinal relationship with plants could have been very different today. Nothing about the nature of plants or the demands of modern science, for example, dictates the present-day emphasis on finding the single active molecule, using only one chemical from a plant. Reliance on the single active molecule began to emerge in the late 19th century, largely as a result of the need to have medicines whose contents could be tested, standardized, and patented. This has precluded most use of plants, which can contain dozens of bioactive substances (see Chapters 4-8).

But approaches other than relying on the single active molecule were possible. Modern science could have built upon China's multimillennial experience with plant remedies, including those using numerous plants. Testing, documenting, and refining these remedies could have provided society with medicines at least as safe and predictable as the Western medicines we have today. Emphasis could have been placed on cultivation techniques, improving standards for quality and measurement, and studying dosage and toxicity. All of this could have been accomplished via low-tech techniques, relying on observation, empirical testing, measurement, and record keeping.

China, however, kept turning inward, further refining the complicated and often mysterious medicinal recipes outsiders encounter today. In 1552 Li Shih-chen, the son of a physician and a physician himself, started to compile information on medicine as practiced in China. He finished his work more than a quarter century later. It consists of 52 volumes documenting 1,892 medicinal substances. Of these about 60 percent come from plants; the others, from minerals and animals.

————

STRIKING, AT LEAST FROM THE WESTERN PERSPECTIVE, is how Ayurvedic and Chinese medicine share major characteristics and raise similar issues. This kinship is crucial to understanding medicinal plants as potential sources of modern pharmaceutical drugs, as well as botanical remedies that are increasingly popular in the West. Both Chinese and Ayurvedic medicine have a strong spiritual component. For outsiders this often raises the question of whether the patient must believe in the plant remedies for them to work. Does the placebo effect—healing generated by the patient's body and not a pharmacologically active substance—lie at the heart of analyzing all botanical remedies? This question is particularly important for Westerners who try to discover if Ayurvedic and Chinese plant remedies offer medicinal benefits. To be deemed valid—especially to be judged scientifically valid—the Asian treatments must work even if the patient rejects all the spiritual assumptions upon which their formulation has been based.

The two systems use one plant to treat many different conditions and different plants for the same condition. They also employ many plants at the same time—utilizing virtually every plant part—and they have complicated ways of preparing them.

Each system is split between formal teachings and folk medicine, which often translates into a rift between those with access to professional medical care and those who rely on village healers. Whatever their background, healers emphasize that medicine, including plants, should promote wellness and not just treat disease.

Chinese and Ayurvedic medicines grew and remained vibrant through intercultural contact, and they have flourished without knowledge of germs and other agents that often cause disease. They sometimes share roughly similar views of the human body: It consists of a balance among basic elements that also define the natural world.

This same view of the human body dominated European medicine, which called the basic elements humors, for more than 2,000 years—from the time of Hippocrates until the advent of modern science.

Hand-colored drawings on rice paper in the archive of the Academy of Traditional Chinese Medicine illustrate four plants from the parsley family in a 1655 volume, a reprint of one of China's first herbal texts. Written Chinese medical texts date back to at least the third century B.C. and contain remedies still used today.

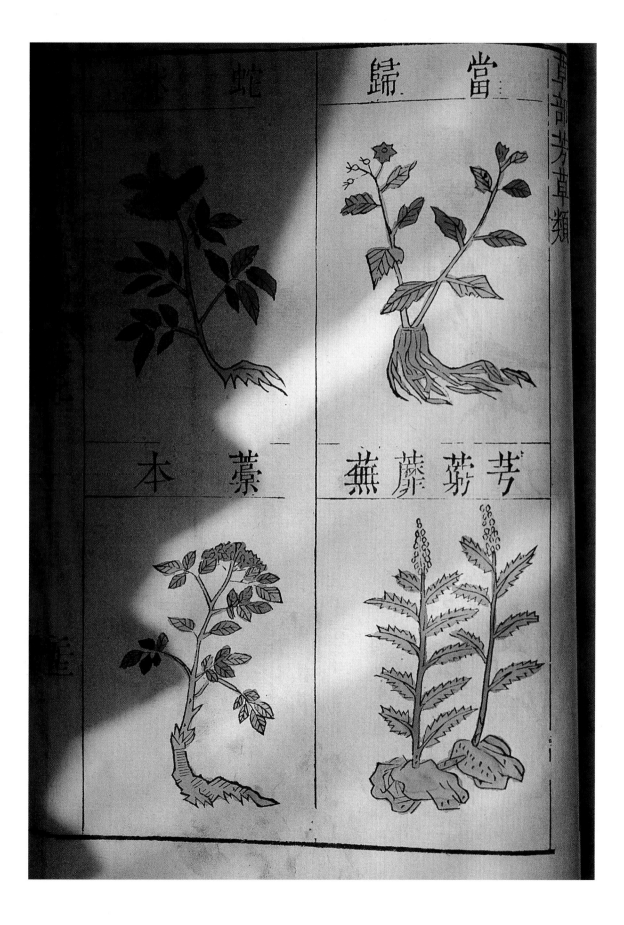

CHAPTER TWO

Plants Begin to Serve the Four Humors

An influential English medical treatise, John Gerard's *The Herball or Generall Historie of Plantes*, published in 1597, was based on the then dominant philosophy that four humors ruled human health. To keep those humors in balance when someone was poisoned, the *Herball* advocated the use of antidotes. These remedies were called mithridates, after Mithradates VI. The ruler of Pontus, in present-day Turkey, from 120-63 B.C., Mithradates feared being poisoned and worked with physicians to devise an antidote. The eventual concoction was so complicated it took six months to prepare, and in subsequent centuries experts expanded the number of ingredients to more than a hundred. These items, set to verse to help people remember them, included rhubarb, ginger, black pepper, anise, fennel, red roses, and licorice. By Gerard's time doctors used mithridates to treat headache, shortness of breath, spitting of blood, nausea, liver ailments, epilepsy, stress, and tetanus.

For more than 2,000 years Western doctors believed that a balance of four humors defined human health. In a medieval manuscript people reflect the humor dominant: Black bile contributed to melancholia, phlegm made people slow and stolid, yellow bile made them choleric, and blood made them sanguine. The word "humor" derives from the Latin *humere*, to be moist; most doctors used herbs to eliminate fluid from the body.

Bettmann/CORBIS

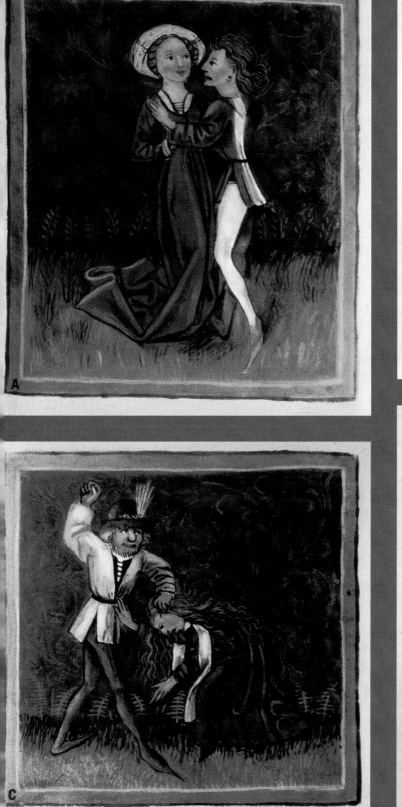

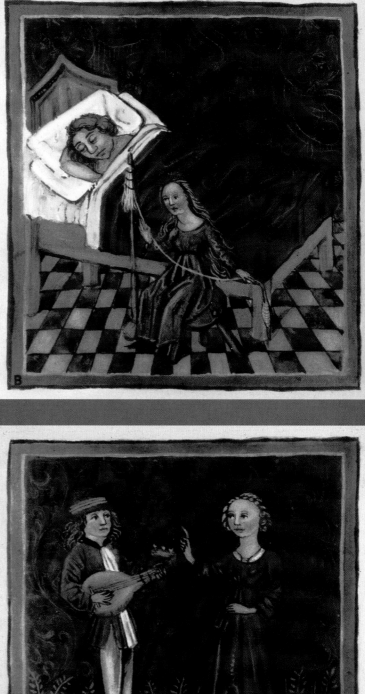

By the fifth and sixth centuries B.C., as Indian and Chinese medical texts were being written down, important roots of what we now call modern medicine were developing in present-day Greece. At the time, Greece consisted of city-states whose populations totaled approximately 140,000 people. Their principal economic activities were farming and commerce. Trade in medicinal plants between the Mediterranean and India and China was well established. Ayurvedic medicine, for example, used pepper, a perennial climbing shrub native to India and Sri Lanka as a stimulant in cholera cases and for fevers and coma; the Chinese treated stomach problems with it. Use of spices such as pepper in the Mediterranean already had a long history. In 2600 B.C., for example, slaves building the great pyramid of Cheops were fed spices to enhance their energy.

Just how significant such foreign influences were on Greece remains unclear, but they may have contributed to the basic idea that all illness and health come from an imbalance or balance of fluids, or humors, within the human body. That philosophy dominated European medicine and the use of medicinal plants until the late 19th and early 20th centuries. The word "humor" derives from the Latin *humere*, to be moist.

In Europe the first known written version of humors came from Empedocles, a Sicilian-born philosopher who lived from 490 B.C. to 430 B.C. Empedocles attacked the traditional Greek belief that two elements—fire (heat, life, and knowledge) and night (cold, death, and ignorance)—make up the world. He asserted that the physical world consists of four elements: air, fire, water, and earth, but many of Empedocles' scientific views were what we now call modern. His belief that natural selection plays a role in the formation of animals influenced Charles Darwin (1809-1882).

Hippocrates (460-377 B.C.), famous as the author of the oath now taken by many physicians, believed in maintaining a balance of body humors. He thought that primary efforts to promote health should come from diet and exercise, and that the use of medicines was unimportant. The writings of Hippocrates address medicines only briefly. Toward the end of his *On Regimen in Acute Diseases*, he writes: "If you think it necessary to give medicines, you may purge upwards [cause vomiting] by hellebore [dried powder from a perennial shrub]." The brief discussion of medical treatments that follows includes use of plant products such as beans, fig juice, marjoram, cumin, almonds, and madder. But Hippocrates placed no particular emphasis on plants. For the use of cantharides, which are dried beetles, he specifies that after "removing their head, feet, and wings, crush their bodies in three cupfuls of water" and have patients drink this until they "complain of pain...."

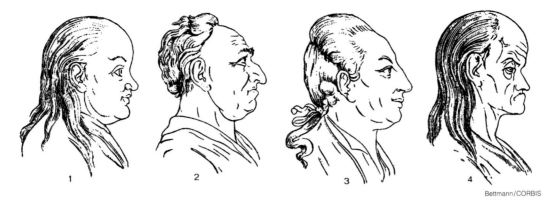

Facial features, emphasized in an undated illustration, purportedly reflected a person's tempera-ment and psychological characteristics. The dominant humor was believed to determine an individual's temperament. Doctors used herbs, bleeding, and other measures to restore balance to the four humors and thus return the patient to good health.

Whose idea was it to use insects this way? Presumably, such medical treatments were not devised at random or on a whim. Was the practice based on experience, on see-ing such prescriptions help sick people, or was it a myth that people such as Hip-pocrates simply repeated?

No one knows. But we do know that today's written version of Hippocrates' thoughts comes from scholars doing research at the ancient world's most extensive library, the one in Alexandria, Egypt, during the first and second centuries B.C. These scholars probably based their work on things they heard and on written fragments that had survived from the time of Hippocrates. Whatever their sources, some of the wis-dom the Egyptian scholars attributed to Hippocrates does sound strange. The "mode of distinguishing persons in an hysterical fit," for example, is to "pinch them with your fin-gers, and if they feel, it is hysterical; but if not, it is a convulsion."

Greek philosopher Aristotle (384-322 B.C.) corroborated the emphasis on the ele-ments and decreed that four corresponding qualities—hot, dry, wet, and cold—make up the human body. Basing his ideas on observation and inference rather than on exper-imentation, Aristotle concluded that health is a balance among these qualities and that disease is an imbalance. Such views mirrored Indian and Chinese concepts of disease.

———————

BY FAR THE MOST INFLUENTIAL advocate of the humors was Galen (A.D. 131-200). Born in the city of Pergamum, in present-day Turkey, Galen studied anatomy in Alexandria, Egypt. Returning to Pergamum, he served as surgeon to gladiators and then went to Rome, where his reputation as a healer earned him the position of personal physician to Emperor Marcus Aurelius.

Following Aristotle's lead, Galen divided the human body into the four humors: Blood, associated with the heart, corresponded to air and was warm and moist; phlegm, associated with the brain, corresponded to water and was cold and moist; yellow bile, associated with the liver, corresponded with fire and was warm and dry; and black bile, associated with the spleen, corresponded to earth and was cold and dry.

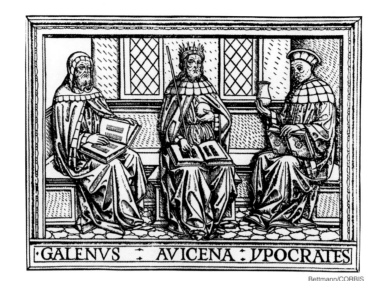

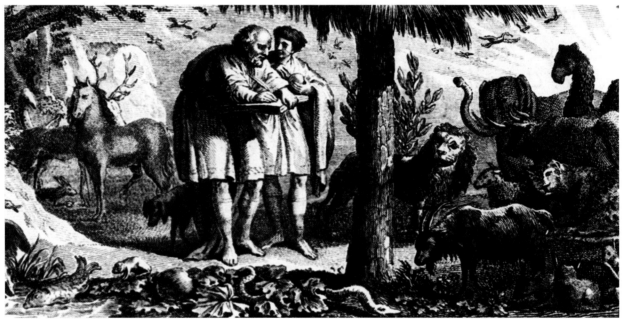

An illustration from a 1791 French natural history text depicts Aristotle taking notes as he studies nature (above). He based his conclusions on observation rather than experimentation. Perhaps the most influential Greek philosopher and scientist, Aristotle believed that disease results from an imbalance of four basic humors found in nature and in the human body. Three other strong advocates of the humoral approach—the fourth-century B.C. Greek Hippocrates, the first-century A.D. physician Galen, and the tenth-to-eleventh-century A.D. Islamic physician Avicenna—compare notes in a 1511 woodcut from a medical text (top). Galen's influence was so strong that most Western physicians called themselves Galenists until the early twentieth century. An illustration from a fifteenth-century Hebrew translation of Avicenna's *Canon of Medicine* depicts pharmacists preparing prescriptions (opposite). Plants for such remedies came from Asia, Africa, and Europe.

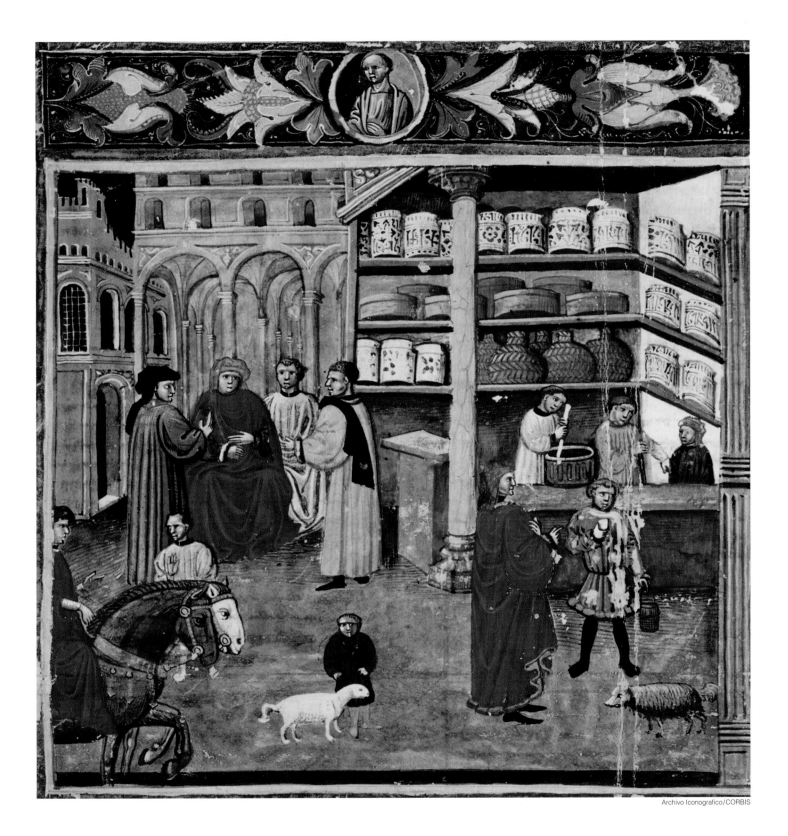

As Galen explained, health was a normal balance of humors, and illness occurred when something upset the balance. This view of medicine, Galen believed, was self-evident. "Now in reference to the *genesis of the humours*," he explains, "I do not know that any one could add anything wiser than what has been said by Hippocrates, Aristotle….and many other among the Ancients. These men demonstrated that when the nutriment become altered in the veins by the innate heat, blood is produced when it is in moderation, and the other humours when it is not in proper proportion."

Galen cites empirical evidence to show how and why his statement is true: "All the observed facts agree with this argument. Thus, those articles of food, which are by nature warmer are more productive of bile, while those which are colder produce more phlegm." After discussing what he calls "scientific proofs," Galen seems aware that all his readers may not yet be convinced. His assertions, he says, are also "based on prolonged experience." We can almost hear Galen's frustration with anyone who doubts his self-evident truths: "There is not a single thing to be found which does not bear witness to the truth of this account. How could it be otherwise?"

Galen's work with gladiators, who often received horrendous wounds during their to-the-death combat, presumably provided knowledge about human anatomy otherwise not available in a society that did not permit human dissections. He did dissect monkeys, pigs, sheep, cats, lions, wolves, an elephant, and other animals, conducting experiments that were rough, yet scientific. Galen fed pigs different foods and opened their stomachs to see what happened during digestion. He tested the prevalent belief that fluids in the body always flowed both ways. "Before the animal urinates," Galen wrote, "one has to tie a ligature round his penis and then to squeeze the bladder all over; still nothing goes back through the ureters to the kidneys."

Calling himself and his followers "the Moderns," Galen exhibited many attitudes and attributes that do seem very modern. The Galenists were intelligent, well-informed, and solidly based in the scientific knowledge of their time. They placed great faith in empirical observation. Galen, indeed, urged young people to question and doubt the highly respected scholars he himself praises as the "Ancients." Instead of accepting what the Ancients say, he asserted, a Modern "must test and prove it, observing what part of it is in agreement, and what in disagreement with obvious fact; thus he choose this and turn away from that."

However, Galen never applied any of this skepticism to his faith in humors. Nor did he conduct experiments that examined the effects of hellebore, pepper, scammony, and other plants he frequently recommended. Such experiments would have been

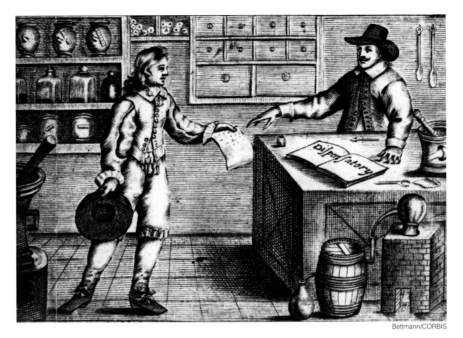

A 17th-century pharmacist receives a doctor's instructions on which remedy to prepare. Western apothecary shops with drawers and shelves full of ingredients for medicines did not change until the mid-20th century, with the advent of modern pharmaceutical drugs.

limited by the technology available to him, essentially knives and fire. But he could have given some patients one herb and others with similar symptoms another herb to see which worked best.

Instead, Galen based his conclusions about plants on clinical observation and information he received from healers, many of whom had discovered plants via the doctrine of signatures. According to this doctrine, the Creator (or creators) endowed plants with signs of their medicinal usefulness: Lung-shaped leaves were useful for breathing problems; yellow leaves were helpful against jaundice; bladder-shaped leaves helped with urinary problems. Inherent in the doctrine of signatures is an implied belief in intentionality on the part of the plant: It grows a certain way to offer a specific service to humans.

The Roman scholar Pliny (A.D. 23-79), who preceded and influenced Galen, described a bushy plant called the erynge. "Marvellous is the characteristic reported of it," Pliny wrote, "that its root grows into the likeness of the organs of one sex or the other; it is rarely so found, but should the male form come into the possession of men, they become lovable in the eyes of women."

Most cultures believe in some variation of the doctrine of signatures. It has lasted, in modified form, into the modern era because it helps people find what they're looking for. If you want a medicine for stomach problems, it is not difficult to find some parts of some plants shaped like stomachs.

Closely related to the doctrine of signatures was the belief in astrology. Medical astrologers built upon basic astrology, which assigned certain attributes to major heavenly bodies. For example, the planet Jupiter was associated with, among other things,

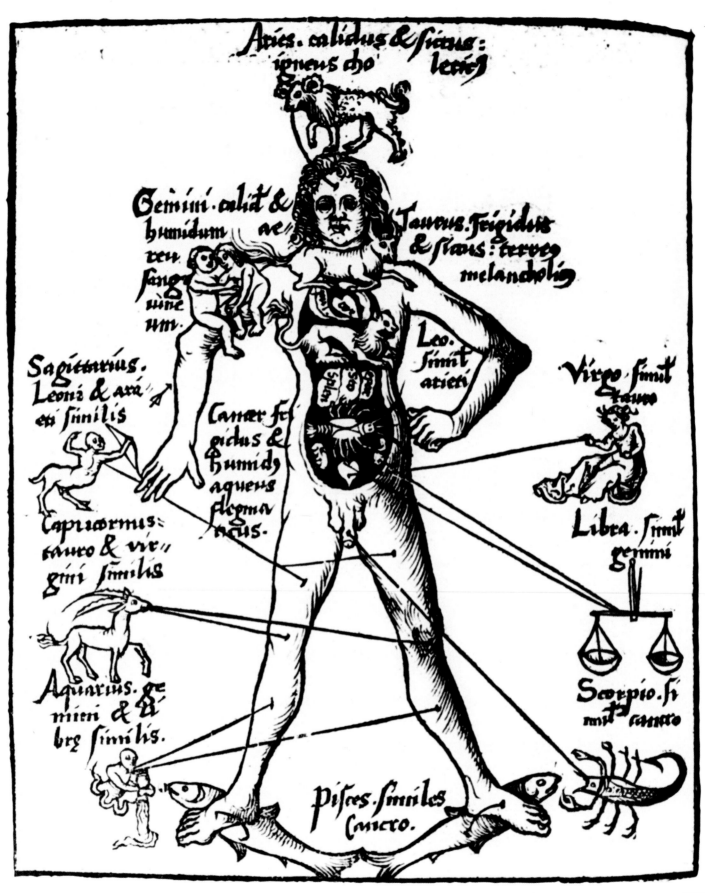

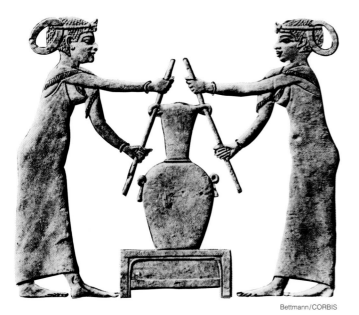

Astrological signs, shown in a 1517 medical diagram (opposite), influence various parts of the body—according to beliefs that date back thousands of years. Many leading physicians also believed that medicinal plants worked best when collected under certain astrological conditions. Such beliefs keep many people today from taking herbal remedies seriously, even though the remedies often contain plant chemicals now known to have powerful effects on the human body. In an ancient portrait two women prepare an herbal medicine (left). One Egyptian remedy from the plant bishop's weed led to the development of a pharmaceutical drug now used to treat asthma. In a 16th-century illustration (below) injured people line up to have their blood taken. Herbal remedies probably filled the jars shown in what was called the "leech's chamber."

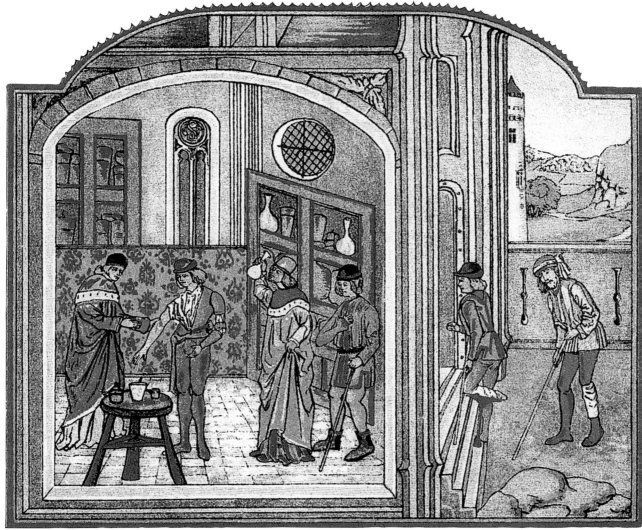

science and scholarship; the planet Mercury was associated with gardens. The application of such beliefs to medicine dates back at least as far as the ancient Egyptians and required that healers know both a patient's birth horoscope and the position of the stars when he fell ill. Medieval experts ascribed astrological characteristics to medicinal herbs, which were collected according to presumed dictates from the planet governing them. Herbal books and other documents thus recorded information about astrological positions associated with particular plants, and physicians often relied on abbreviated tables to help with bedside calculations.

According to Galenic thinking, a doctor must diagnose a humor imbalance and take measures to correct it. The standard approach was to treat a specific imbalance with a drug opposite it in quality. A hot complaint, for example, would require a cold remedy. Central to most diagnoses was the need to remove fluids from the body. Doctors thus wanted people to urinate, sweat, vomit, salivate, or develop diarrhea.

With our present knowledge, Galen's notion of humors sounds strange. How could making patients sweat, or giving them herbs to make them vomit, cure disease? The Galenic belief that a poison had to pass from the body to restore humoral balance, however, was logical. Although no one knew that bacteria and other disease-causing microbes existed, they did know that something in the body had to be eliminated. This approach fit well with the medicinal use of plants because finding a plant that makes someone urinate, sweat, vomit, salivate, or develop diarrhea is not difficult.

The focus on fluids also helps explain why Galen's ideas about humors dominated medicine until relatively recently. Humors made Galenic medicine flexible because so many plants could be used to affect fluids in so many ways.

By medieval times the theory of the four original humors was no longer complex enough to fit all the known illnesses and methods to cure them. The notion of degree took hold, with each plant having four degrees of each attribute. Thus, a plant might be "hot near the first degree, and dry in the third."

Galen's ideas about humors also endured because people needed a belief system and a rational approach. In less than 300 years after his death, the Roman Empire had begun to dissolve. Perhaps the absence of a central authority encouraged even the best minds to cling to accepted truths.

————

IN THE CENTURIES FOLLOWING the A.D. 632 death of Muhammad, founder of Islam, Arab civilization saw as a large part of its role translating and reclaiming Greek and Roman contributions that had been lost to "barbarian" conquerors and political anarchy.

Wealthy Muslim caliphs in Baghdad, Damascus, Cordoba, and other cities supported medical schools and pharmacies. These institutions effected medical innovations such as taking pulses and examining urine as means of diagnosis, but they primarily sustained and refined the use of plants to serve Galenic humors.

Although they conquered Egypt in the seventh century, the Arabs did not learn how to read hieroglyphics and never discovered an Egyptian medical papyrus. Anything the Muslims might have learned about ancient Egyptian medicine had been transmitted orally over the centuries.

Turning to their pre-Muslim roots in the desert—which has a relatively narrow range of plants—the Arabs had a strong interest in the use of metals in medicine and in alchemy, defined as the practice of employing plants and chemicals to change one metal to another. Most ancient cultures practiced some form of alchemy, which often included efforts to transform lead and other metals into gold.

Mastery over metals had been a serious part of medicine in China, where ancient alchemists had attempted to formulate a "pill of immortality," as well as in India and ancient Greece. Muslim contributions to the science of chemistry and its application to medicine were so significant that the word "alchemy" comes from the Arab *al-kīmiyā*.

In their work with plants Arab chemists used acid preparations and equipment that permitted evaporation, as well as filtration, crystallization, distillation, and other procedures. They experimented with remedies, refined dosages, simplified prescriptions, applied mathematical calculations to medicines, and emphasized the need for precision in using medicines.

Influential Muslim physicians included Ibn Sina, who lived in present-day Spain from about 980 to 1036. Called Avicenna in the Western world, Ibn Sina wrote *Canon of Medicine*, based on Greek and Roman classics. Translated versions of his book influenced the curriculum of European medical schools until the mid-17th century. Arab botanist and pharmacologist Ibn al Baitar (1197-1248) wrote several books that discuss about 1,400 medicines. Included are some 300 plants—such as dragon's blood and tamarind—from Mesopotamia, Arabia, India, and China that had not been used in Mediterranean medicine.

————

ONE MEDICAL COMMODITY that the Arabs helped popularize was sugar. The pharaohs' battle surgeons had used mixtures of sugar and honey to stop bleeding from wounds, a technique used by Europeans until the advent of antibiotics. Sugar promotes new tissue growth by drying the bed, or bottom, of a wound, weakening the bacteria present there by dehydrating them. Some surgeons today have started using sugar to help heal deep wounds.

The Muslims learned about sugar from the works of Galen, who said it was equal in value to silver. They imported sugar from India, where it had been cultivated since at least 3000 B.C. Growing it first in Sicily and Spain, Arab farmers then took sugar to northern Africa. Its use in medicine fueled the demand for it. Apothecaries needed sugar because it not only had medicinal properties but also helped people take the so often foul-tasting mixtures that were prescribed.

According to legend the first nonmedical use of sugar in Europe came around 1200, when a French apothecary coated almonds with it. Sugar remained an expensive medicine until large-scale production began in North America after the arrival of Europeans.

Most striking about Arab influence is its range. The Arabs disseminated medicinal plants and knowledge from China and India to the west coast of Africa and present-day Spain—a sphere of influence larger than had been embraced by any previous civilization. Arabs who traveled through these regions were among the first ethnobotanists. Ibn Battuta, an Islamic scholar, journeyed between Beijing and Tombouctou in the 14th century. While in Arabia he witnessed uses for plants, such as betel and coconut, that were not well-known in other regions. Nuts of betel, Ibn Battuta wrote, "sweeten the breath and aid digestion, prevent the disagreeable effects of drinking water on an empty stomach, and stimulate the faculties." He called coconut palms "one of the strangest of trees" whose nut "strengthens the body, fattens, and adds redness to the face." One century later another Arab traveler, known as Leo Africanus, reported tales from Africa; he described the "priests of Angola," who have power over life and death because of their "knowledge of medicinable hearbes, and of deadly poisons…."

Leo Africanus was born in Granada in present-day Spain and lived for many years in Italy. He never visited England, but an English translation of his three-volume *The History and Description of Africa and of the Notable Things Therein Contained* was published in London in 1600. William Shakespeare, then at the height of his popularity, could have seen this work. In *Henry IV, Part II* Shakespeare cited Africa as a place of "olden joys." He also demonstrated an eclectic knowledge of medicinal plants.

————

SHAKESPEARE'S WORKS CONTAIN 712 medical references; 32 are to doctors, apothecaries, and quacks; and 25 are to medicines and poisons. In *A Midsummer Night's Dream*, Lysander tells one of the young women, "Get you gone, you dwarf; You minimus, of

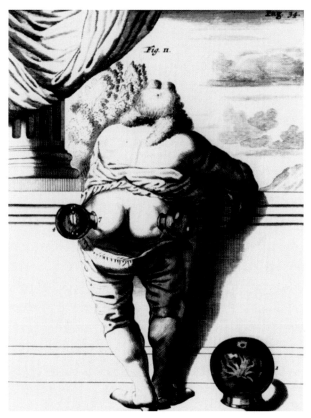

Until the emergence of modern medicine in the 20th century, most Western doctors believed that extracting a patient's blood could remove contaminants and help restore a healthy balance. In this 17th-century Dutch engraving, glass cupping bells collect blood as it is being drawn from a patient's buttocks.

hind'ering knot-grass made...," a reference to the belief that eating knotgrass, an herb now used to treat sore throats and respiratory problems, stunted the growth of young children. In *Othello* Iago refers to opium and mandrake, whose root serves as a sedative, when he predicts Othello's reaction to news of Desdemona's supposed infidelity: "Not poppy, nor mandragora, Nor all the drowsy syrups of the world, Shall ever medicine thee to that sweet sleep Which thou owedst yesterday." In *Much Ado About Nothing*, Margaret advises the ailing Beatrice, "Get you some of this distill'd Carduus Benedictus, and lay in on your heart: it is the only thing for a qualm." *Carduus benedictus* is a yellow-flowered plant, now known as *Cnicus*, that was used to stimulate the appetite.

———————

A REVEALING GLIMPSE OF MEDICINE as practiced in Europe at the time—the beginning of the scientific revolution (see Chapter 4)—comes from the case notes of Shakespeare's son-in-law, John Hall. Eleven years younger than Shakespeare, Hall married Shakespeare's oldest daughter, Susanna, in 1607.

Hall practiced medicine in Stratford upon Avon from 1611 to 1635. A country doctor, he had no known medical degree and called himself a master of arts. Some physicians at that time studied for ten years and were educated at Oxford, Cambridge, or in Scotland and continental Europe. Both Oxford and Cambridge had established professorships of medicine, and an effort was under way in England to limit medical practice to authorized persons. Despite his lack of a formal medical degree, Hall must have enjoyed a good reputation: Among his patients was William Compton, the Earl of Northhampton, who lived more than 40 miles away—several days on horseback.

In 17th-century Europe, the ailing who had money saw a doctor; others saw a neighbor, friend, or family member. Most villages had at least one self-trained healer who usually dispensed "simples," remedies using only one plant. These folk healers used remedies whose origins lay in what were called old wives' tales. Some also relied upon widely held beliefs in plant lore. One popular notion was that the juice of a flower known as love-in-idleness caused people to fall in love with the first person they saw upon awakening. Another belief was that any woman who washed with water distilled with cowslips would become more beautiful. According to a third story, the mandrake plant grew naturally under gallows and shrieked when plucked, killing anything and anyone who heard it. How much such stories reflected the actual beliefs of folk healers or, alternatively, how much they reflected how opponents of "old wives" might have spread the tales to denigrate them is impossible to determine.

The distinction between folk healers and doctors like Hall is sometimes difficult to discern. Their ideas about medicine were similar. According to one folktale, for example, basil caused the spontaneous generation of life-forms such as worms and scorpions. Like most European doctors of the time, Hall shared this belief in spontaneous generation, which originated with Aristotle. Hall thought that worms and other visible manifestations of disease arose from a combination of heat and wind.

Hall believed in the Greek system of humors. His case notes document his efforts to restore each patient's proper humoral balance. A patient's balance of humors was affected by diet, climate, exercise, emotions, and sleep patterns. Hall also relied heavily on purges and diuretics as tools. Galenists, as men like Hall called themselves, believed that taking a patient's blood could resolve humoral problems. Hall extracted blood by cutting veins under the tongue or in the ear, and by attaching leeches. While some doctors in Hall's time resisted such practices, others used even more extreme means to extract blood. Cuts were made in the patient's body, and hot cups were placed around the cuts to collect blood. Fontanels, or small fountains—cuts kept open by putting peas or other small round objects under the skin—were supposed to help keep humors in balance. Sometimes a patient had open sores for months or years.

Physical examinations reflected Hall's concern for the blood and other humors.

Signs of "excess" blood included red skin, swollen veins, headaches, and a fast pulse. Trouble with the phlegm resulted in indigestion, slow pulse, and a runny nose. Nightmares, fears, or dementia indicated the presence of too much black bile.

Hall purchased about 300 plant drugs, 39 animal drugs, and 38 drugs made from minerals such as mercury, arsenic, copper sulfate, iron, and sulfur. To determine which medicines to use, Hall consulted herbal books consisting primarily of statements, claims, and complicated prescriptions. Some of these herbs and recipes, which had their origins in Chinese, Indian, Greek, and Roman civilizations, dated back thousands of years.

The most popular herbal book in England at the time was *The Herball or Generall Historie of Plantes* by John Gerard (1545-1612). Gerard, a barber-surgeon who later became herbalist to King James I, did no original research. Translating the work of others, he described each plant's "vertues." Gerard's book and other herbal books reflected little awareness that different species of plants existed. They failed to note that even if one obtained the correct plant, its medicinal properties could depend on variables such as what time of day the plant was picked—variables often well understood by traditional folk healers.

———

HALL LEFT 178 CASE NOTES. One patient, Lady Esther Rous, suffered from daily intermittent fevers that were probably caused by malaria. Hall prescribed a drink to be taken two hours before the next bout of fever was expected. The draft consisted of diascordium, an opiate, mixed with pearl and coral to strengthen it. Hall mixed in water made from the flower *Carduus benedictus*. He chose this potion because it was "hot and dry" and would counteract the "cold wet phlegm" of her illness.

Another disease common in Hall's England was tuberculosis, which we now know is caused by bacteria and is best treated with antibiotics. Hall's prescription—"cooling" meats, including snails, frogs, crayfish; drinks of warm barley; and an enema made of chicken broth and herbs—was designed to reduce the imbalance of the humors. For a migraine headache Hall's treatment—which he said was successful—included a pill made from amber, clove, cinnamon, camphor, rosemary, sage, and musk. He also gave the patient an emetic and bled her.

Hall prescribed enemas that contained cassia, tamarind, senna, and rhubarb for his wife's colic. He applied a plaster to her stomach made with labdanum, resin from a shrub grown in Crete; caranna, a tree resin from South America; and oil of mace. These, too, he said, worked. When Hall's daughter, Elizabeth, had "convulsions of the mouth," he used nutmeg, cinnamon, cloves, and pepper. When an "erratick" fever threatened her, he responded with sarsaparilla, sassafras, and guaiacum, and concluded that "she was delivered from Death, and deadly Diseases for many years."

Hall claimed success in his recorded cases. Some of the benefit he provided may have come from the placebo effect, a phenomenon in which patients who receive medical treatment can improve, not directly due to the treatment, but because belief in it stimulates healing action by their own bodies.

Many of the plants Hall prescribed, however, do have scientifically proven effects similar to those he sought. These include winter cherry and marshmallow for urinary difficulties; wormseed, to help expel worms; mugwort for uterine problems; nettles as a diuretic; and chicory to aid digestion.

Whatever the effectiveness of particular herbs, among the people most satisfied must have been the suppliers of Hall's medicines. Clearly, one of the products of such complicated—and often esoteric—remedies was the profit made by the people who supplied them. Someone had to catch the frogs and crayfish and import the precious stones. Hall bought locally grown herbs, which provided steady business to growers and suppliers, and he also used plants imported from as far away as the Middle East, Africa, Asia, and the Western Hemisphere.

With the possible exception of tobacco, which Hall used as a medicinal plant, none of his herbs came from British colonies in North America. The Jamestown colony had been founded in 1607, the Plymouth colony in 1620, and the Massachusetts Bay colony in 1629 to 1630. All three settlements were still tenuous and generated little trade. About 100,000 Spaniards, however, were living in Mexico and Central and South America and had established cities, schools, monasteries, mines, and haciendas.

Despite conflict between England and Spain—the Spanish Armada had attacked in 1588, and war between the two countries had continued until 1604—Spain's colonies in Central and South America exported large amounts of medicinal plants to England. Among those Hall used were caranna for stomach pain, jalap as a purgative, sassafras and sarsaparilla to induce sweating and cause diarrhea, rhubarb to cause vomiting, and China root as a laxative and to cause sweating. Trade in such medicinal herbs generated extraordinary revenue and prompted much of the desire to explore the New World.

A sign advertises medical services available from an English doctor in 1623. Such physicians used hundreds of herbal remedies, many adopted from old wives' tales and other folk traditions. The herbs were mostly homegrown, but some came from as far away as Asia and North America.

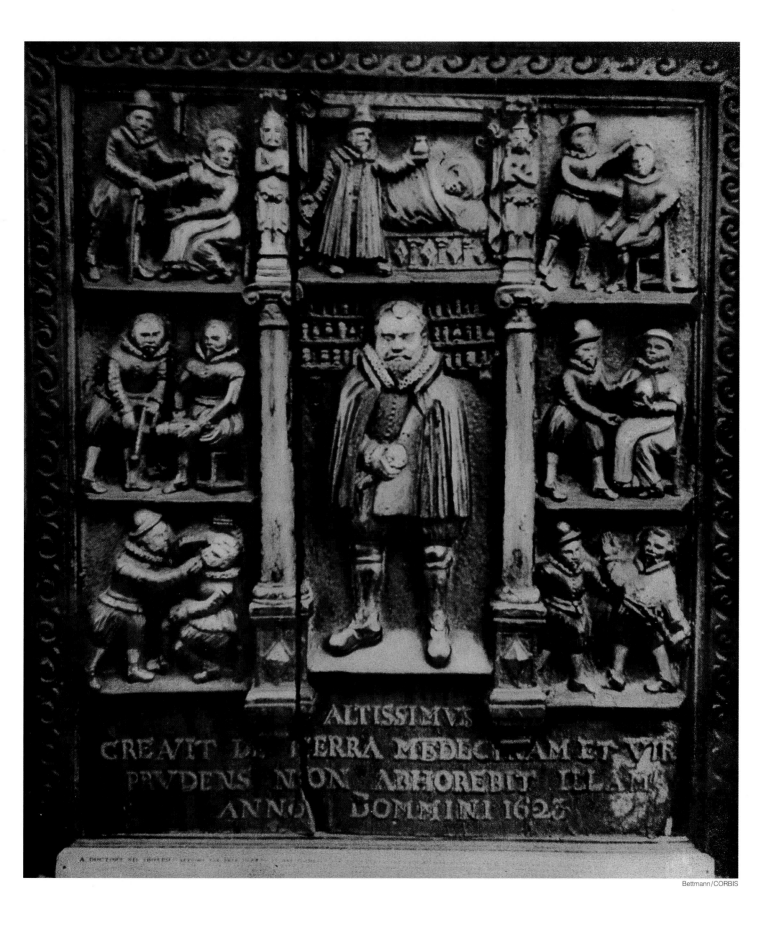

ALTISSIMVS
CREAVIT DE TERRA MEDECINAM ET VIR
PRVDENS NON ABHOREBIT ILLAM
ANNO DOMMINI 1623

CHAPTER THREE

Learning From the New World

In the winter of 1535 to 1536, the three ships of French explorer Jacques Cartier were frozen in the Saint Lawrence River at Sainte Croix. A disease began to spread among his 110 men. Putrid gums, purple blotches on the skin, pains throughout the body, ulcerations, swollen legs, and fatigue debilitated all but three Europeans. Dozens were dying. Cartier, who for unknown reasons was not among the ill, noticed that a Native American who had been extremely sick with the same illness had suddenly recovered. Cartier asked what was responsible for the cure and learned that the native women had given him bark of the white cedar tree. As the women directed, Cartier's men ground the bark and leaves, then boiled them in water. After drinking this concoction, the men felt better immediately, and after a few more treatments, they were fully recovered. They had been suffering from what we now call scurvy, and the white cedar had provided them with Vitamin C.

In the remote village of Milagro, Peru, on the eastern slope of the Andes, Alcides Quinchuya Quinshima uses a plant from the Piperaceae family to treat severe pain caused by an unidentified illness. Quinshima's son pours water, in which the plant was boiled, over his father. The water still contains pieces of torn leaves. Cinchona tree bark from Peru and Ecuador led to the most effective known treatment for malaria.

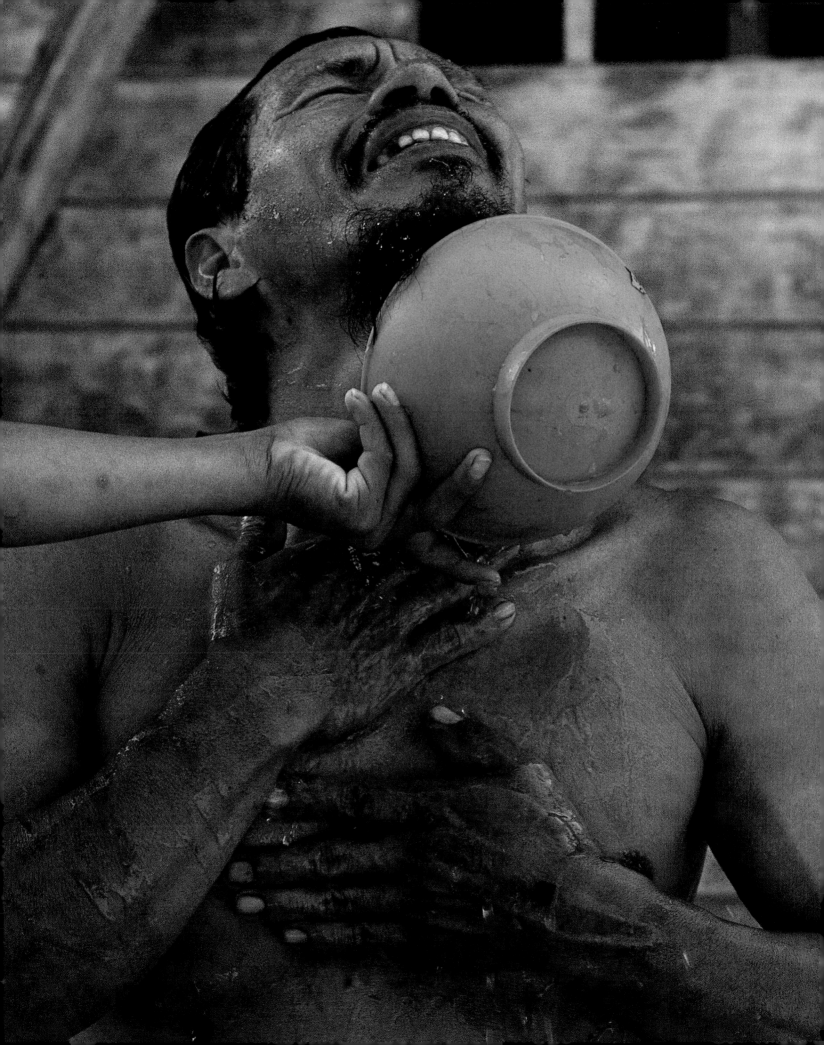

At the same time that Chinese treasure ships were touching east Africa and then withdrawing, Portuguese sailors were edging their way south along the coast of western Africa. They sought slaves and gold, but their prime purpose was to reach the Spice Islands, the present-day Moluccas, to obtain saffron, ginger, clove, turmeric, anise, cardamom, and cinnamon.

Most of these spices served as food preservatives and flavor enhancers, but their main function was medicinal—which is the reason that nutmeg, for example, increased 60,000 percent in value after its journey to Europe. Doctors used spices to treat, among other things, coughs, colds, flatulence, dysentery, and the plague. Some of the most expensive medicines combined up to 15 spices.

Portuguese explorers reached India by 1498 and the Spice Islands by 1512 to 1513. Like other Europeans, they were vaguely aware of civilizations in Asia but had little interest in learning medicine from them, even narrow lessons such as how to use particular plants. Nor did they envision finding new plants. They simply wanted to get spices they were already using and bypass Venetian traders whose merchant galleys had dominated the spice trade for several centuries. The Venetians were vulnerable in the late 15th century because the recently formed Ottoman Empire was disrupting Europe's Asian trade routes.

Similar motivation sparked the Spanish, who funded Christopher Columbus's efforts to reach China and the Spice Islands by sailing west across the Atlantic. Columbus, too, demonstrated no curiosity about new medicinal plants. Possible sightings of Chinese herbs such as rhubarb excited Columbus, but, like the Portuguese, he was looking only for herbs whose reputations were already established.

Landing on the island of present-day Jamaica, Columbus found tropical forests that he later described as "the most beautiful thing that I have seen....nor can I tire my eyes looking at such handsome verdure, so very different from ours." He recognized immediately that this greenery had "in it many plants and many trees which are worth a lot in Spain for dyes and for medicines of spicery; but I do not recognize them, which gives me much grief."

Columbus wished he had brought a botanist with him from Europe, but this regret could not have been strong because he did not include a botanist on any of his subsequent three voyages, which spanned the next 12 years.

During all of these expeditions, Columbus did nothing to learn about medicines from the native peoples, whom he perceived as savages. He believed that whatever health benefits they derived from local plants came to them without any thought or

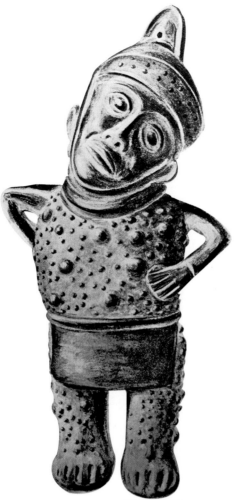

Bettmann/CORBIS

Pustules indicative of syphilis erupt on an Inca clay figure, its date of origin unknown. In the 16th century newly arrived Europeans believed—incorrectly—that native peoples used bark from the guaiacum tree to treat syphilis. The popularity and price of guaiacum in Europe soared, even though the treatments provided absolutely no benefit.

intelligence on their part. The natives, according to Christopher's brother Diego, who accompanied him on his voyages, dwelled in a "golden world, without toil, living in open gardens…contented with such simple diet, whereby health is preserved.…"

For 50 years after Columbus's arrival in the New World, few botanists crossed the Atlantic. But Spain's leaders clearly understood the economic value of medicinal plants. Their interest in plants continued after the early 1500s, when the Spanish realized that their explorers were in a New World rather than in Asia.

———

MUCH OF THE POPULARITY of New World drugs in Europe came through the work of a Spanish physician named Nicholas Monardes (1493-1588). Monardes never visited the Western Hemisphere, but he studied plants arriving in Seville, the home port for Spain's expeditions. In Seville he maintained a large garden replete with New World plants and interviewed returning explorers and the natives they brought back to Europe with them. *(Continued on page 76)*

71

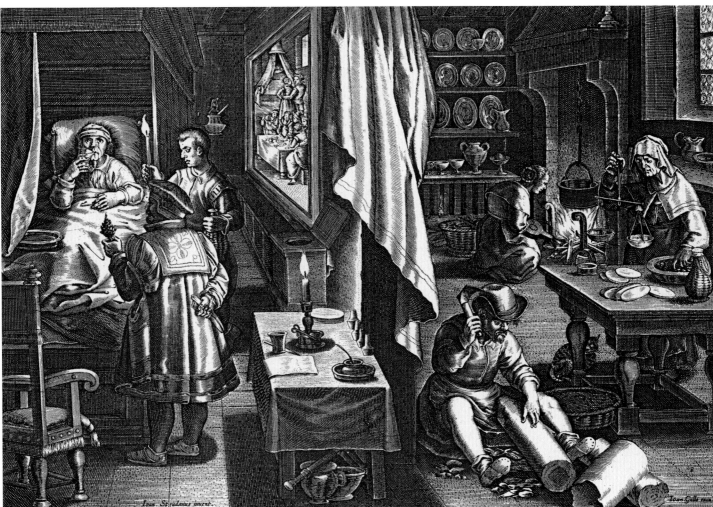

A syphilitic patient drinks a guaiacum-bark remedy in an undated drawing as his physician looks on; the decoction was warmed over the flame of the candle. Workers in the next room prepare and weigh the bark. Faith in guaiacum remained strong into the mid-to-late 16th century, when Europeans reverted to using mercury as their principal medicine against syphilis.

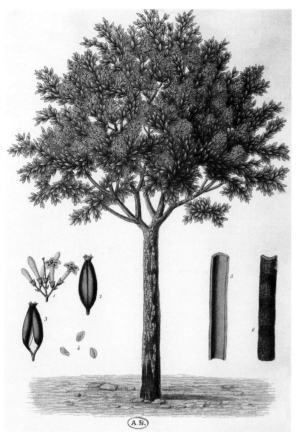

A botanical print from the Library of Decorative Arts in Paris (left), details characteristics of a cinchona tree. Cinchona bark contains quinine, a plant compound that kills the parasite responsible for malaria. Prior to World War II workers on the island of Java, in present-day Indonesia, dried cinchona bark in the sun (below), pulverized it, and exported it for use against malaria. When combat and Japanese occupation disrupted trade with the Indies, Allied scientists used quinine that had been synthesized. Synthetic drugs are now the chief source of modern antimalarial medications.

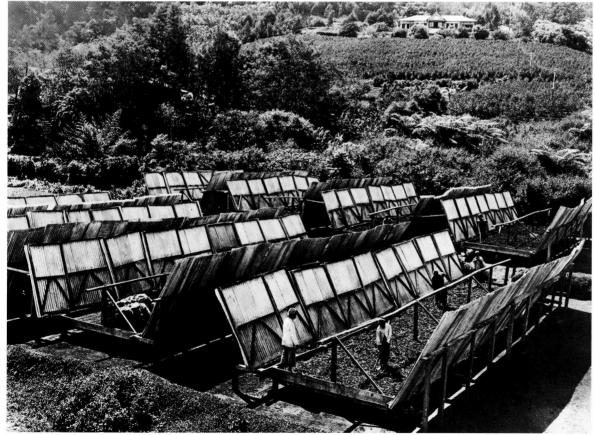

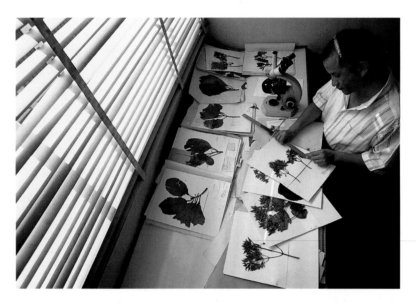

Professor Percy Zevallos Pollito, one of Peru's leading experts on cinchona, studies the tree's leaves (above). Several centuries of over-harvesting have put cinchona on Peru's endangered species list. Growing resistance to synthetic antimalarial compounds has sparked renewed interest in cultivating cinchona trees. The herbal tradition that gave the world quinine continues as Antonio Ramirez, a member of the Shipibo-Conibo people, prepares a remedy that will eventually include 15 ingredients (right). Such remedies, most untested by modern science, may disappear as local cultures and languages give way to the lure of technology and urban life. The Shipibo-Conibo, whose population numbers about 35,000, live on the Ucayali River near the headwaters of the Amazon River and have had minimal contact with the outside world.

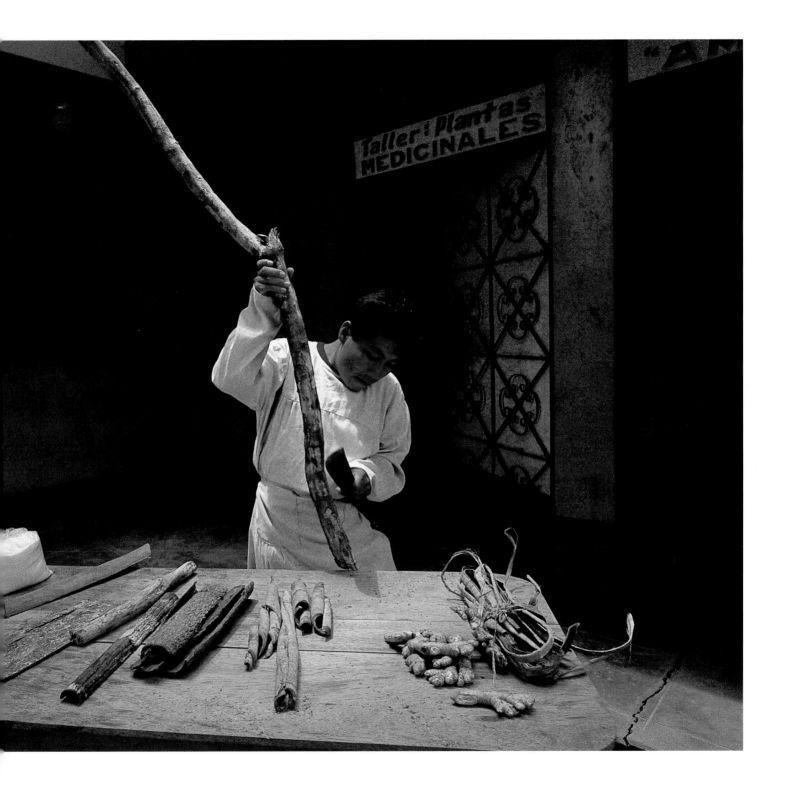

In 1536 Monardes published a book proclaiming that New World drugs were inferior to those of Spain.

For reasons Monardes never made clear, he then changed his mind. His three subsequent books, published between 1565 and 1574, reported that New World plants had great therapeutic powers. John Frampton, a British businessman who translated Monardes' work into English in 1577, published it under the title *Joyfull Newes out of the Newe Founde Worlde*. Both Shakespeare and his son-in-law, John Hall, could have seen this book.

Monardes reported that "our Occidental Indias doeth sende unto us many Trees, Plantes, Herbes, Rootes, Joices, Gummes, Fruites, Licours, Stones that are of greate medicinall vertues…." Among the medicinal plants Monardes praised were tobacco, coca, sarsaparilla, and sassafras.

In 1570, prompted in part by Monardes' writing, Spanish ruler Philip II told his men in New Spain to find "information on the herbs, aromatic plants the Indians use to cure themselves…." He also named one of his personal physicians, Francisco Hernández, as royal physician for the New World. Hernández's instructions were "to gather facts from all physicians, surgeons, Spanish and native herbalists, and other inquisitive persons with such abilities who can possibly know something, and, in general, obtain an account of all medicinal herbs, trees, plants, and seeds" in New Spain.

Hernández spent seven years in Mexico, collecting and describing 1,200 plants and conducting clinical trials in Mexico City, using native inhabitants as subjects. Like other European doctors, he saw the plants in humoral terms. Often influenced by taste and smell, he tried to categorize all plants in terms of hot or cold, wet or dry.

A key part of Hernández's effort was to question native healers who accompanied him to what was left of Aztec botanical gardens at Huaxtepec. These gardens, established by Aztec emperor Moctezuma I in 1453, included thousands of medicinal plants that had been collected from throughout his empire. The Spanish had not destroyed the gardens because they were near a new Spanish hospital. Hernández considered most of what the healers told him magical-religious nonsense and criticized them for merely repeating what their parents and grandparents had told them. He believed that the healers' use of plants was crude and incorrect because they had no knowledge of the writings of Galen. Hernández perceived himself to be among the *gentes de razon*, the people of reason, who were vastly superior to the superstitious natives.

Ironically, the people of Mexico did hold views roughly similar to Galen's. Illness, to them, was due largely to the accumulation of heat in the body. They believed that differ-

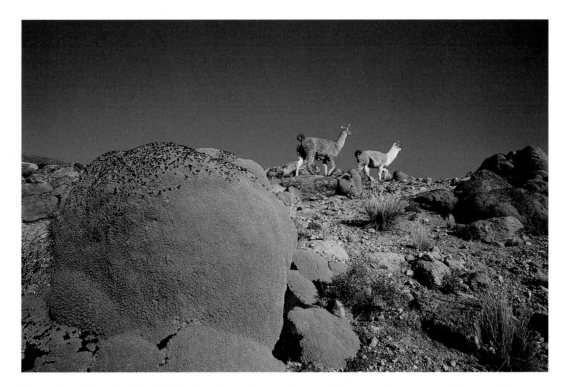

In southern Peru's Colca Valley local people use the woody *yareta* plant as a medicine and as a fuel. Since the arrival of the conquistadores, outsiders have usually considered the use of such remedies to be magical-religious nonsense.

ent phlegms put pressure on the heart and nerves, and that the most effective medicinal plants cause fluids to leave the body.

Even though Hernández and other physicians did not recognize it at the time, this similarity between the views of the Mexicans and those of the Galenists in Europe contributed to the swift transfer of specific New World drugs into the European pharmacopoeia. Guaiacum, jalap, sassafras, sarsaparilla, and other plants crossed the Atlantic and quickly won enthusiastic acceptance—as their use by John Hall demonstrated.

GUAIACUM, ONE OF THE most popular New World plants, was used to treat syphilis. No one knows the origin of syphilis, which is debilitating and often fatal, but by 1495, the first documented epidemic spread across Europe. Written records and radiocarbon analysis of pre-1492 bones indicate earlier instances of what could have been syphilis, but clearly a new and virulent disease arrived in Europe from the Western Hemisphere. One possibility: In the era before extensive world travel, European people's immune systems were unprepared for the syphilis-causing bacteria that crossed the Atlantic.

Coming only 150 years after the Black Death devastated the continent, syphilis shocked Europeans. They quickly realized that sexual intercourse spreads the disease. The most commonly accepted explanation of its presence at the time was that prostitutes in Barcelona had spread syphilis to Spanish troops under the command of French King Charles VIII. These troops had marched to Naples in 1495, put the city under siege, and then conquered it. Syphilis was thus soon called *(Continued on page 82)*

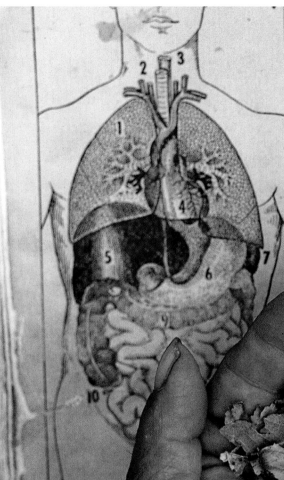

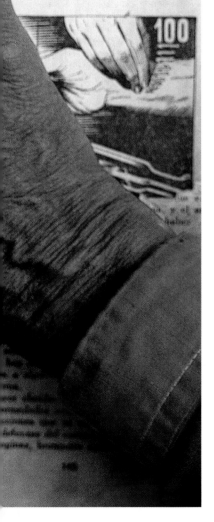

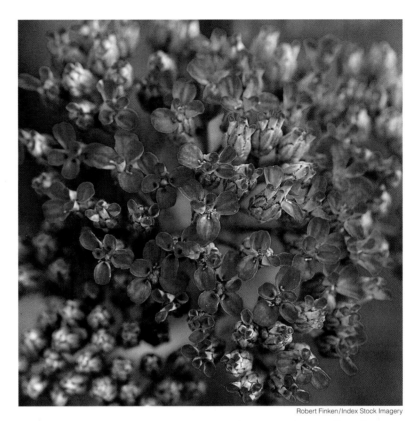

The work-calloused and knowing hand of an herbalist cradles plants he pressed and dried in an old text. Master herbalists and their knowledge are lost daily as people abandon traditional medicine for pharmaceutical drugs. The *Achillea millefolium rosea,* or pink yarrow, boasts bright pink blossoms. Yarrow has a proud pedigree as a medicinal plant. Pollen remnants in a 60,000-year-old burial indicate that Neandertal people used it, and an ancient Chinese pharmacopoeia recommends it. Legend says that Achilles used yarrow to cure wounds during the Trojan War. Scientific evidence indicates that it can curtail internal and external bleeding and can serve as an anti-inflammatory.

Nuts from the *uxi* tree surround medicinal roots and leaves in Belém, the seaport capital of the Brazilian state of Pará and a major distribution center for the Amazon Basin. Local people eat the grainy meat of the uxi nut and make juice from it, saying it increases their strength. As the Amazon rain forest is cut and burned in response to relentless economic and social pressures, countless species of such plants as the uxi tree face possible extinction before science has the opportunity—and the ability—to assess their potential medicinal properties and to document how humanity might continue to benefit from them.

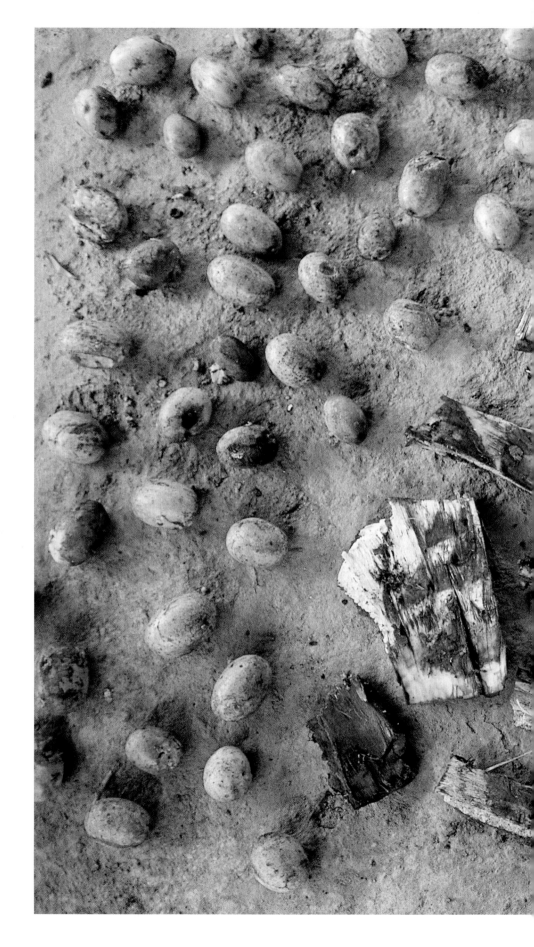

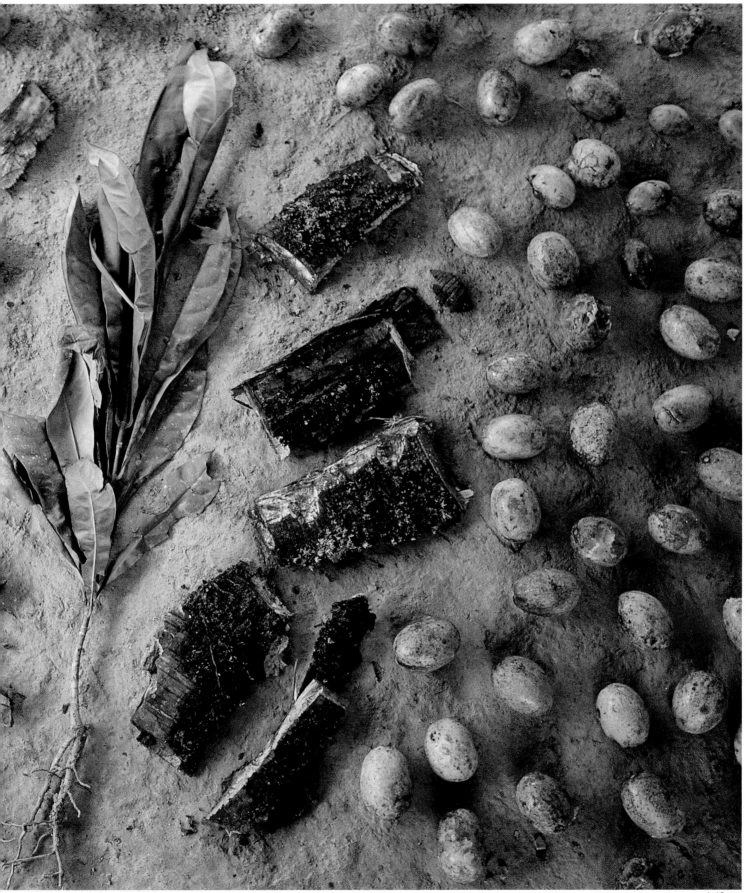

the "French disease" and the "Neapolitan disease." By the early 16th century syphilis could have been called the "American disease," because people then believed sailors returning from the New World and the natives they brought with them had initially introduced syphilis to Spain's cities.

————

GALEN HAD SAID NOTHING about any disorder resembling syphilis, but 16th-century European doctors soon announced humoral treatments for the disease, treatments that included bleeding, purging, decoctions, and bitter herbs. For the skin ulcers that accompany syphilis they prescribed ointments of goose grease, linseed, honey, and daffodil roots. Principal treatments for syphilis centered on mercury, particularly mercurial ointments and pills made from mercuric chloride.

While the exact origins of this method of treatment remain unclear, one of the first manifestations of syphilis can be skin lesions, and mercury as a treatment for such skin problems had been a legacy of Arabic medicine.

Galen had advised against using mercury because it can be very poisonous. But applied to syphilitic abscesses and absorbed through the skin, mercury might have killed the spiral-shaped bacterial spirochetes that cause syphilis.

Doctors often insisted that patients being treated with mercury spend weeks in an extremely hot room. The heat, too, may have helped kill the disease-producing bacteria. But doctors, thinking in Galenic terms, advised the heat because they believed that sweat eliminated poisons that caused the skin lesions.

To judge the validity of numerous claims of successful mercury cures is impossible because the natural progression of syphilis often resembles a cure. Swelling and ulcers disappear, but flare-ups that produce rashes, sores, or pains in the bones may occur as the bacteria spread. Again, the symptoms can clear up on their own. A person can feel well for months, or even years. Then the disease returns, even more intensely. Eventually, it hits the heart, brain, or nervous system.

In addition to extreme pain, side effects of mercury treatment usually included tremors, general paralysis, ulcerations, loosening of the bones, choking, and throats so constricted with mucus that people wanted to vomit but could not. The effect of mercury often caused a stench to fill the homes of those being treated. Doctors often prescribed a starvation diet and mercury salve, which made the patient salivate, on the assumption that extreme salivation would eliminate more poisons.

"Many people," an early 16th-century writer noted, "preferred to die of the disease rather than be cured this way."

In the midst of much fear and frustration, word spread throughout Europe that to cure themselves of syphilis, Native Americans used wood from the guaiacum, an evergreen shade tree with beautiful foliage and flowers. According to these stories, the local people sprinkled themselves with water infused with guaiacum, their "sacred tree"—which they believed their gods gave them to combat this vicious disease. Friar Ramón Pane, who accompanied Columbus on his second voyage, studied local folklore and wrote about Guagugion, a mythological hero. Guagugion saw a woman he desired and "with her took great pleasure, and immediately he sought many salves to cleanse himself, being infected with that plague which we call *mal francese.*"

This salve was the so-called natural guaiacum cure, which was immediately popular all over Europe. It had few side effects, an obvious advantage over mercury, and fit somewhat with Galenic thinking because it caused people to sweat. Another major reason for guaiacum's success was that Europeans contracted syphilis around the same time as the printing press came into use. Books, pamphlets, and newspapers written in the vernacular as well as in Latin (the language of the educated classes) began to extol the effectiveness of guaiacum.

GUAIACUM ARRIVED IN SPAIN by 1508. By 1516 patients were paying a prominent spice dealer for a treatment mixture made according to a secret recipe. By 1517 the mixture was used throughout the continent amid numerous stories of miracle cures. People began to hang pieces of what they called the "Indian cure" in churches, and guaiacum became, at least unofficially, *lignum sanctum,* or holy wood. Anyone who could not afford to buy the wood, people said, could pray in front of any lignum sanctum they saw in a church and be cured.

Due in part to huge demand, the price of guaiacum soared. Also pushing prices upward was the virtual monopoly held by the Fuggers, a German merchant and banking family prominent in the 15th and 16th centuries. The Fuggers, who also controlled most of the supply of mercury, received their monopolies from the Spanish royal family in exchange for a loan. Their role in spreading news about the efficacy and virtues of guaiacum remains unknown. Because high prices meant only the wealthy could afford this holy wood, fake guaiacum, mostly European cypress, pine, and fir, flooded the market. Guaiacum sold by weight, so a favorite trick was to fill wormholes in decayed guaiacum with red clay.

Despite such problems, more and more guaiacum recipes for syphilis cures appeared, some attractive because of their simplicity. Said one: Grind the wood; soak

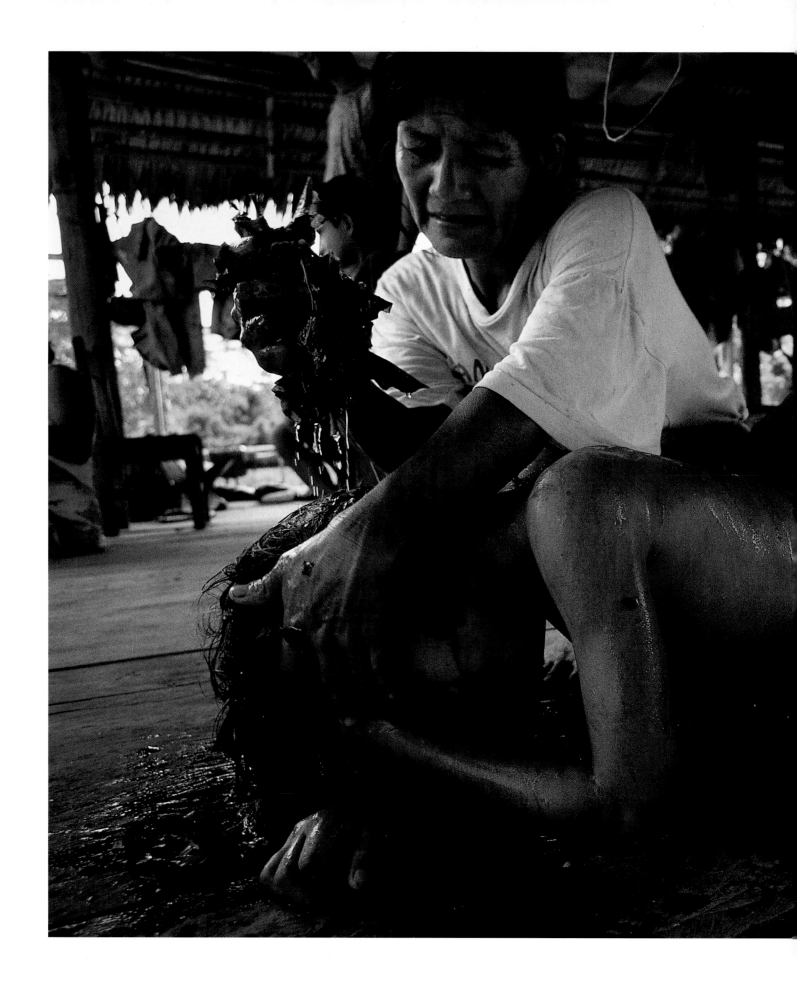

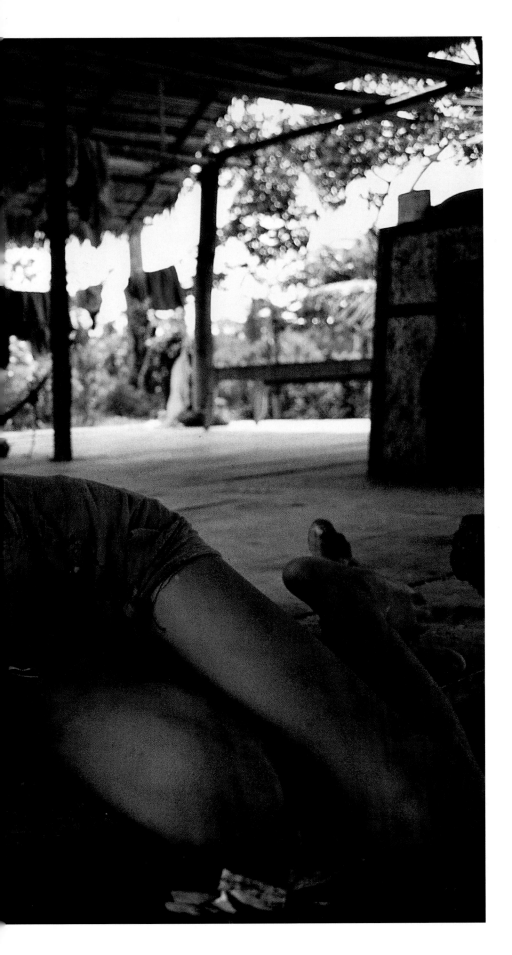

Maria Pena Lucas gives her daughter, Luz Maria Santos Pena, an herb bath to help reduce a fever. The women live in Milagro, Peru, where such use of herbs is an everyday occurrence—and the chief source of medical care. Villagers simply strip a handful of leaves from a shrub or tree and boil them in a pot of water over an open fire. Whether such remedies offer curative powers not found in Western pharmaceuticals—even if families in villages such as Milagro could afford them—remains an unanswered question. Clearly, however, the plants often contain powerful bioactive compounds.

the ground wood in water overnight; cook slowly, but do not boil, for six hours. Remove the foam and dry it. Apply the powder to dry syphilitic sores, and drink the water.

————

SIMPLICITY LAY AT THE HEART of guaiacum's appeal. Native Americans used it, Europeans reassured each other, so the drug must be as simple as they were. Ulrich von Hutten, a German knight whose 1519 book on guaiacum was translated into numerous languages and became a standard reference on syphilis treatments with holy wood, noted that "in that barbarian land where guaiacum originates there are no doctors, no exotic plants, no canons, no aphorisms [statement of principles]." In 1539 a Spanish surgeon reported with great scientific certainty that guaiacum worked best on natives of the New World because it is less harsh than mercury, and they were "delicate [and] effeminate" compared with the "more robust" Christians.

Europeans maintained a philosophic, almost spiritual, faith in the "Indian cure." Plants work best, they thought, where they originate, and God had placed every plant that poor people need around them. They did not need to pay excessive amounts to plant importers or doctors.

Thus, according to popular belief, if God put syphilis among the poor natives, he must have put the cure there also. Guaiacum, which is slow growing but can reach heights of 40 to 60 feet, seemed to prove this belief to be true because it was so plentiful throughout the West Indies and the northern coast of South America.

In part because they assumed that guaiacum would work best where it grew, some rich and adventuresome young European men infected with syphilis sailed to the Caribbean. Two of them wrote letters home describing how a local woman collected twigs, chewed them, spit the pulp into water, and made the foreign patients drink it. The woman made the Europeans work up a sweat and drink the special remedy again. After six weeks of this twice daily routine, the foreigners felt cured and returned home.

Europeans continued to believe in this cure even though they saw little else in the natives' medical arsenal worthy of emulation. The Europeans, furthermore, believed that the natives could outsmart syphilis even as those same natives continued to die helplessly at the hands of smallpox, measles, diptheria, and other infectious diseases that the Europeans had introduced.

————

EUROPEAN USE OF GUAIACUM was based on a fallacy. Although Native Americans may have used guaiacum to treat yaws, an infectious tropical disease that produces skin lesions roughly similar to those of syphilis, there is no evidence that they ever used it to

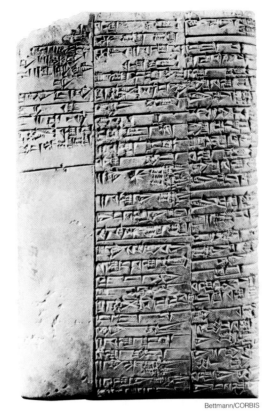

Wedge-shaped cuneiform letters of a 4,000-year-old Sumerian clay tablet represent the world's oldest known medical handbook. A portion of the right column reads: "White pear tree, the flower of the 'moon' plant, grind into a powder, dissolve in beer, let the man drink." No herbal remedies from the Sumerian civilization, which was the first to introduce revolutionary ideas such as writing and the wheel, have had an impact on modern medicine.

combat syphilis. When taken internally, guaiacum seems only to cause sweating, nausea, and a warm feeling in the stomach. A rash that itches can also appear.

The failure of guaiacum treatment soon became impossible to ignore. Ulrich von Hutten had suffered from nine years of ineffective treatment for syphilis and then claimed to be cured by 40 days of intense guaiacum treatment. But less than four years after the supposedly successful treatment and the 1519 publication of his book praising the New World bark, von Hutten was dead of syphilis.

As guaiacum fell out of vogue by the mid-to-late 1500s, Europeans turned to other syphilis treatments from the New World. These included sarsaparilla, sassafras, China root, and tobacco—all of which, like guaiacum, caused people to sweat. As prices for these herbs shot upward, Europeans continued to take guaiacum as an adjunct to mercury, which once again became their principal treatment for syphilis.

Faith that natives of the Western Hemisphere relied on guaiacum as a syphilis cure persisted, however. The Abbé Corneille de Pauw, a leading French scholar in the latter part of the 18th century, wrote in 1768: "The ultimate proof, without possible contradiction, that venereal disease came from America is the quantity of remedies [such as guaiacum] used by its natives to combat its fatal progress. They used more than sixty different elements that urgent danger had forced them to *(Continued on page 92)*

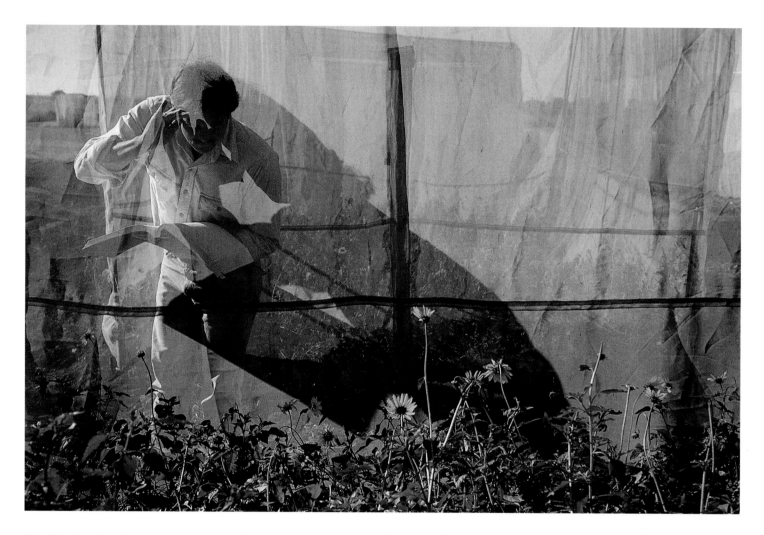

Shielding his face from glare, a worker checks the growth of sunflowers at a research facility in Ames, Iowa. Native Americans used sunflowers for food, as well as for a wide range of medicinal purposes, including treatment of lung problems, spider bites, rheumatism, and stomach worms. Sunflower seeds contain chemicals that fight rheumatism and relieve pain.

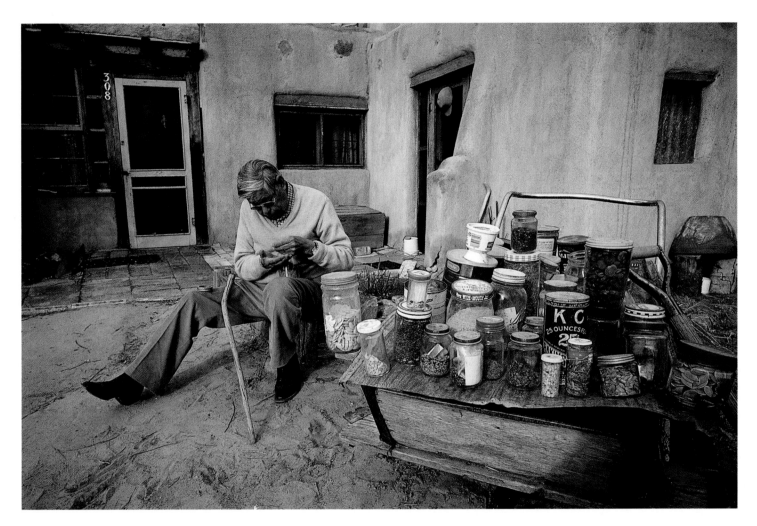

Collecting and maintaining seeds is especially important in a world economy that increasingly relies on hybrid plants. Ben Talachy of Espanola, New Mexico, keeps a collection of rare seeds, some of which have been passed from generation to generation, by taking the best seeds from each year's crop.

FOLLOWING PAGES: Cranberries, harvested by John McMahon and his son at their farm in Oregon, contain chemicals that prevent disease-causing bacteria from attaching themselves to the walls of the urinary tract. Native Americans ate cranberries as a food and used them for a variety of medicinal purposes, including treatment of nasal and respiratory infections.

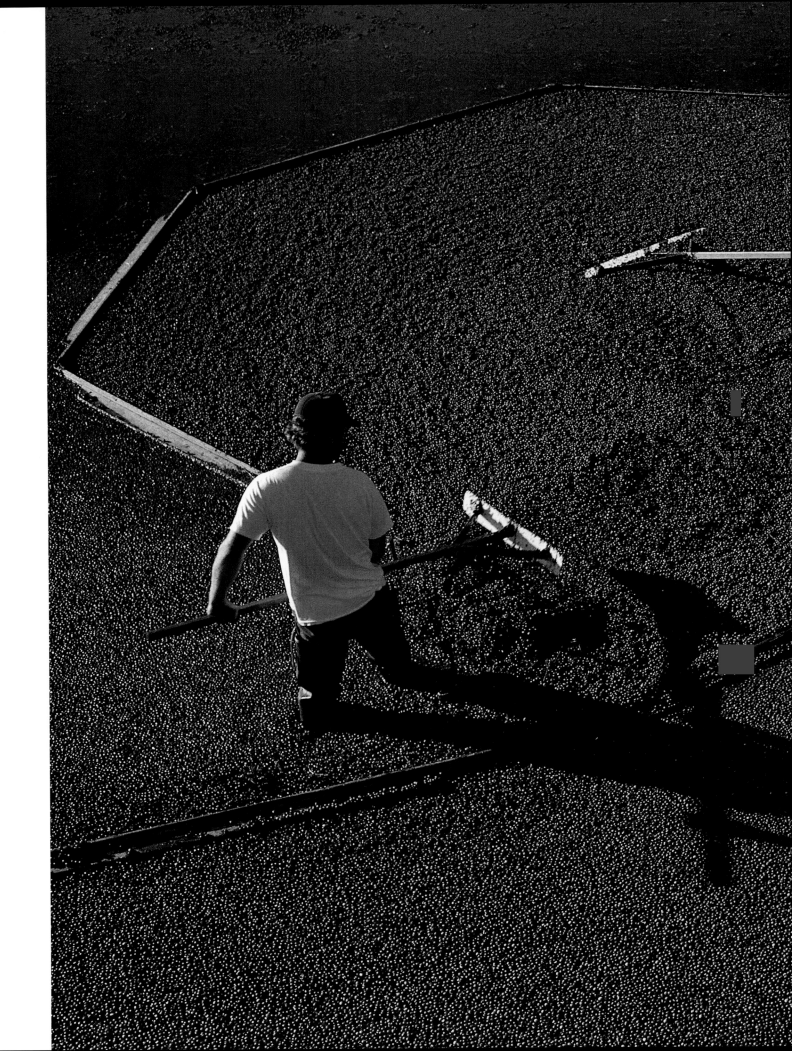

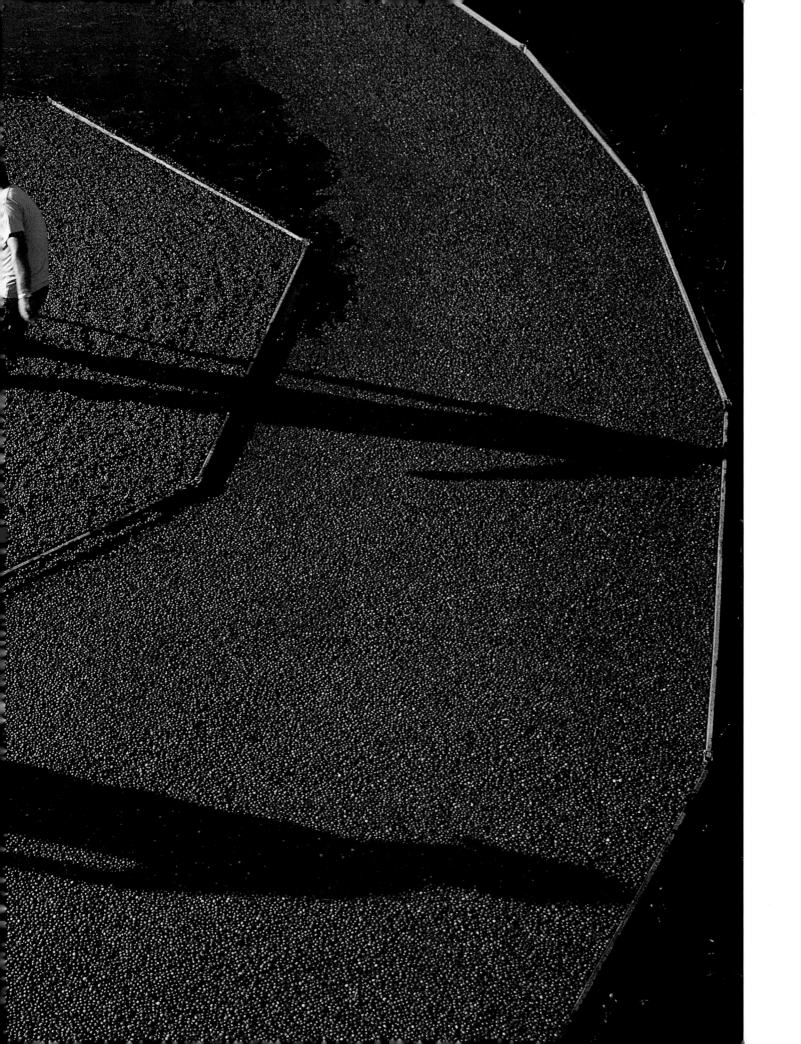

discover. It would be supremely absurd to say that Americans had sought so many cures for a malady unknown to them."

During this period doctors began to use guaiacum to treat other illnesses. Writing in the mid-1500s, Monardes had said that guaiacum is "good for the Dropsy [severe swelling in the legs caused by congestive heart failure and the heart's subsequent inability to circulate the blood well], for the shortnes of breath, for the Falling sicknes, for the evill of the Bladder...."

In England, Shakespeare's son-in-law, John Hall, combined guaiacum with sarsaparilla to treat skin diseases. He also used guaiacum in a remedy that he kept secret until his death. To treat problems of the uterus, he combined guaiacum, spring water, and horse dung. Hall sweetened and "aromatized" the mixture to the patient's taste.

Guaiacum remained popular among doctors into the 20th century. When first published in 1820, the *Pharmacopoeia of the United States*, a medical compendium gathered by scientists, doctors, pharmacists, and others interested in health care, included five different preparations of guaiacum. The herb remained in the U.S. pharmacopoeia until 1910.

———

ONE OTHER NEW WORLD medicinal plant, the cinchona tree, quickly became popular in European medicine. It provided an effective treatment against a disease, named malaria by the 18th century, that is caused by parasitic protozoans that enter human red blood cells.

Identifying malaria in ancient written sources can be difficult. The premodern diagnostician often focused on symptoms such as high fever and chills that actually describe many illnesses. Contemporary analysis of blood samples from hundreds of people in Africa with fevers and chills shows that less than half of the blood has the protozoan that causes malaria.

Malaria in ancient times can be identified, however, because malarial fevers usually occur in distinct cycles. After entering a human red blood cell, the one-celled protozoan that causes malaria divides into smaller entities called merozoites. The number of merozoites grows until the red blood cell bursts apart, releasing them. They then find and enter other red blood cells, and the cycle starts over. Fevers and chills occur when red blood cells rupture, releasing the merozoites. This cycle repeats on a regular basis, resulting in recurring attacks of fever and chills that last from four to ten hours. These attacks usually come daily in the early stages of the disease, and then every 48 hours or every 72 hours, depending on the type of malaria. Malaria epidemics, furthermore, are

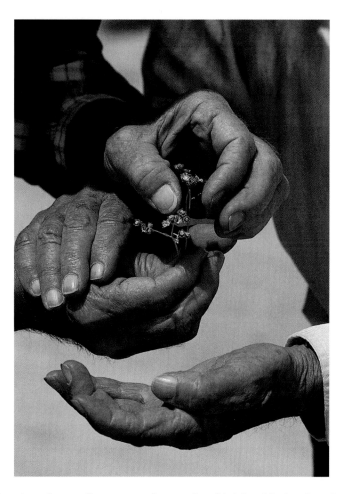

Stained hands of caring plant collectors cradle a sprig of jojoba. Native Americans use the jojoba plant, a desert-dweller indigenous to the Sonoran Desert of Arizona, California, and northern Mexico, to treat certain skin problems. Some tribes dry and pulverize the jojoba seed and then apply it to sores. Other tribes dry the fruit and char it over a fire before rubbing it into the skin.

seasonal. Ancient writers often described this seasonality, although they did not seem to understand that it occurred because mosquitoes spread the malaria-causing parasite.

Sumerian medical tablets dating from the sixth millennium B.C. mention a malaria-like disease, as do ancient Chinese texts. Chinese healers saw malaria in terms of yin and yang; the chills and fever were evidence that something was out of balance. Malaria seems to have reached Europe via trade with Asia by the sixth century B.C. Writing in the fifth century B.C., Hippocrates described the patterns of fevers characteristic of malaria. He saw it, as he saw all disease, as evidence that the humors were out of balance. Hippocrates associated malaria with black bile, presumably in response to depression that can accompany bouts of the disease.

Shakespeare mentions ague, the contemporary word for the fever and chills we now call malaria, in at least ten places. In *Macbeth*, written in 1606-07, Macbeth believes that the witches have assured him he will never be defeated until Birnam wood moves to his castle at Dunsinane. Of his approaching enemies, Macbeth says, "Hang out our banners

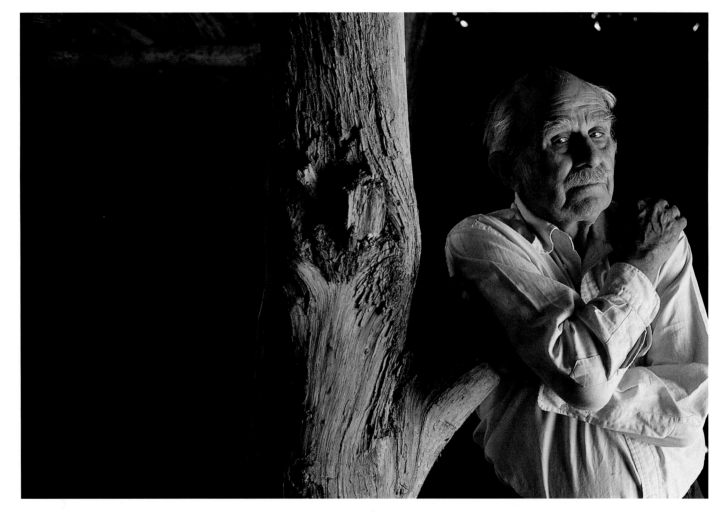

One of the world's experts on medicinal plants, the U.S. Department of Agriculture's Howard Scott Gentry spent more than 60 years traveling the world and gathering seeds. The National Seed Storage Laboratory in Fort Collins, Colorado, which conserves seeds and conducts research on how best to preserve plant genetic diversity, houses his collection.

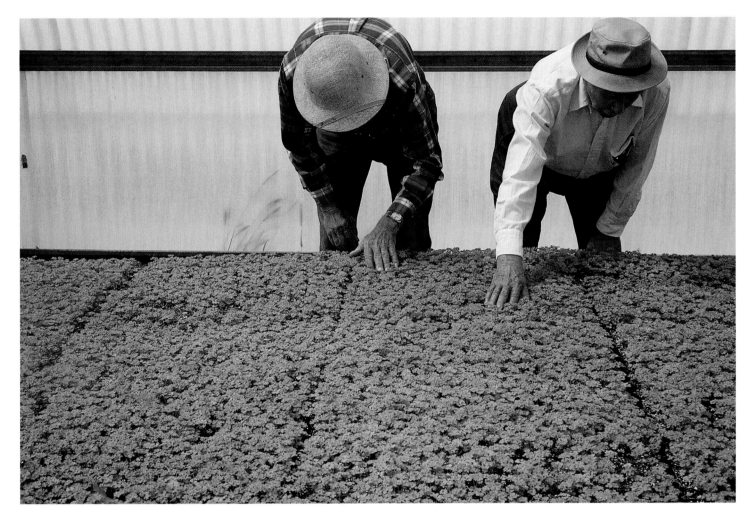

Seed collector Howard Scott Gentry, in the yellow shirt, and friend and plant breeder George Able examine jojoba seedlings. Their efforts at preserving such plants will allow future generations, perhaps armed with better technology and understanding, to study the plant's medicinal properties. Gentry, who died in 1993, believed that the healing potential of jojoba has yet to be explored.

on the outward walls; / The cry is still 'They come!' our castle's strength / Will laugh a siege to scorn: here let them lie / Till famine and the ague [malaria] eat them up...."

Although Asians crossing the Pacific in rafts could have brought malaria a millennium before the arrival of Europeans, evidence indicates that the disease did not exist in the Western Hemisphere until after Columbus's arrival. Maya and Aztec medical records discuss nothing like it, and early explorers do not mention encountering it. Why would malaria exist everywhere but the Western Hemisphere? A good guess: Thousands of years ago, when humans first crossed the Bering Strait that separates Siberia from Alaska, the protozoan that causes malaria could not survive the cold temperatures.

Neither Hippocrates nor any European doctor ever developed an effective treatment for malaria. Hall treated it with, among other things, maidenhair ferns, snails, and China root. For a woman suffering from malarial-type fever just three days after childbirth, he advised something that would cause little vomiting: a sweetened alcoholic drink made with hart's horn, as well as a milk-and-sugar enema and an herbal compress applied to the stomach.

Another malaria remedy popular in England at the time was to sit knee-deep in milk that was as hot as the patient could endure, while sipping a steaming drink made of sweetened and spiced milk curdled with ale or wine.

———————

FINALLY, AN EFFECTIVE MALARIA remedy, one essentially still used today, arrived from the supposedly "primitive" people of the New World.

The most commonly accepted story about the discovery of this remedy may or may not be true. Around 1640, Francesca de Ribera, the Countess of Chinchon and the second wife of the Viceroy of Peru, became very sick with fever and chills. Nothing her physicians did seemed to help, and her condition worsened. Desperate to save her life, the doctors sent out word that they were looking for a cure. In response, people in a distant Andean village north of Lima provided a particular kind of bark.

The natives, descendants of the Inca who ruled an Andean empire, left no written record of what instructions they sent, but Spanish priests ground the bark into a tea and tested it on patients in a hospital. The brew was effective, so it was given to the countess, curing her fever and chills. In honor of this moment, the bark was called chinchona after the countess. The first *h* in her name was dropped by mistake when the tree was first classified. When the viceroy's term ended and he returned to Spain, he took with him the bark, whose power he had confirmed by testing it on other people after his wife recovered.

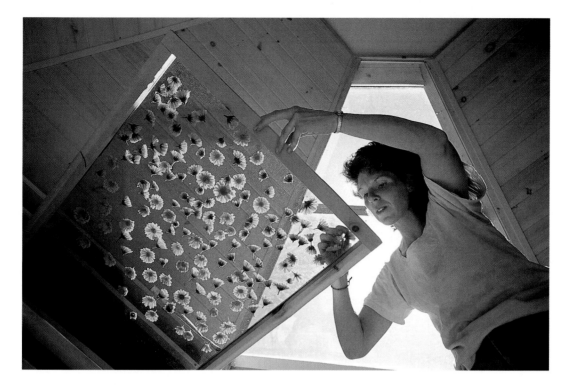

In the drying house of Avena Botanicals in Rockport, Maine, a worker spreads calendula blossoms to dry on a special screen. Native to Europe, calendula is now a common garden flower that has antiseptic properties. Although it can be taken internally, its most common use is for skin problems such as cuts, rashes, stings, and bites.

We know the story of the countess because of an account written by a missionary, Father Antonio de la Calancha, the year of her supposed cure, and published in Barcelona. Father Antonio failed to mention perhaps the most amazing fact: At most about a hundred years after their first exposure to malaria, the Inca people had accomplished what the Greeks, Romans, and thousands of years of European civilizations had failed to do.

Another version of the malaria-cure story reports that Jesuit priests observed natives in the most remote part of the province of Quito using cinchona bark to combat chills after wading through cold mountain streams. The Jesuits, according to this scenario, then took the bark to Lima with them. Trials conducted by the Jesuits in the mid-1600s resulted in endorsement of the bark by Pope Innocent X. According to one contemporary account, "The miracles of the bark in restoring the sick were exalted." It was so closely associated with the Jesuits that the strongly antipapal Oliver Cromwell, who briefly ruled England in the mid-17th century, called cinchona bark "the powder of the devil" and refused to touch it, even though he himself suffered from malaria.

Despite such resistance, cinchona became part of the Jesuits' public relations-diplomatic repertoire. Founded in 1539 by Ignatius of Loyola, the Society of Jesus sent missionaries throughout the New World and Asia. Although these men took an oath of poverty, their knowledge and use of medicinal plants enhanced their power and influence. In 1692, when China's Emperor K'ang Hsi became sick, Jesuit missionaries offered a pound of cinchona bark they had recently received from India. Three other malaria-sufferers took the bark as a test. When they were quickly cured, the emperor also took cinchona, was cured, then ordered public celebrations honoring the Jesuits.

USE OF CINCHONA BARK does not appear to have been widespread among the inhabitants of the New World, in contrast to their supposed reliance on guaiacum. Europeans left no indication they were aware of this discrepancy, or that they wondered why a malaria treatment emerged only to help the Countess of Chinchon.

Countless plants kill the parasite that causes malaria, and if Europeans had been paying attention, they could have seen malaria cures all around them. Portuguese sailing along the west coast of Africa since the mid-to-late 1400s, for example, had contact with local tribes using malaria-fighting herbs. Modern tests have proven these plants to be effective. One example is the scrub bush *Cryptolepis sanguinolenta*, which is found in present-day Ghana.

That a medicinal plant from a remote village in the Andes got noticed in Europe was extraordinary. No one knows how many New World plants the Europeans tested as possible treatments for malaria. Cinchona bark succeeded for several reasons. It was effective, and it had a simple recipe: Boil the bark in water and then drink it. Cinchona also traveled well. Many, perhaps most, medicinal plants change chemically after being picked, but cinchona bark was stable. It could be stored and transported without noticeably changing its chemical make-up or physical state. Cinchona maintained its antimalarial potency during the long eastward journey across the Atlantic.

Credit should go to the Jesuits for noticing the bark. If people in Ecuador were like traditional people virtually everywhere, each tribe employed dozens of plants against fever and chills. They almost certainly also used these same plants to treat countless other unrelated problems. To an outsider the possibilities for malaria treatments must have seemed endless, confusing, and overwhelming. The Jesuits, furthermore, played a vital role in testing and disseminating information about cinchona bark. Without the backing of a respected organization like the Society of Jesus, medical authorities might never have noticed that a remedy so effective was available.

To have identified a medicine like cinchona bark, the Andean natives must have devised effective methods for gathering data via trial and error. However, there is no evidence that Europeans tried to learn from them. No one, apparently, went back to the Andes and said, "This cinchona is fantastic. How did you discover it?" And apparently no one asked, "Do you have anything else we could take a look at?"

This lack of interest characterized most European dealings with the Inca, whose civilization dated from at least 1200. Measured by control of land, the Inca had the largest empire in the New World and the third largest in the world, ranking behind only the Ts'ing Dynasty and Ottoman Empire. The Inca Empire spanned roughly 2,600 miles, from what is now southern Colombia to central Chile. The Inca had sophisticated art, especially ceramics, textiles, and architecture. Although they had no writing, trained scribes used knotted cords called quipus to keep numeric records.

All of this had been quickly destroyed. In 1532 conquistador Francisco Pizarro attacked the Inca. Their empire immediately collapsed, and the people, like natives elsewhere, were soon serving as slaves in Spanish gold and silver mines. In the meantime, the Spanish, who clearly did not perceive the Inca as capable of contributing anything of value, called the new fever medicine Jesuit bark and Jesuit powder, rather than Inca bark or Inca powder.

Nor did the Spanish try to learn from the other major civilizations they encountered. The Maya civilization, centered primarily on the Yucatán Peninsula, began roughly at the same time as the Christian era. The Maya developed cities, ceremonial centers, hieroglyphic writing, astronomy, and a calendar. Spanish officials burned their books, including medical texts, as the work of the devil.

Research is now beginning to show what might have been lost. The highland Maya people currently living in Chiapas, Mexico, use at least 38 species of plants to treat gastrointestinal problems. These plants seem effective against disease-causing pathogens and in relieving symptoms.

————————

ANOTHER NEW WORLD GROUP, the Aztec, lived mostly in the vicinity of present-day Mexico City. Like the Inca, the civilization of the Aztec dates from about the 12th century. Aztec achievements were primarily agricultural and included irrigation systems, breeding new plants, and the cultivation of large botanical gardens.

The Aztec used pictographs to keep records but had no formal writing. They spoke the Nahuatl language and transmitted knowledge about medicinal plants orally

FOLLOWING PAGES: The coneflower, often known by the first word of its scientific name, *Echinacea*, contains compounds that fight viruses and stimulate the human immune system. The plant is indigenous to North America, where native healers have used it to treat snakebites, toothaches, burns, enlarged glands, colds, and headaches. No one has identified a single active compound that is responsible for the coneflower's medicinal actions.

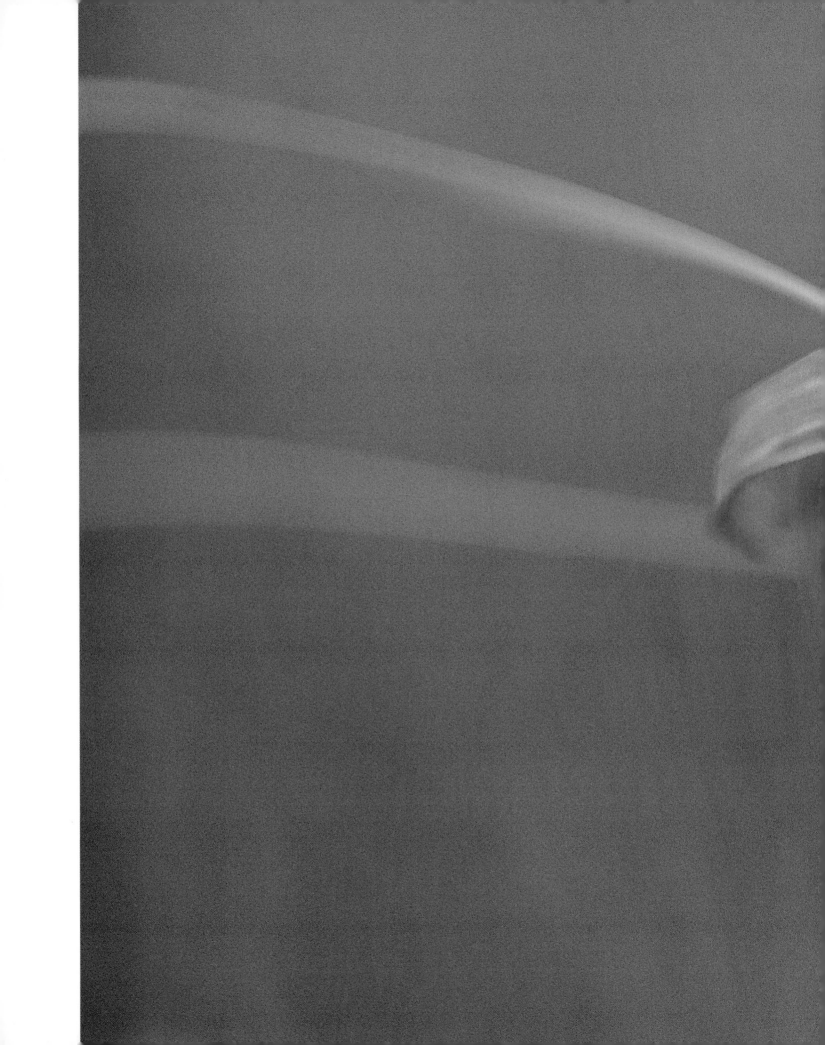

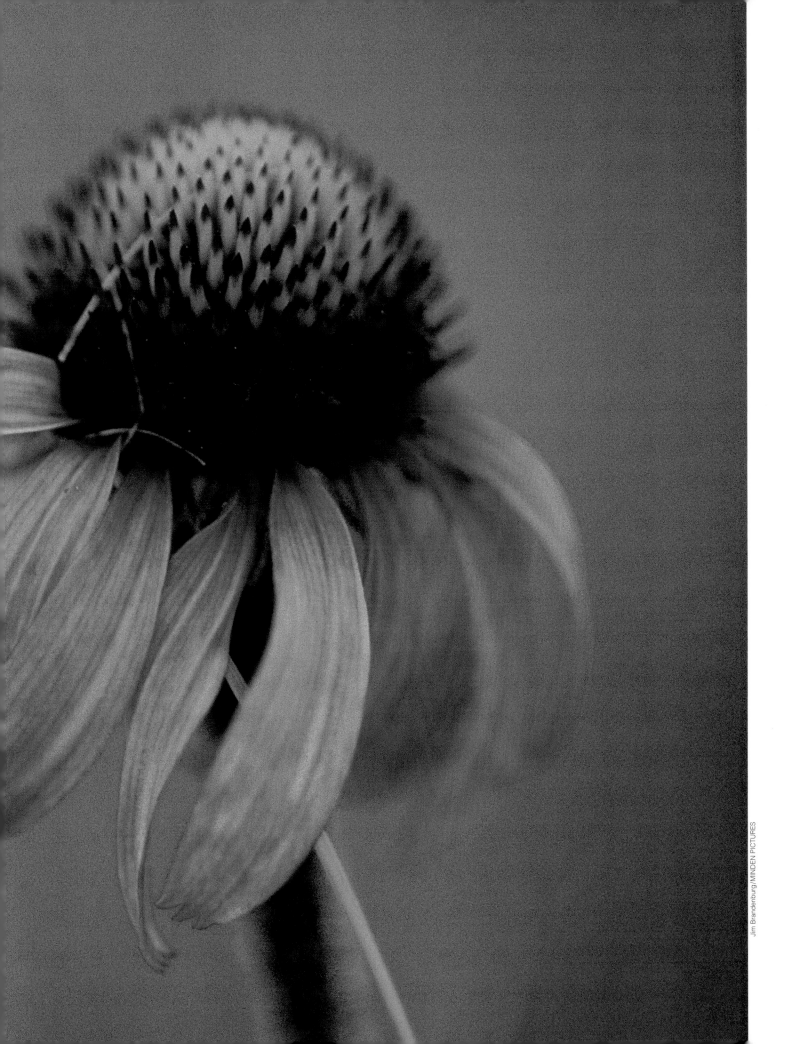

from one generation to the next. Much of what we know about Aztec medical treatments is contained in a book called the *Aztec Herbal of 1552*. In Latin and found in Vatican archives in 1929, this text on herbal medicine had been commissioned by the son of the Viceroy of Mexico in 1552, 31 years after the Spanish conquest. An Aztec seminary student, Martin de la Cruz, had written the book in Nahuatl, saying he had received his information from "old men." Another student had translated the book into Latin.

The book's young author clearly wanted to impress the Spanish, to appear sophisticated, and to show the old ways in a bad light. In the preface de la Cruz told his readers that his Aztec sources had "no formal reasonings but [were] educated by experiments only." "Remember," he wrote, "that we poor and unfortunate Indians are inferior to all mortals, and thus our insignificance and poverty implanted in us by nature, merit forbearance."

The "old men" who provided the information upon which the book was based may not have wanted to divulge ancient secrets. Presumably, they knew that they would not be held accountable for what they told the Spanish-oriented students, and they may have made up many details.

Some of the prescriptions are straightforward: "The *iztaqc-patli* plant is to be crushed in a little clear water and the juice dropped into the nostrils of one suffering from headache." *Patli* is a general Nahuatl term for medicinal plants, and iztaqc-patli translates to "white medicine," so the identity of this plant, like other plants in the *Aztec Herbal of 1552*, remains unclear.

To stop bleeding, the book recommends "the juice of nettles" from *a-tzitzicazli* "crushed as a lotion, with milk infused into the nostrils…." Other treatments are more complicated. One recipe has seven varieties of flowers, twelve varieties of leaves, a bark, a fruit, a stem, and blood from six different animals. Hair loss "is to be stopped by a lotion of a dog's or deer's urine, with the plant called *xiuh-amolli* boiled with reeds and the *avat-tecolotl animalcula*." A "broken head is to be smeared with plants growing in summer dew, with green-stone, pearls, crystal and the *tlacalhuatzin*, and with wormy earth, ground up in the blood from a bruised vein and the white of egg; if blood cannot be had, burned frogs will take the place." Against "stupidity of mind" the book prescribes: Take a drink made of roots, vomit; a few days later, take a drink made of roots and flowers; stones from the stomach of birds, gallbladder of a night owl; then be "anointed with the brain of a raven and a dove's feathers crushed and put in water with human hairs." Those hit by lightning are told to anoint the body with a potion made from leaves of trees and bushes struck by the lightning.

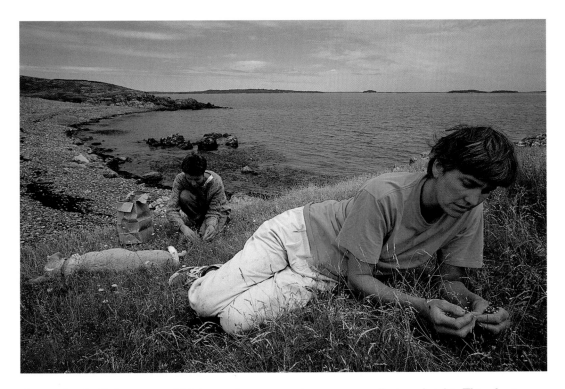

On an island off the coast of Maine, a dog naps as two women collect eyebright. This plant, whose Latin name is *Euphrasia officinalis*, helps treat conjunctivitis and other ailments of the eye. The flower looks like a bloodshot eye, which premodern healers who believed in the doctrine of signatures would have seen as a sign indicating its medicinal applications.

Spanish leaders, perhaps fearing the effect of Aztec thinking on impressionable readers and apparently seeing nothing of value in the *Aztec Herbal*, locked it away in the Vatican Library.

––––––––

THIS SAME ATTITUDE, essentially that barbarian natives have little to offer, dominated the thinking of European colonists in North America. Like the Spanish and Portuguese to their south, explorers of North America's Atlantic coast wanted medicinal plants but expected nothing new. Giovanni de Verrazano, a Florentine exploring the eastern coast of North America on orders from the King of France, wrote in 1524 of the new territory, "It cannot be devoid of the same medicinal and aromatic drugs" already in use.

In 1603, before any colonists settled in Massachusetts, English explorers looked for sassafras, which the Spanish had introduced to Europe as a treatment for rheumatism, syphilis, and dropsy. The plant does, in fact, grow as far north as Ontario.

Colonists obviously had contact with Native Americans and saw their medical practices. But members of the Plymouth colony and the Massachusetts Bay colony demonstrated little interest. In 1630 John Winthrop, Governor of the Massachusetts Bay colony, took pharmaceutical supplies, including plants, with him from England. He provided medical treatment to the settlers and natives according to written instructions from doctors in London. "For the stopping of the urine, or the stone," ran one typical instruction, "give the party to drinke of the Decoction of Maiden hayre, fennell rootes, and parsley rootes. Let him Drinke great quantitie. But before let him drinke 2 or 3 ounces of the oyle of allmonds, newly extracted, or more…." For diseases of the bladder, treatment included "make injections of the decoction of Hypericon, the bark of a young oak (the outward black skin being taken off) and linseede…."

Winthrop and most of his fellow colonists believed that the Native Americans had little worthwhile knowledge. In their estimation local people used primarily roots, had no capacity to store medicinal plants, and relied on sorcery and witch doctors. The natives' medicine ceremonies, such as midwinter gatherings aimed at renewing all the plants' medicinal qualities, seemed strange, as did the practice of lighting a feather and thanking the Creator when picking a medicinal herb.

The colonists, furthermore, considered the natives to be barbarians because they never developed cities, writing, or European-style art, which the colonists perceived as essential for culture. The issue seemed uncomplicated: How could what some colonials called "speaking apes," who lacked the ability to read or write, have medical knowledge of any value?

———————

NATIVE AMERICAN HEALERS, in fact, had sophisticated knowledge of plants derived from generations of trial and error. Like the Maya and other peoples to the south, they also thought somewhat in humoral terms. They believed, for example, that only vomiting, sweating, and other excretions could remove poisons from the body.

The colonists, however, continued to rely on imported plants. "I beg you to send some medicinal seeds, purgatives, for instance, and similar seeds," a Jesuit missionary on Lake Huron wrote to his brother in 1641. The records of a Boston apothecary shop from 1698 to 1701 show that the only homegrown herb it offered was sassafras. Medicines that George Washington ordered for his plantation included what he called "modern" ones such as antimony, sulfur, and spirits of turpentine, but no plants that grew locally. Indifference to native use of plants continued after the United States achieved independence.

In 1804 one botanist noted, "among these people the art of medicine is truly in a shapeless and an embryo state." Medicine chests of American naval ships into the early 19th century contained all imported herbs except for senega root.

Of course, some exceptions existed. Cotton Mather (1663-1728), a Boston minister famous for his support of the Salem witchcraft trials, believed that God put medicinal plants where they are most useful. Praising unique cures available only from local plants, he wrote that "our Indians do cures many times which are truly stupendous."

Although surviving letters, diaries, and journals rarely mention use of native plants, some do record instances born of necessity. A Jesuit priest wounded by an unfriendly member of the Huron tribe described treatment provided by a friendly native. He took a "pointed stone," the priest wrote, "to make an incision in me by which he tried to drain out the discolored blood and then he poured cold water on the top of my head in which he had put some boiled root. He took his medicinal liquor in his mouth and squirted it on the sore and on the incision he made. This cure was so good than in quite a short time I was healed."

Most contact with local plants and native healing traditions may have occurred via colonial women. As in all agricultural societies, their responsibilities usually included growing and collecting medicinal herbs for their families. They certainly must have exchanged ideas and plants with Native American women. Letters, diaries, and journals indicate, however, that colonial women believed that English herbs worked best for English people.

Of the 212 plants in the *Pharmacopoeia of the United States* published in 1820, nearly 100 had been used by Native Americans. But all the book's explanations for how to use the plants were based on European humoral interpretations. None was based on Native American knowledge or practices.

Modern medicine continues to ignore Native American experience. Native American uses of plants contributed virtually nothing to modern pharmaceutical drugs. A possible exception is the mayapple, a perennial flower that Native Americans used to cause sweating and vomiting and to treat what they called skin cancer. In the 1970s and 1980s scientists derived the chemical podophyllotoxin from the mayapple and tried it as an anticancer agent. Podophyllotoxin proved to be too toxic for safe use, but it led to two other drugs, etoposide and teniposide.

These drugs are called semisynthetic because they are made by modifying compounds found in nature, in this case a plant species related to mayapple and grown in India and Pakistan. A fully synthetic drug is one whose original formula comes from human ingenuity in a laboratory, not from a naturally occurring entity such as a plant. Both etoposide and teniposide are used to treat various forms of cancer. Resin from the mayapple has also proved to be an effective treatment for genital warts, which may explain its use by Native Americans for their "skin cancer."

———————

THE JOURNEY OF NEW WORLD plants to Europe demonstrates how a culture learns, and resists learning, about new medicines. It also reveals the power of economics and of wishful thinking, and the delicacy of the ongoing balance a society must make between its empirical evidence and the dictates of its belief system.

Had European doctors and medical researchers been quicker to listen, they would have learned about dozens of plants—including senega root, Indian pink, *Collinsonia*, *Sanguinaria*, lobelia, American ginseng, joe-pye weed, mayapple, echinacea, goldenseal, and black cohosh—that are among the most commonly used medicinal plants in the United States today.

Goldenseal is a typical example of what Europeans missed. It grows naturally through much of the United States east of the Mississippi. Most of its medicinal uses come from the rhizome, a long underground stem, and rootlets. Native Americans prepared goldenseal in various ways, sometimes mixing it with other ingredients. Among other things, goldenseal served them as an insect repellent, diuretic, and stimulant; as a wash for sores and inflamed eyes; and as a treatment for jaundice, stomach ulcers, and colds.

Meriwether Lewis, who served as doctor for the 1803-to-1806 Lewis and Clark expedition that explored America's Louisiana Territory, called it "a sovereign remedy for sore eyes." He treated eye infections by infusing the rhizome in hot or cold water. Claims by 19th-century authors included goldenseal as a treatment for rattlesnake bites, cancer, dropsy, sore legs, fevers, and loss of appetite. It was used, among other things, to stimulate the flow of bile into the small intestine and to control sweating.

Goldenseal was listed in the *Pharmacopoeia of the United States* in 1830, 1860 to 1920, and 1945. Major U.S. pharmaceutical companies sold it until 1960. People currently use it as an antiseptic, an antimicrobial, and as an immune stimulant. Berberine, one of the chemicals in goldenseal, seems to activate macrophages, white cells that are a powerful part of the human immune system.

Whether modern science will now document, utilize, and build upon the medicinal chemicals found in plants such as goldenseal remains unclear (see Chapters 7 and 8). To do so, scientists would have to overcome attitudes toward plants and expectations about what constitutes a medicine that have their origins 500 years ago in the vague beginnings of what we call the scientific revolution.

Thomas Jefferson's garden book includes an accounting of plants and their locations on the grounds of Monticello. Jefferson, who collected seeds from around the globe, did not differentiate between food and medicinal crops. He knew that many plants, such as garlic, capsicum, and tarragon, serve both functions.

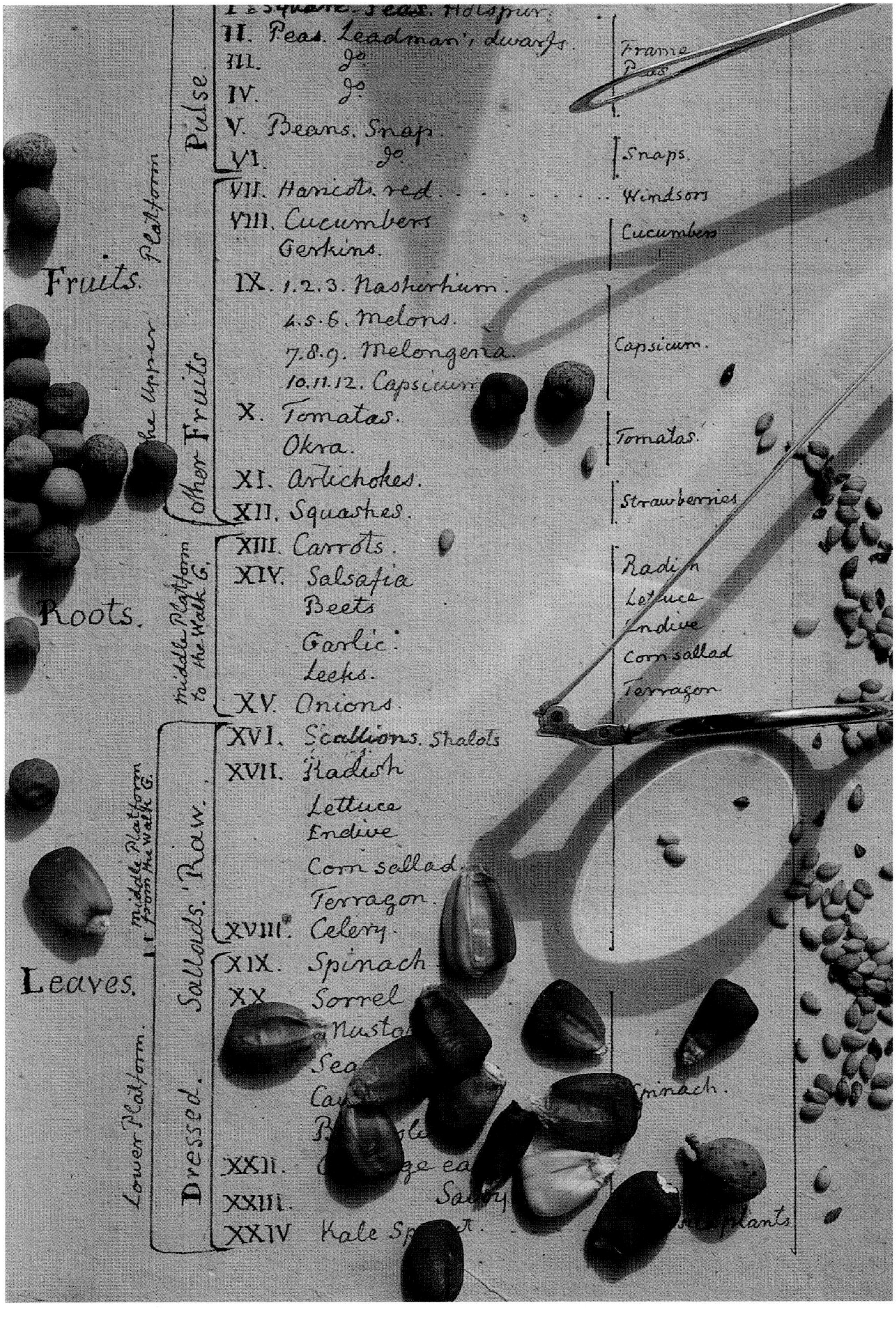

Fruits.

Pulse

The Upper Platform

I. ... squash Peas. Holspur.
II. Peas. Leadman's dwarfs.
III. Do
IV. Do
V. Beans. Snap.
VI. Do
VII. Haricots. red . . . . .
VIII. Cucumbers
    Gerkins.
IX. 1.2.3. Nasterhum.
    4.5.6. Melons.
    7.8.9. Melongena.
    10.11.12. Capsicum
X. Tomatas.
    Okra.
XI. Artichokes.
XII. Squashes.

other Fruits

Frame
Peas.

Snaps.
Windsors
Cucumbers

Capsicum.

Tomatas.

Strawberries

Roots.

middle Platform to the Walk G.

XIII. Carrots.
XIV. Salsafia
    Beets
    Garlic.
    Leeks.
XV. Onions.

Radish
Lettuce
Endive
Corn sallad
Terragon

Leaves.

Lower Platform.

middle Platform from the Walk G.

Dressed.   Sallouts. Raw.

XVI. Scallions. Shalots
XVII. Radish
    Lettuce
    Endive
    Corn sallad.
    Terragon.
XVIII. Celery.
XIX. Spinach
XX. Sorrel
    Mustard
    Sea
    Cay...
    B...
XXII. O...ge ea...
XXIII.   Savory
XXIV. Kale Sprout.

Spinach.

...plants

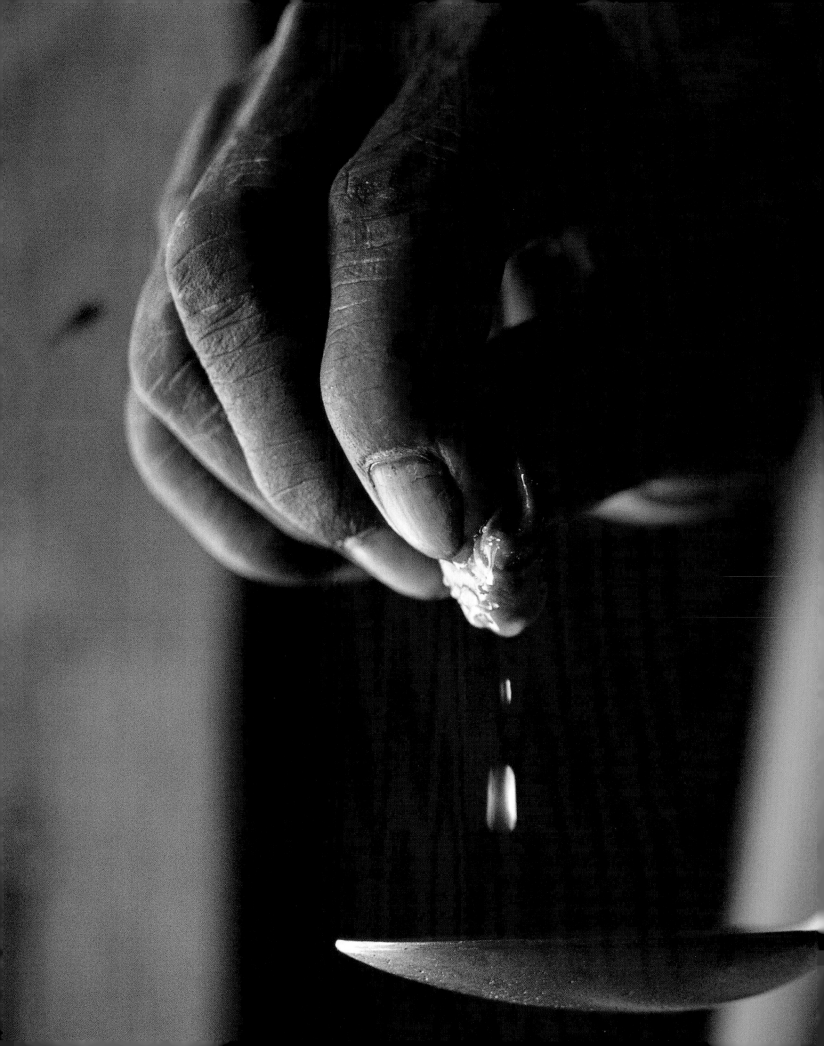

THE BIRTH OF MODERN SCIENCE

TO THE

END OF THE 20TH CENTURY

CHAPTER FOUR

Modern Science Embraces Medicinal Plants

Before the advent of modern science in Europe, women there maintained herb gardens and served as village healers. Beginning in the 17th century, as the male-dominated scientific and medical professions sought chemicals from plants, they relied on remedies from these women but pressured governments to prevent them from seeing patients. Among the charges against Margaret Jones in 1648, one of the first women in New England to be hanged as a witch, was that she practiced medicine that went "beyond the apprehension of all physicians and surgeons." Traditional healers had devised more than 14,000 remedies for problems associated with fertility, childbirth, and menstruation. During his childhood in Missouri nearly two hundred years later, Mark Twain noticed that "every old woman was a doctor, and gathered her own medicines…."

Munni Bibi of Lucknow, India, has spent most of her life collecting medicinal plants. The neem and basil she holds possess strongly bioactive chemicals.

PRECEDING PAGES: A healer in Madagascar squeezes sap from a leaf. The juice, still readily available despite destruction of much of the island's rain forest, will ease the pain of an earache.

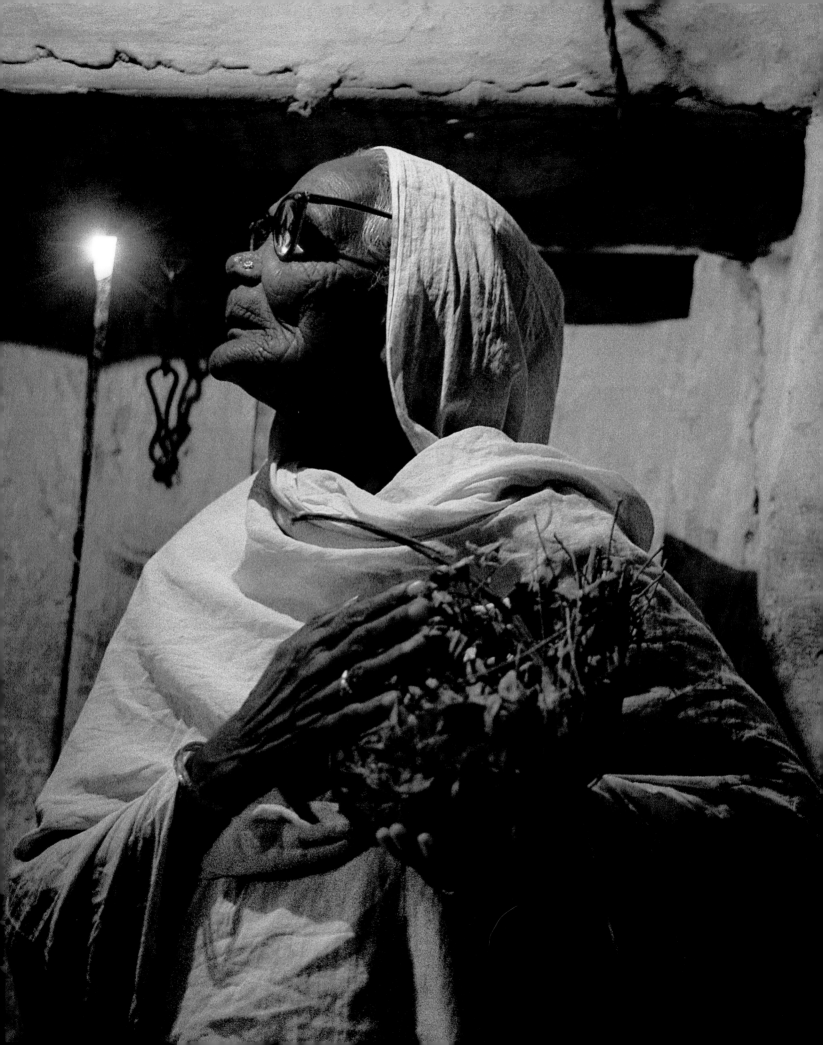

The beginnings of a change in attitude toward medicinal plants can be seen in the legacy of Philippus Theophrastus Bombast von Hohenheim, who was born in 1493 near Zurich, Switzerland. His father, a doctor, made sure that Philippus was well educated in the classics. But he rebelled, joining the large group of adolescents who wandered from university to university looking for inspirational professors.

It is unclear whether Philippus ever earned a medical degree, and his main reaction to formal higher education was negative. He wondered, as expressed in his later writing, how "high colleges managed to produce so many high asses." To truly learn medicine, he believed, "a doctor must seek out old wives, gypsies, sorcerers, wandering tribes, old robbers, and such outlaws and take lessons from them." Knowledge needed by the doctor, he said, "lies in the mysteries of Nature," not in secondhand learnings "borrowed from books."

Roaming throughout Europe, Philippus lived by this creed. Captured by nomadic Tartars from the Asian steppes, he learned about medicinal roots and herbs from what he called their "spiritual healers." Executioners taught him anatomy. Early in his travels Philippus took the name by which he is famous today, Paracelsus. In Latin it means "surpassing Celsus," who was a first-century A.D. Roman medical writer. Paracelsus' *The Great Surgery*, published in 1536, was one of the first medical books printed in Europe. Its discussions of diet, medicines, and surgery made Paracelsus famous.

Paracelsus was handsome, dashing, and unmarried, and his travels as a healer and itinerant teacher inspired stories of romantic medical miracles. In one such story Paracelsus encountered the 23-year-old daughter of the owner of an inn in Ingolstadt, a city in Bavaria on the Danube. The young woman had been paralyzed since birth. Paracelsus gave her Azoth of the Red Lion, a remedy made of mercury, his favorite medicinal substance, and told her to take it with a spoonful of wine after every meal. She began to sweat heavily, and that very same day found herself able to walk. Crying with gratitude, she threw herself at his feet.

Other Paracelsus myths survive: He could twirl his fur-trimmed cap and cause a hurricane; three of his hairs in a locket would dispel evil spirits; when he wrapped his cloak around himself, he became invisible.

In Paracelsus' judgment the ideas of Galen and other classical experts came from "histories, poets and old women." All were "useless," he told his audiences, as was a more recent book on herbal remedies, which he called "rumors which are fun to read" and "a work to empty the peasant's pockets."

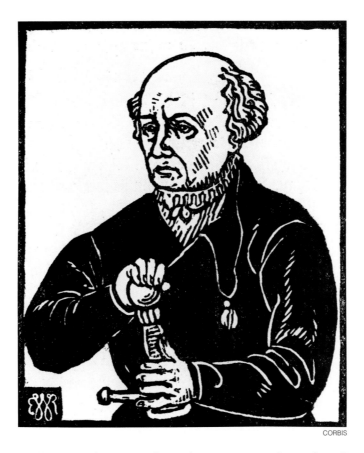

An undated woodcut depicts 16th-century Swiss doctor-scientist Paracelsus. Paracelsus helped introduce some of the basic ideas that now dominate modern medicine: that bioactive compounds can be extracted from plants, and that elements such as mercury and lead should replace herbal treatments.

On June 24, 1527, at a public bonfire in the marketplace of Basel, Switzerland, Paracelsus dramatized his challenge to accepted medical wisdom by burning volumes written by the famous Arab physician Avicenna. The students surrounding him cheered, but such actions made enemies. Less than a year later, due to the threat of jail, Paracelsus had to sneak out of Basel in the middle of the night.

PARACELSUS ATTRACTED ATTENTION in large part because of such dramatic actions, but he is remembered today because he argued that the medicinal value of plants came from the chemicals in them—the perspective that dominates modern science. Paracelsus emphasized that the most desirable parts of plants are not their leaves, bark, stems, or roots. A plant works best, he said, if you extract or distill its essence in the form of tinctures. He called this the "quintessence," or fifth essence, of the plant—the other four being earth, air, fire, and water. This idea was not unique to Paracelsus. The notion of chemical precision in the use of plants had existed in medieval Europe for hundreds of years. But Paracelsus popularized it. His work was a major step toward the present-day pharmaceutical approach toward plants: Isolate the pure form of plant constituents, particularly the active ingredient. Paracelsus also helped introduce the idea that non-plant

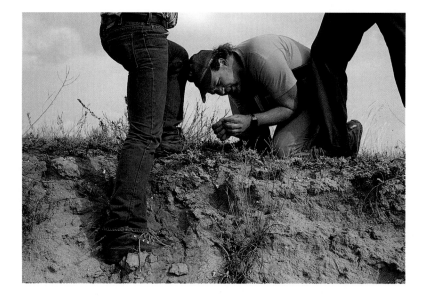

On the vast, and mostly uninhabited, Russian steppe, a team of botanists from the United States collects seeds. The value of this material may not be known for years. Collecting from such remote areas ensures that seeds will be chemical free and that outside influences such as agricultural hybrids have not modified their genetic structure. These plants must survive periods of extreme and extensive cold, so they are likely to possess unique chemicals—chemicals that could have medicinal applications.

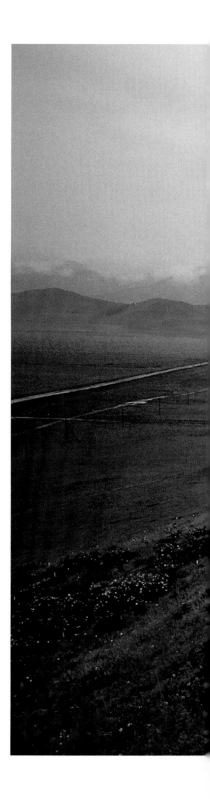

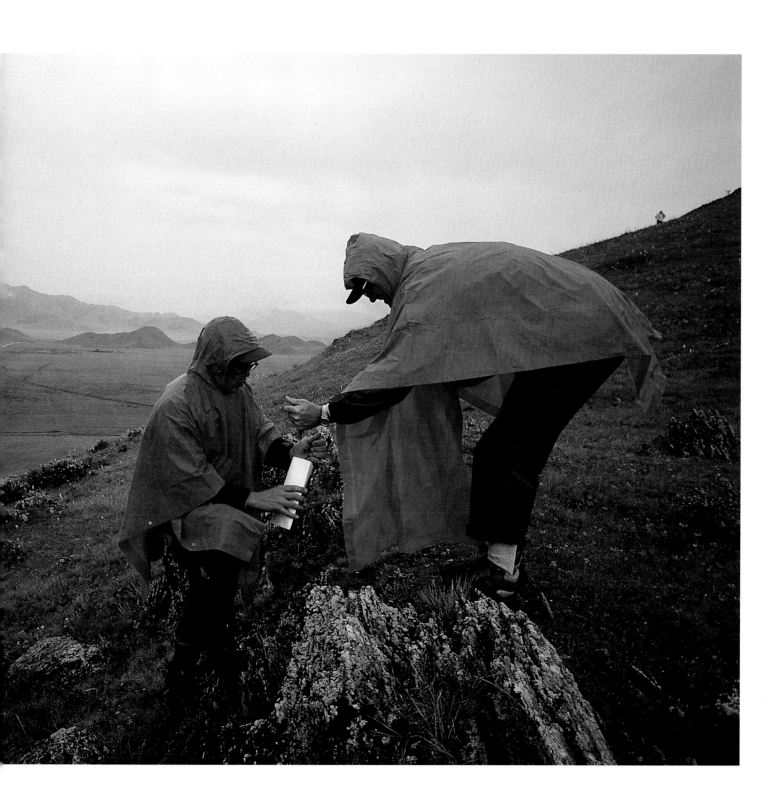

remedies—elements and compounds such as mercury, lead, sulfur, iron, arsenic, antimony, copper sulfate, and potassium sulfate—should replace herbal treatments.

As one treatment, Paracelsus recommended letting wine sit in a cup made of antimony, a poisonous metal that modern medicine uses to kill some parasites. After the wine had absorbed large amounts of metal, a patient taking Paracelsus' prescription would drink it. Ingestion of the metallic poison would cause immediate vomiting as the body tried to rid itself of the antimony. Metal not vomited out entered the bloodstream, causing sweats, violent shaking, and a burning sensation.

———

PARACELSUS LIVED AT THE SAME time as Nicolaus Copernicus, whose proof that the Earth revolves around the sun was one of the major steps toward what we now call modern science. Science had existed for thousands of years in a wide range of cultures, but something new began to develop in Europe in the early 16th century—the time of Paracelsus and Copernicus. The new philosophy relied on experimentation, not on citations from ancient authorities, as the source of truth. Everything became open to question: Posit a hypothesis; conduct experiments to determine its validity; confirm the experiments' results by replicating them. Quantification, counting, and comparing numerical results began to dominate thinking. Fundamental to this new approach was a belief that the unknown surrounds us, a frontier awaiting conquest.

One of the principal changes in science, often overlooked in analysis of the scientific revolution, was the systematic organization of empirical efforts. Scientific journals, which began to be published in the mid-17th century, led to rejection of the mystical. They bred an insistence on descriptions and reproducible experiments, generating the expectation that no finding would be accepted until reviewed and approved by the experimenter's peers. It was a philosophy that called all knowledge into doubt.

Technological advances, such as the development of the microscope in the late 16th century, also played a huge role. Modern science for the most part went in the direction of finding what technology, such as improved microscopes that permitted the viewing of smaller and smaller entities, made possible.

The study of plants had existed in ancient China, India, and Greece. Aristotle and his pupil Theophrastus (370-285 B.C.), for example, had devised a logical system for describing various plant types. Building upon this system, the first university chair in the study of plants was established in the Italian city of Padua in 1533. Slowly, the herbalist became a botanist, a profession distinguished by studying the function of plants beyond their immediate medical applications. Essential to this

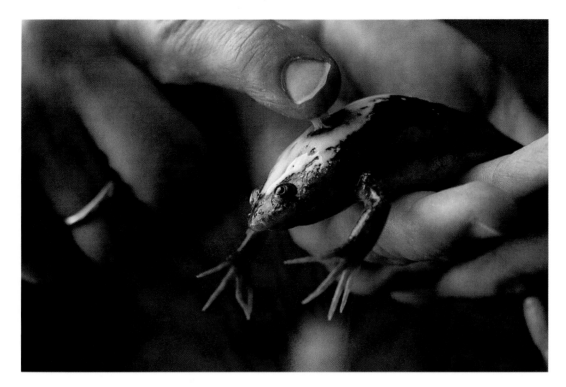

When threatened, the African clawed frog, held by Dr. Michael Zasloff of Magainin Pharmaceuticals, exudes a protective white mucus containing chemicals that are closely related to defensive compounds produced by plants. These frog-derived chemicals offer new ways to devise antibiotics and other pharmaceutical drugs.

study was standardization in the naming of plants, the formal science of plant taxonomy. In 1753 Carolus Linnaeus published *Species Plantarum*, which established standard scientific nomenclature.

––––––

CLOSELY RELATED TO BOTANY was the development of the science called "chemistry," a term in use by the end of the 16th century. Chemistry emphasized notions of uniformity, consistency, and testing for purity. Using concepts and techniques borrowed from chemistry, botanists began to isolate the exact part of each plant that gave it its medicinal qualities. Those parts then could be homogenized, standardized, and measured. Driven by the beliefs that specific chemicals in a plant account for its medicinal effects and that the best medicine consisted of standardized, predictable dosages, scientists began to isolate the active principle in plant-based medicines.

In the early 19th century a French scientist found an unknown type of plant component, which he called "a new, quite peculiar vegeto-animal matter." Named an alkaloid in 1818, it would soon become central to plant-based medicine.

Alkaloids are distinguished by organic—that is carbon-containing—compounds constructed around rings of nitrogen atoms. Although about 60 percent of all plant families have no known alkaloids, many have dozens or hundreds of them. To date, more than 10,000 alkaloids have been discovered. Most are in plants, but some are in mammals, salamanders, frogs, marine organisms, mosses, and fungi.

To put the discovery of alkaloids in context: At roughly the same time that they first identified alkaloids, scientists were learning about the basic functions of plants. In 1817, for example, scientists isolated chlorophyll and deciphered the mechanisms of photosynthesis—the process by which a plant converts solar energy into energy it stores via chemical bonds.

Most medicines from plants contain alkaloids. Throughout the 19th and 20th centuries, however, scientists discovered that other plant chemicals and compounds also have medicinal effects. These substances are all secondary metabolites (see Introduction), which fall into two general categories. The first are phenolics, compounds that have a hydroxyl group attached to a ring of carbons containing double bonds. Discovered in 1872, phenolics exist in most plants and plant parts. The least known of the secondary metabolites, phenolics include flavonoids, water-soluble pigments that help maintain the walls of small blood vessels in humans (see Chapter 8).

The second and largest group of plant chemicals and compounds with medicinal effects consists of terpenoids, commonly known as terpenes. These were discovered in 1933. What primarily defines them is a number of "isoprene units," cells from carbon dioxide that photosynthesis has recently reconverted to organic compounds. Terpenes include cardiac glycosides, discovered in 1930, which affect the heart muscles of higher animals (see Foxglove on page 134).

Scientists in the early 19th century began their search for alkaloidal drugs by making a powder of plant parts and mixing it with water, alcohol, or dilute acids. They then purified and filtered this mixture, extracting the alkaloids with a solvent. Alkaloids were separated from one another through differences in their solubility and their salts.

Throughout the 19th century, scientists scoured old herbal books and followed leads suggested by local doctors, apothecaries, and herbalists. Hundreds, and perhaps thousands, of plants were pounded, diluted, and distilled in an effort to find isolated compounds with medicinal value.

———

ONE PLANT THAT RECEIVED considerable attention was tobacco. Europeans arriving in the New World found that natives from North to South America were using this leafy plant for ritualistic purposes. Smoke, they believed, carried prayers to the Great Spirit. Even tribes that relied primarily on hunting for food cultivated tobacco. The plants seemed to vary in effect; certain species of tobacco induced hallucinations. Some shamans blew smoke over the body of a sick person; others spit tobacco on open wounds. Tobacco was applied directly to painful teeth and was used to treat snakebite.

The Spanish physician Monardes, who helped popularize New World plants, said tobacco was hot and dry to the second degree and cured 20 ailments. It could, he wrote, bind wounds, counteract poison, dissolve stomach obstructions and kidney stones, treat inflammation or swelling, kill worms, fight pain in the joints, and cure headaches, toothaches, and bad breath.

Hernández, the Spanish expert on New World plants, classified tobacco hot and dry in the fourth degree. One of its principal medical benefits, he said, was causing the patient to cough up phlegm—an important goal in Galenic medicine. This was accomplished by taking in irritating smoke through the mouth.

Tobacco became popular in Europe as a cure for these and other illnesses sooner than it caught on as something pleasurable to smoke. Juan de Cardenas, a Spanish physician, wrote in the 1570s, "To seek to tell the virtues and greatness of this holy herb, the ailments which can be cured by it, and have been, the evils from which it has saved thousands would be to go on to infinity...." Thomas Harriot, a British scientist who explored the Carolinas in 1585, reported that tobacco "purgeth superfluous phlegm and other gross humours, and openeth all the pores and passages of the body."

Tobacco growing in Lisbon herb gardens, and stories about its virtues, impressed Jean Nicot, the French ambassador to Portugal in 1559 to 1561. Nicot, who became a great advocate of tobacco's medicinal benefits, wrote to a friend that tobacco had cured an ulcer of a type usually cancerous that physicians were unable to heal. Nicot sent tobacco plants and instructions on how to cultivate them to members of the French royal family and forwarded powdered tobacco to Catherine de Medici for her persistent headaches. Members of French royalty, in turn, proclaimed its proven effectiveness in treating diseases such as asthma. Prominent people, including church officials, began to distribute tobacco as a medicinal miracle.

In the late 17th century, Francesco Redi, a Florentine physician, conducted scientific tests by injecting oil of tobacco into animals. All died. This did not impede growing faith in the plant, which remained a key subject for researchers. In 1828 the alkaloid nicotine, named after Jean Nicot, was discovered in tobacco leaves. Scientific journals reported that nicotine had successfully treated urinary diseases, nervous disorders, hemorrhages, malaria, and other ailments. Earlier studies had confirmed that nicotine is highly toxic.

Isolation of nicotine helped in the eventual development of tobacco-based insecticides. This makes sense because nicotine's natural function is to repel bugs by jumbling their nervous systems. But none of the research on tobacco led to any modern drugs.

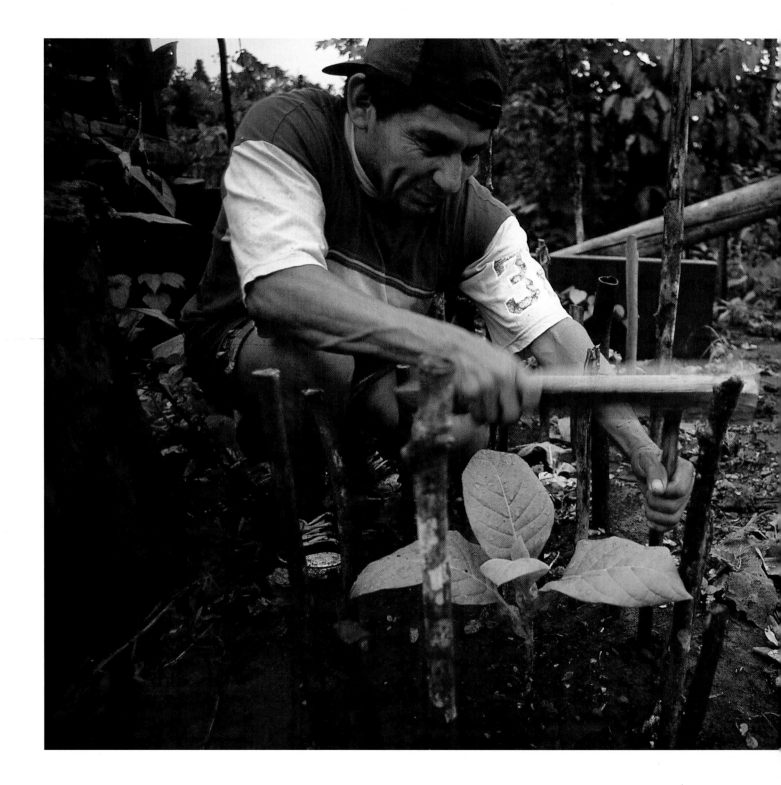

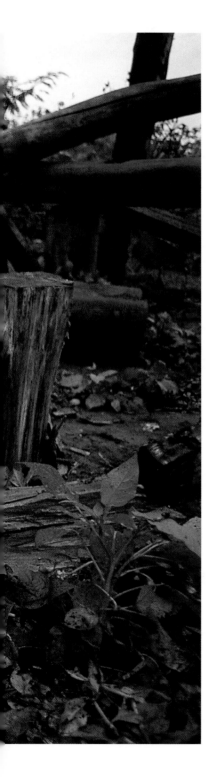

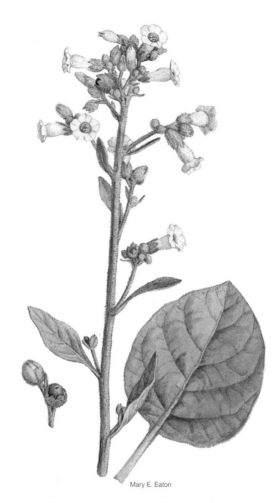

Mary E. Eaton

Near the Piches River in east-central Peru, a farmer erects fences to protect his tobacco. He cleared an area the size of six football fields and planted it with a variety of moneymaking crops. Traditional healers use tobacco smoke to communicate with the Great Spirit, and Spanish settlers used it to treat ailments ranging from kidney stones to bad breath. A botanical illustration delineates the dainty yellow flowers and broad leaf of this plant. Aztec and other New World peoples smoked tobacco to purify themselves and to achieve a trance state—both of which they considered essential to healing. Of 60 known species of tobacco, two have been cultivated. Both have higher concentrations of nicotine than do species that grow in the wild.

The tobacco experience was typical. Of all the plants studied in the 19th century, only perhaps a dozen yielded drugs still used today.

Although important to the people who benefit from them, some of these drugs are used infrequently. One example is bromelain, an alkaloid from pineapple, that breaks down proteins and can dissolve blood clots and clean away dead tissue after burns. Colchicine, an alkaloid from meadow saffron, is sometimes part of treatments for gouty arthritis; some countries use it to fight cancer. Atropine, an alkaloid from belladonna and other members of the nightshade family, is used to relax smooth muscles and as an antitoxin.

A few alkaloids discovered in the 19th century became pharmaceutical drugs that modern medicine has since dropped. Examples include piperine, from black pepper, which is now used as an insecticide; and brucine from *Strychnos ignatia* and *S. nux vomica*. Both piperine and brucine were used as circulatory stimulants and were listed in the *Pharmacopoeia of the United States* into the 20th century.

In the 19th century, however, only six plants—ipecac, opium poppy, coca, foxglove, cinchona, and white willow—yielded medicines that are widely used today.

————

IPECAC   In 1682, as the son of King Louis XIV of France lay dying of dysentery, the king learned that a doctor in Paris was prescribing a secret cure.

In 1680 a Parisian merchant had purchased 150 pounds of the root and rhizome of ipecac, a small, shrubby plant that grew in present-day Brazil and Bolivia. Told that its common use there was to treat dysentery and amoebic dysentery, he, in turn, had informed the doctor, who used it to make a medicine. No one knows who first brought the plant to Paris. Presumably, it was a traveler in the New World who noticed the plant's efficacy.

When the medicine, also called ipecac, saved his son, Louis XIV gave the Paris doctor exclusive rights to sell the plant in France. A few years later the French government purchased the ipecac formula for 1,000 louis d'or, about 5,000 dollars in today's money. The ingredients of the medicine remained secret until 1688, when the government made them public.

Why Louis XIV revealed the formula remains somewhat unclear. His troops at the time were invading German cities and slaughtering their inhabitants. While poverty was rising throughout France, he was investing tax money in ventures such as his palace at Versailles. Although France was not experiencing one of its periodic epidemics of dysentery, the king may have simply wanted to curry public favor.

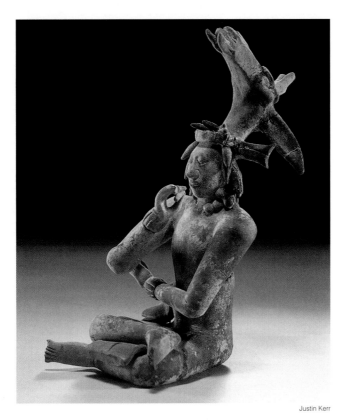
Justin Kerr

Fine details stand out in a pre-Columbian Maya figure of a man wearing a large deer headdress and smoking a cigar. He may have been participating in a religious ritual. Ceremonies, usually part of medical treatment in Maya and other traditional societies, often make it difficult for outsiders to appreciate the empirical trial-and-error process that determines much of traditional societies' use of herbs.

Galenic doctors began to use ipecac to promote vomiting, and an early 18th-century remedy popular in England combined it with opium to cause sweating. In 1817 French researchers discovered emetine, an active alkaloid in the ipecac root. Growing demand and rising prices in the mid-to-late 1800s prompted continued research, and emetine is now synthesized from cephaeline, another alkaloid in ipecac. Doctors continue to give emetine to treat dysentery and amoebic dysentery. At a higher dose, it is also still used to induce vomiting when certain toxins have been swallowed.

OPIUM POPPY　　Two plants extensively studied by scientists in the 19th century—the opium poppy and coca—contain alkaloids that are used as painkillers; they are addictive drugs.

Ancient Sumerians called opium, derived from the seedpod of a poppy, the "joy plant." Indians, Chinese, Egyptians, Greeks, Romans, and (Continued on page 128)

FOLLOWING PAGES: Coca leaves attract buyers at a highland market in Huasao, Peru. Locals still use coca to reduce fatigue and hunger and to produce a sense of well-being. Ingesting the leaves enables the people to walk long distances and work at high elevations. Modern science has derived synthetic drugs, used as anesthetics, from coca.

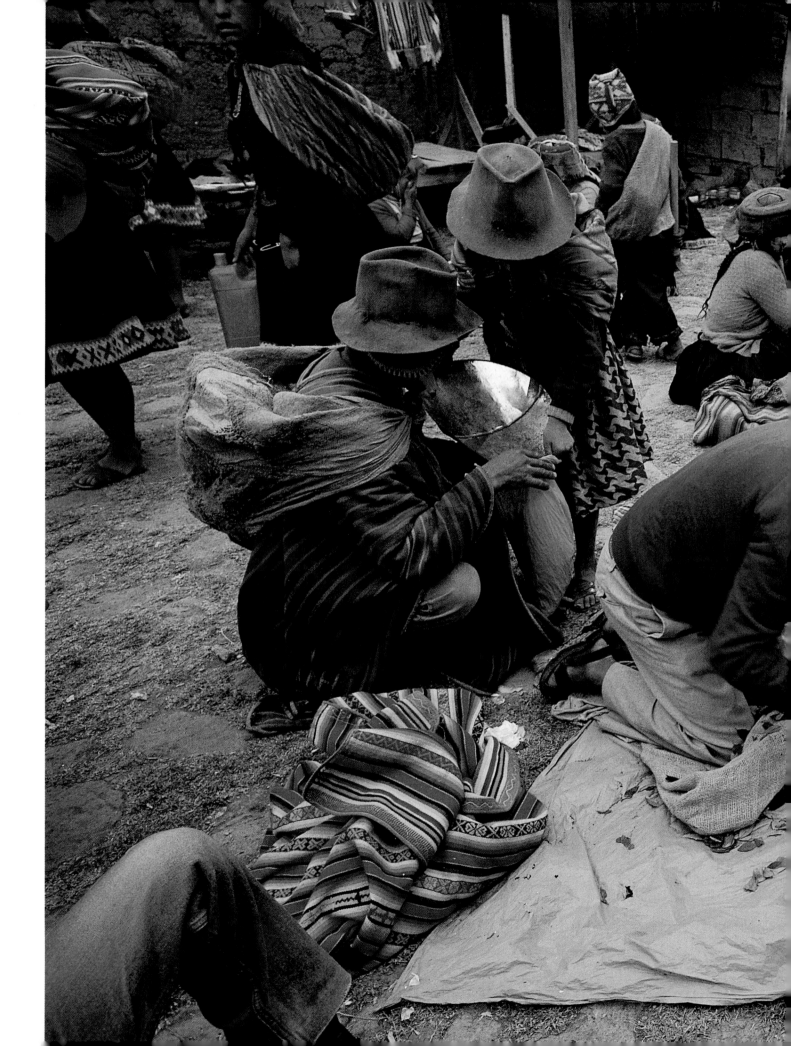

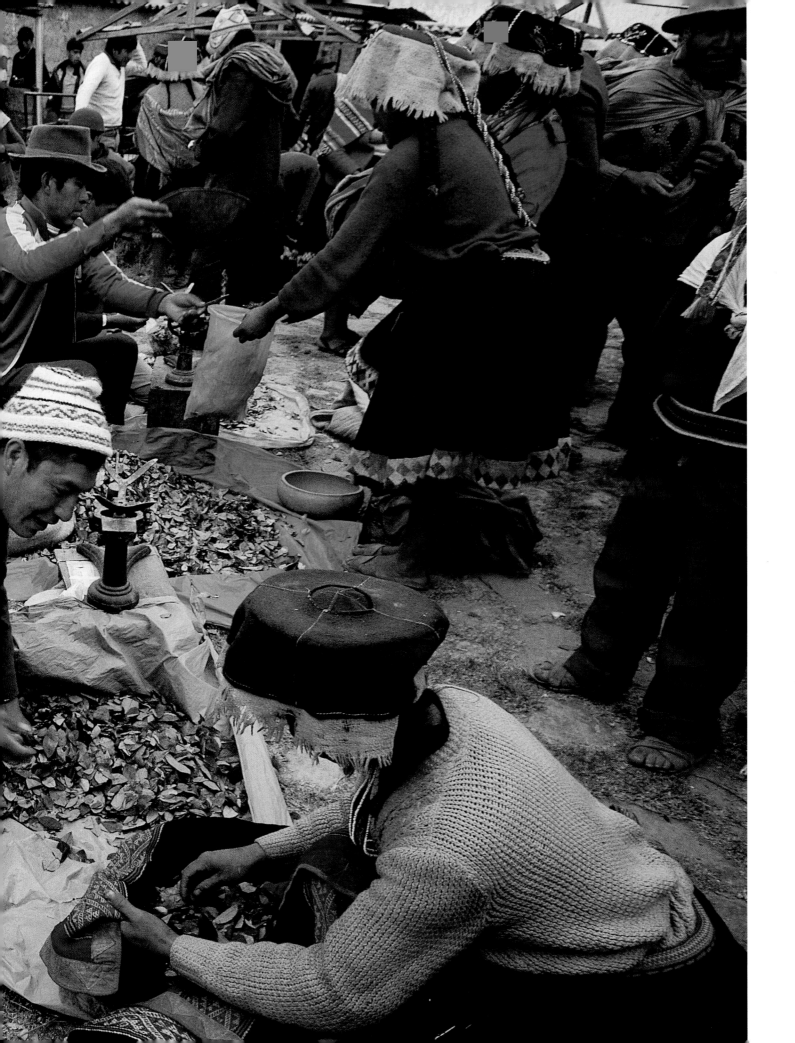

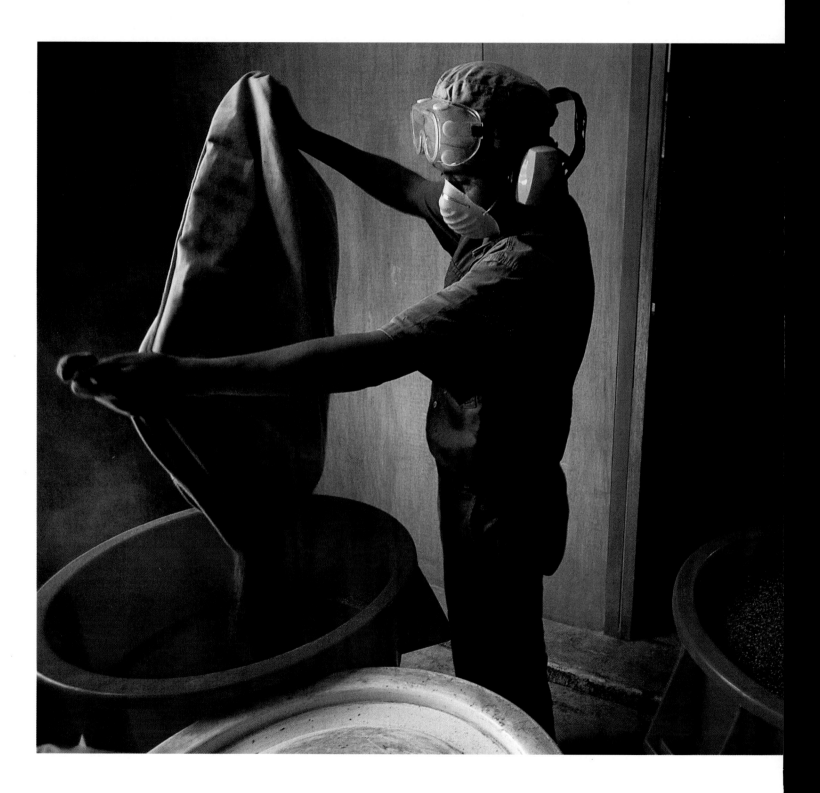

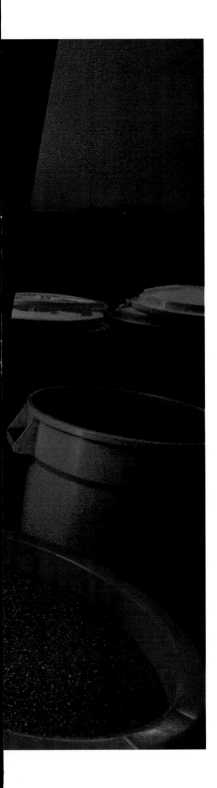

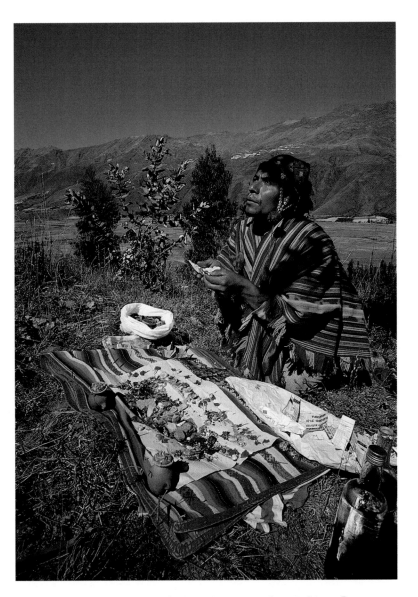

At a government-sanctioned coca-processing plant in Lima, Peru, a worker pours shredded leaves into a barrel for shipping (left). Peruvians will chew most of it. Until the early 20th century, many U.S. patent medicines contained cocaine extracted from coca leaves. Bacilio Garcia Guispe, a healer outside Huasao, Peru, holds coca as he prays for a bountiful harvest (above).

Arabs used opium for pain and dysentery. The drug is woven throughout Western literature. Some believe the potion Homer describes in the *Odyssey* that Helen of Troy used "to quiet all pain and strife, and bring forgetfulness of every ill" was opium. People continued to think of opium as a painkiller in the early 19th century, when John Keats wrote in his poem "To Sleep": "Or wait the 'Amen,' ere thy poppy throws / Around my bed its lulling charities."

Europeans used seeds of the opium poppy as a sedative and to control pain. Benjamin Franklin relied on laudanum, the term used for various preparations of opium, to ease the pain of kidney stones. One popular laudanum recipe devised by a prominent physician consisted of opium in sherry, flavored with cinnamon, cloves, and saffron. Opium often served as a treatment for cholera, asthma, fever, dysentery, and coughs.

In 1803 Friedrich Sertürner, a 20-year-old pharmacist's assistant in Germany, began looking for whatever gave the poppy its power. Three years later he published his initial findings. He had identified the active part of opium, an alkaloid. In 1817 he named it morphine.

Before the isolation of morphine, people had chewed opium or had soaked it in alcohol and eaten it. They had thus ingested all the chemicals in opium. But morphine was something new for the human body: an active element from opium without all the other chemicals to moderate it.

Curious to determine the exact effects of morphine on humans, Sertürner and three volunteers each ate a half grain of morphine. This caused a reddening of the face and what he described as "enhancement of the vital forces." After two more half-grain doses over the next half hour, the four men each felt sharp stomach pains and sleepiness. Alarmed that the men were being poisoned, Sertürner had them all drink vinegar, which caused violent vomiting that probably saved their lives.

Morphine blocks sensory nerve cells in the cerebrum and decreases respiration. In sufficient dosages, it can kill. It also can serve as a painkiller and a stimulant, creating feelings of euphoria and dispelling fears and tensions. By mid-century, people began to realize that morphine is addictive. Fueling further addiction was the hypodermic syringe, which came into common use by the mid-1800s.

Morphine quickly became a drug of choice as the medical profession began to see it as a panacea. During the American Civil War, the most effective way to help wounded men was by injection, but needles were often not available. Morphine was frequently placed directly on flesh wounds. Under the stress of combat conditions, the military also had to rely on raw opium. The Union Army used 2.8 million ounces of opium tincture

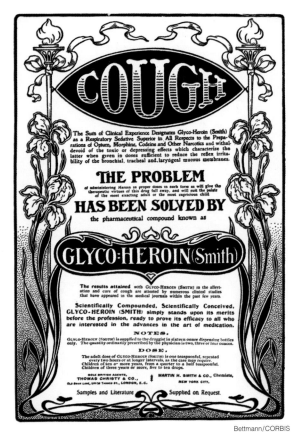

Flames and flowers embellish the label of a cough syrup made with heroin, which was first extracted from morphine, a chemical found in the opium poppy plant, in 1874. People could buy such heroin-containing drugs without a doctor's prescription well into the 20th century. Various extracts from the poppy plant still serve as important painkillers.

and powder and nearly 500,000 opium pills. One officer sometimes sat on his horse while men licked opium off his glove. Morphine, however, seems to have generated the most addiction. By the end of the war so many wounded veterans had become dependent on morphine that the addiction was known as "soldiers' disease."

Known natural receptor sites for morphine exist in the brain, spine, and intestines. The human brain seems to have a tendency toward addiction—a condition of chemical dependence resulting in severe discomfort if the addictive substance becomes unavailable—to plant materials. These include fermented plants (alcohol) and a range of plant alkaloids: nicotine, morphine, heroin, codeine, and cocaine (see Coca on page 130).

Humans do get addicted to non-plant substances such as synthetic chemical depressants like benzodiazepines (Valium) and barbiturates and stimulants such as amphetamines. People also become addicted to certain behaviors, including gambling, risk-taking, and sex. But most addiction is to plants.

In 1874 a London pharmacist, seeking a nonaddictive form of morphine, boiled it with acetic anhydride—an acid then being used in the development of aspirin (see White Willow on page 149). This gave him a new substance, which by the end of the century had been named heroin for its heroic qualities as a painkiller. Its potency was well-known, but its addictive nature was not immediately clear. A major pharmaceutical company, for example, was soon selling Glyco-Heroin cough syrup.

————

THE OPIUM POPPY HAD even more to offer. It contains at least 21 alkaloids, which constitute about one-fifth its total weight. Alkaloids found in opium include codeine, which serves as a pain reliever and cough suppressant, and papaverine, a muscle relaxant used for stomach and respiratory spasms.

In the 1960s researchers derived another chemical from morphine. Named etorphine, it is about 10,000 times more powerful than morphine. Then, in the late 1990s, researchers developed a form of heroin that is much more potent and addictive. Such discoveries indicate that modern science will continue to extract and develop chemicals from the opium poppy. Whether these will have medicinal applications and the degree to which they will generate and exacerbate addiction problems remain unclear.

All of opium's alkaloids come from unripe seedpods. None are present when the opium seedpods ripen, and their role may be to somehow defend the seeds as they mature. Clearly, however, these alkaloids do stimulate an alliance between the opium plant and humans. In evolutionary terms, this alliance serves the poppy plant well. A few of the 200 known species of poppy generate the most alkaloids. They, like all poppies, require rich and moist soil, a good deal of sunlight, and a clear place in which to grow. They do not do well in the wild or when competing with other plants for nutrients; hence, the partnership with humans. The poppy provides alkaloids in exchange for good growing conditions, more land, and the removal of competing plants.

————

COCA   A similar alliance exists between humans and coca, a shrub that grows in mountainous regions of present-day Peru, Bolivia, Ecuador, and Colombia.

People in areas under Inca control in South America had worshiped the coca plant since pre-Inca times, using it as they used tobacco, for ceremonial purposes. This ceremonial use was largely limited to shamans, priests, and the nobility. Other people chewed and sucked on coca leaves to reduce fatigue and hunger and to produce a sense of well-being, enabling them to walk for long distances and to work at high elevations.

Europeans discovered coca shortly after their first contact with the Inca. Although coca quickly entered Europe's pharmacopoeia, missionaries at first decried its use as heathenish, and the conquistadores dismissed it as pagan. Nonetheless, the Spanish realized that natives, whom they enslaved, could be made to work much longer if given coca leaves. This method for increasing worker productivity continued on plantations through the 19th century. By the mid-19th century, researchers had extracted the alkaloid cocaine from coca leaves. Doctors used it to treat sore throats, fatigue, depression, and nervousness; to increase patients' ability to endure mercury during treatment for syphilis; as a local anesthetic; and as a cure for alcoholism.

In the late 19th century one major American pharmaceutical company had 15 products containing coca and cocaine on the market. These included coca cigarettes, cocaine powder for snuffing, and injectable cocaine—which was sold along with a hypodermic needle and three other plant alkaloids: morphine, atropine, and strychnine (derived from species of *Strychnos* and then used as a bitter tonic and circulatory stimulant). This kit, the company promised, "can supply the place of food, make the coward brave, the silent eloquent," and eliminate pain.

In the early 1860s Angelo Mariani, a young chemist from Corsica, began to offer a medicine made with an infusion of coca leaves in wine. Soon, Mariani elixirs, Mariani teas, Mariani lozenges, and a French wine, Vin Mariani, sold well in Europe and the U.S. This wine had one-half grain of cocaine per pint, not a large amount in terms of its physiological effect. Mariani claimed that it "nourishes, fortifies, refreshes, aids digestion, strengthens the system," and that it "prevents malaria, influenza, and wasting diseases." Prominent physicians praised it. Thomas Edison (1847-1931), inventor of the lightbulb and phonograph and author of the statement that "genius is one per cent inspiration and ninety-nine per cent perspiration," said the wine prolonged his workday.

Popular soft drinks containing cocaine included Inca Kola and Coca-Cola. Until 1904 Coca-Cola contained about the same amount of cocaine as Vin Mariani and claimed to be a "Brain Tonic, and a cure for all nervous affections." In an 1886 newspaper advertisement Coca-Cola called itself "The New and Popular Soda Fountain Drink, containing properties of the wonderful coca plant and the famous cola nuts."

As the popularity of cocaine products soared, health officials had begun to recognize it as addictive and poisonous. By the early 1880s they were calling cocaine a "scourge." But researchers who traveled in South America saw, as had the conquistadores, how chewing whole coca leaves helped people at high elevations because it increased respiration. They also noticed that coca seemed far more effective than isolated cocaine and that it was much less addictive.

Around this time a young Viennese physician named Sigmund Freud wanted to advance his career so he could earn enough money to get married. He read about coca and studied accounts of its use by Indian tribes. Excited, he wrote to his fiancée that he thought it might work on "heart disease, then on nervous exhaustion...."

Husband at her side, Cherri Newton of Missoula, Montana, confronts breast cancer with the help of the Chalice of Repose Project, a care program that uses music instead of medicine to help meet the needs of the dying. Such solace can stimulate and harness the body's own painkilling capacities. Morphine-based drugs also helped provide pain relief, but Cherri Newton died in 1997. Opponents of herbal medicine often say—incorrectly—that a patient's own body provides whatever medicinal benefit the patient taking herbal remedies may experience. Plant-derived morphine kills pain in patients no matter what their mental attitudes may be. But physiological effects produced by patients' attitudes can augment and facilitate the morphine's effects.

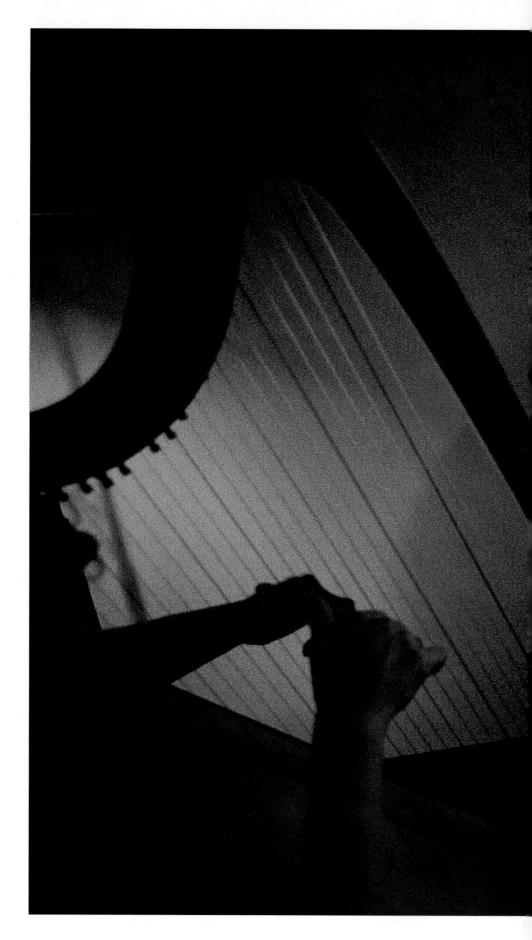

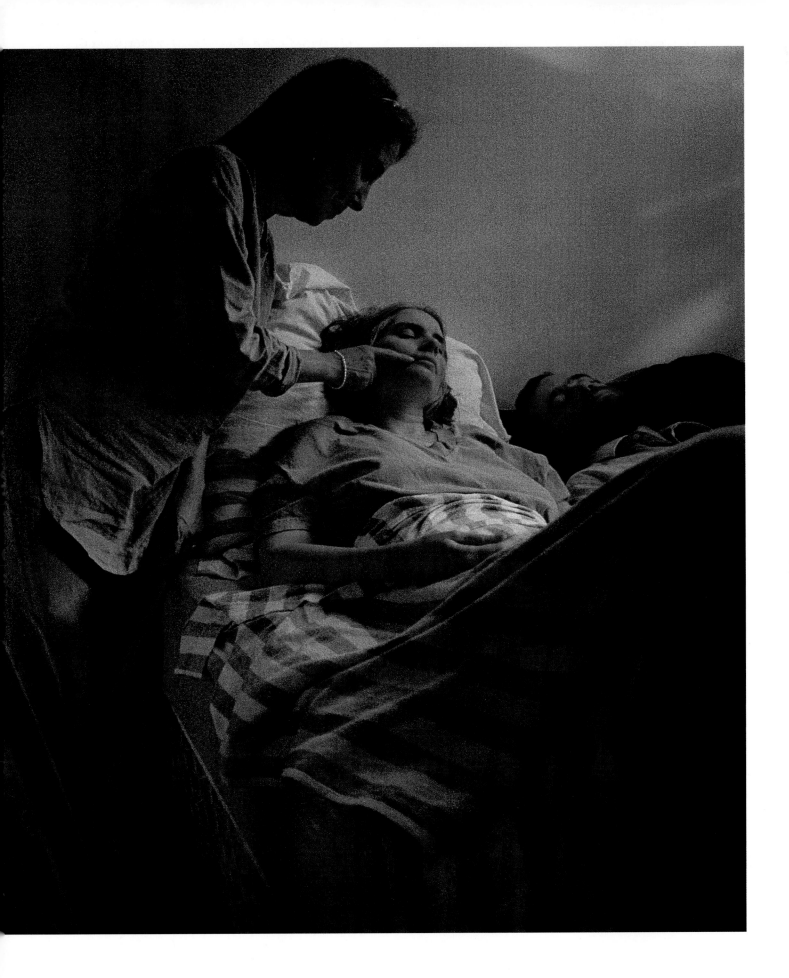

Freud experimented with cocaine by taking some himself. Using a device called a dynamometer, he charted the muscular power of his hands, alone and together. He also recorded the effect of cocaine on his mental reaction time by using a device called the neuroameobimeter.

In 1885 Freud published a paper entitled "Über Coca," which posited that cocaine can suppress the addictive urge for alcohol and morphine. Convinced that cocaine could fight depression and fatigue, increase work capacity, and provide other positive benefits, Freud injected it into one patient as a treatment for morphine addiction.

Carl Koller, a physician who was one of Freud's young colleagues, began to experiment with another use of cocaine. He knew that cocaine numbs the mucous membranes of the tongue and lips, narrows the arteries, and widens the pupils. Consensus within the medical community was that these effects had no practical value, but Koller decided to test cocaine as a possible anesthetic during eye surgery.

General anesthetic for surgery—ether and chloroform—had been in use since 1840, but the only available anesthetic for eye surgery was to spray the eye with ether. Its effects were short-lived, and it worked only for abscesses and other short operations. Unless the patient was given a general anesthetic, most eye surgery was conducted without effective pain fighters. Attempts to use morphine and chemicals such as chloral bromide had failed. Koller put a solution of cocaine in the eye of a frog. "At intervals of a few seconds the reflex of the cornea was tested by touching the eye with a needle," he later wrote. "After about a minute came the great historic moment, I do not hesitate to designate it as such. The frog permitted his cornea to be touched and even injured without a trace of reflex action or attempt to protect himself." Koller repeated the experiment on a rabbit and a dog. Then he and an assistant "trickled the solution under the upraised lids of each other's eyes. Then we put a mirror before us, took a pin in hand, and tried to touch the cornea with its head.…We could make a dent in the cornea without the slightest awareness of the touch let alone any unpleasant sensation or reaction."

Based on Koller's work, doctors began to use cocaine as an anesthetic during eye surgery. In 1905 procaine, a synthetic drug derived from cocaine, became available, and cocaine, which can cause corneal lesions, was dropped as an anesthetic during eye surgery. Today, tetracaine, lidocaine, and bupivacaine—synthetic drugs derived from chemical formulas found in cocaine—are also used.

FOXGLOVE   In 1775, at roughly the same time the Revolution was about to break out in British North America, William Withering, Physician to the General Hospital in

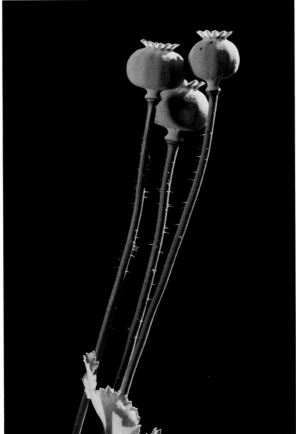

Seed capsules from the opium poppy, which the ancient Sumerians called the "joy plant," yield opium that can serve as a sedative and a painkiller. The role of opium in the plant's development remains unknown; it is present only in unripe seedpods.

Birmingham, England, had a patient with severely swollen legs, a condition then called dropsy. Although this fact was not known at the time, such swelling is often a sign of congestive heart failure. The heart is too weak to pump blood effectively.

Withering had no treatment to offer and thought that the patient, a woman in her forties, would die. A few weeks later he heard she was doing well. Visiting her, Withering learned that she was taking an herb tea provided by an old woman living nearby who helped people whom doctors could not cure. Withering called on the woman and asked for her recipe. The woman, who remains unknown and forgotten by history, could have refused. Her relationships with doctors like Withering were probably antagonistic, and the recipe was a family secret. But she gave it to him.

The woman either did not provide him with any details about where the recipe had come from or he did not write them down. No written records seem to exist. Like

FOLLOWING PAGES: Foxglove plants offer a symphony in color. Digitalis, a complex chemical in foxglove, is widely used as a pharmaceutical drug because it slows cardiac contractions, helping the heart pump efficiently. The chemical formula of digitalis is so expensive to replicate that pharmaceutical companies obtain it directly from plants by making a powder of their leaves.

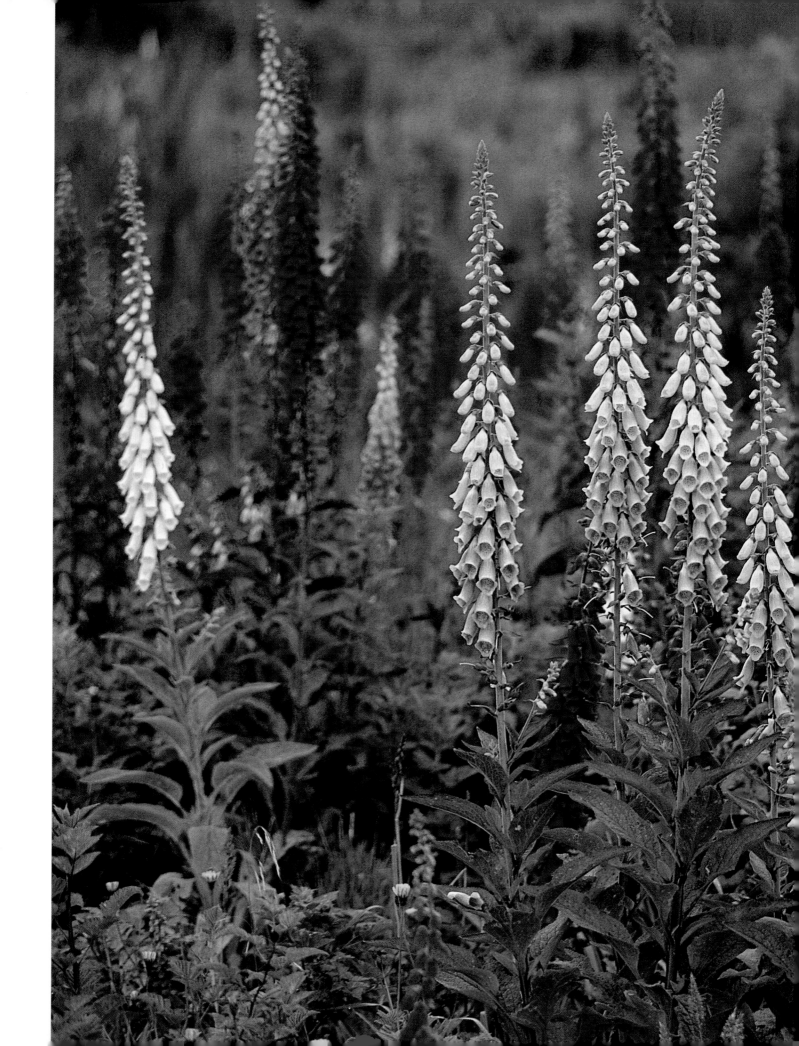

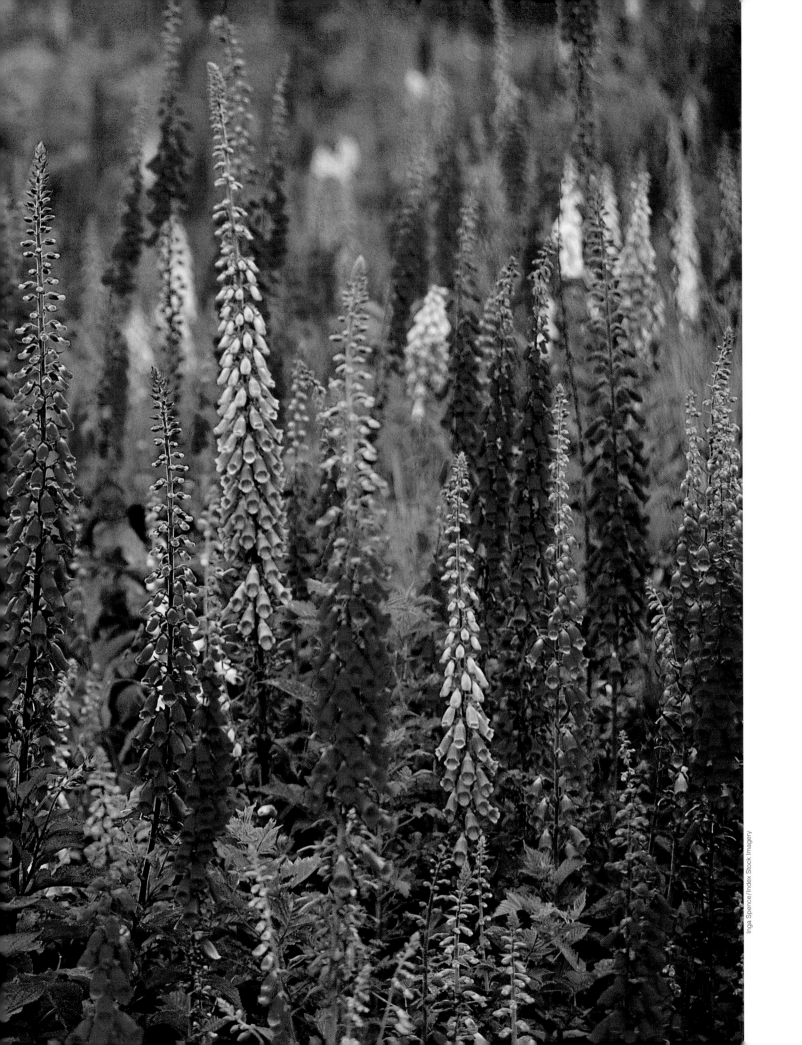

thousands of other family recipes, an unknown number of which may still be in use, the elderly neighbor's remedy for dropsy has never been studied or subjected to scientific scrutiny.

Withering later wrote that he had been told this recipe caused "violent vomiting and purging [diarrhea]." If true, this was unusual, since most home remedies tended to avoid the distressful effects so valued by Galenic doctors. Withering knew only that in cases of dropsy a diuretic is needed to get water out of the system. Looking at what he described as the "twenty or more" herbs in the old woman's medicine, he had no interest in the entire remedy. Based on his knowledge of botany and medicine, he decided: "The active herb could be no other than the Foxglove."

Lost forever is knowledge about the other herbs. All or most of them may have been useless. Some may have been included because of mistakes or misinformation in the generation-to-generation transmission of the recipe in the healer's family. Others may have made the medicinal drink smell good. But some may have acted upon the foxglove, blocking its negative effects or augmenting its positive ones.

Foxglove can grow up to six feet tall and has oval leaves. Its blossoms, which resemble the fingers of a glove, are among the honeybee's favorite. Powdered foxglove leaves had been used as a medicine in Europe for hundreds of years. One herbal book in Withering's time said that "six or seven spoonfuls of the decoction produce nausea and vomiting, and purge." Other books reported foxglove's effectiveness against epilepsy, hereditary deafness, skin ulcers, and eye tumors.

Withering saw poor patients, whom he did not charge, for one hour every day. Deciding to experiment on them, he discovered that foxglove is a "very powerful diuretic." It is unclear whether he told his patients about the experiments. Withering tried several varieties and strengths of foxglove—roots, leaves, leaves in powder, leaves picked when the plant was flowering and when it was dried, green leaves picked in winter, and leaves mixed with small amounts of opium. The plant worked best, he concluded, when people were not vomiting. He also concluded, incorrectly, that foxglove decreased the volume of blood in the body.

Although he believed that digitalis, a word he seems to have used interchangeably with foxglove, only eliminated fluids, Withering recognized that, in his words, the plant "has a power over the motion of the heart to a degree yet unobserved in any other medicine and this power may be converted to salutary ends."

Withering also tried foxglove as a treatment for tuberculosis, ovarian cysts, kidney stones, epilepsy, lead poisoning, and other ailments. It helped with none.

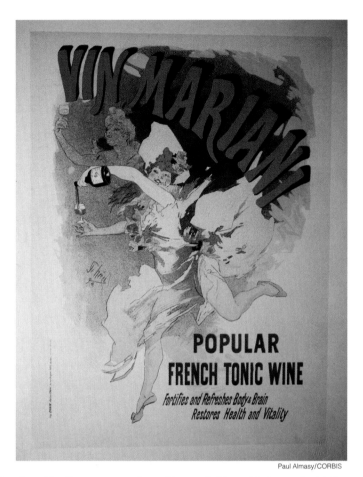

Vin Mariani, introduced in the 1860s and readily available until the early 20th century, featured an infusion of coca leaves in French wine. Vivid advertisements promised that it nourished, refreshed, aided digestion, and strengthened the system.

———————

IN 1785, AFTER TEN years of experimentation, Withering published a book entitled *An Account of the Foxglove*. More and more people were taking foxglove, he wrote in the preface, and he wanted them to benefit from his experience rather than risk harm from improper use of the plant. He also wanted to make sure that "a medicine of so much efficacy should not be condemned and rejected as dangerous and unmanageable." The cases for which he used foxglove, he wrote, were "the most hopeless and deplorable that exist." He did not recommend foxglove until "the failure of every other method compelled me to do it," but said that it saved most of the people treated.

One case of Withering's is typical: He arrived at a woman's house after being called by another doctor. There he found her "nearly in a state of suffocation; her pulse extremely weak and irregular, her breath very short and laborious, her countenance sunk, her arms of a leaden colour, clammy and cold. She could not lye down in bed, and had neither strength nor appetite, but was extremely thirsty. Her stomach, legs, and thighs were greatly swollen."

No treatment her doctor offered had helped the woman except for an herb that made her vomit. The dosage of this herb had been nearly tripled, but after a few days it no longer worked.

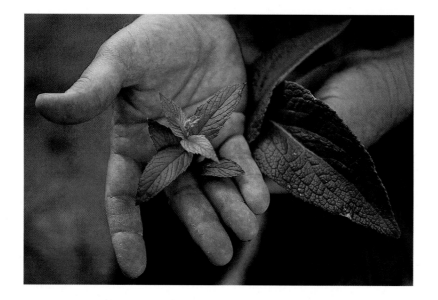

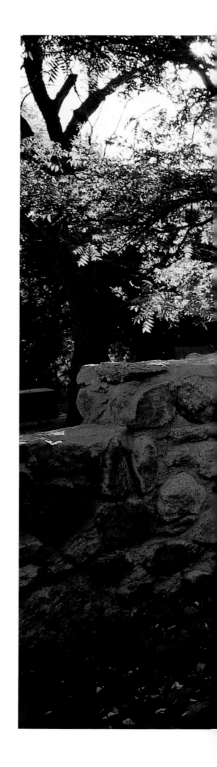

In the hands of Harvard M.D. Andrew Weil, a sprig of spearmint mirrors the shape of larger foxglove leaves. Many people eat spearmint. It can be effective against indigestion, headaches, fevers, and viral infections. Ingesting foxglove is not recommended, but the plant has yielded digitalis, a powerful pharmaceutical drug that strengthens cardiac contractions in cases of congestive heart failure. Weil meditates at his home near Tucson, Arizona (right). Most plant-based healing systems rely on such relaxation techniques, as well as on exercise and proper diet. Belief that health problems can be solved solely by taking drugs is probably found only in modern Western societies.

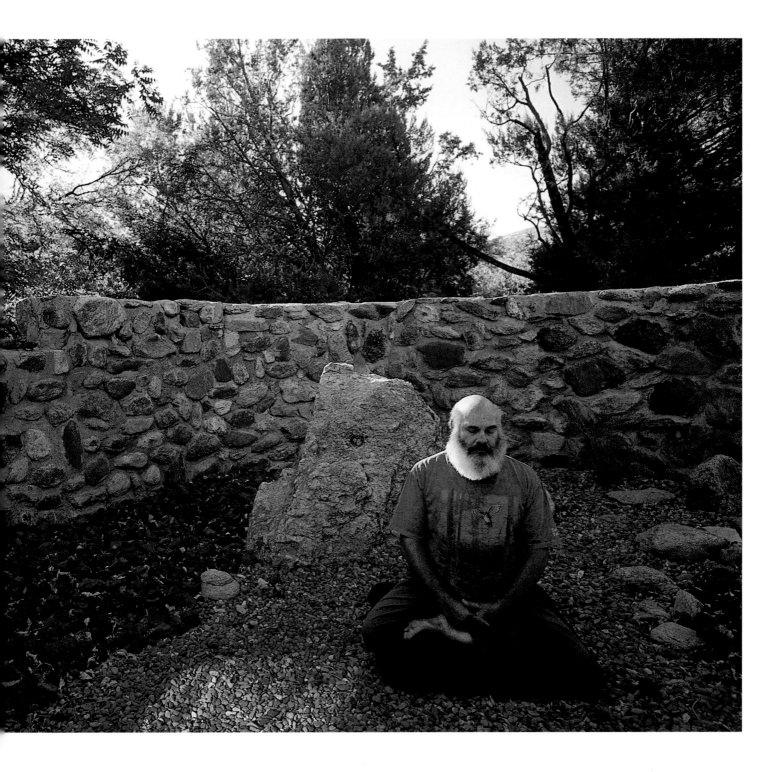

Withering hesitated before giving her his digitalis preparation, believing she would die, and that giving her the new drug would give it a bad name. But with the consent of her regular doctor, he gave it to her. She became very sick. Then she urinated eight quarts of water in the next 24 hours. Her breath came easier, and her swelling subsided.

The woman's regular doctor then gave her repeated treatments with "pareira brava and guaiacum shavings with pills of myrrh" and white zinc sulfate followed by "a pill of calomel and aloes." Calomel, which had been used in Europe since the 16th century, is now known as mercuric chloride and is used as an insecticide and fungicide. Nine years later, Withering reported, the woman still sometimes had dropsy, which the foxglove could not prevent.

Withering warned that "when given in very large and quickly repeated doses" foxglove causes "sickness, vomiting, purging, giddiness, confused vision, objects appearing green or yellow."

This yellow vision has fueled rumors that Vincent van Gogh suffered from digitalis poisoning. Van Gogh, especially in paintings he completed in Arles, France, showed a preference for yellow and an ability to paint numerous shades of that color. In 1890, the year of his suicide, he painted two portraits of Paul-Ferdinand Gachet, a homeopathic doctor, with a stem of foxglove—which homeopathic medicine uses in minute amounts (see Chapter 5). There is no evidence that Gachet gave van Gogh digitalis in any form. Van Gogh, who probably suffered from ailments such as manic-depressive illness and epilepsy, took potassium bromide but no medicines prescribed by Gachet. Van Gogh's letters do not mention foxglove. He had his awakening to yellow, furthermore, years before he met Gachet.

While foxglove entered the *Pharmacopoeia of the United States* in 1820 as a diuretic, not a heart stimulant, we now know that its primary impact is on the heart. It is among a group of plants whose leaves, flowers, seeds, roots, and bark contain glycosides, chemicals that stimulate the heart.

Glycosides act on the contractile force of the cardiac muscle of higher animals, slowing the heart rate and increasing the force of contractions. When the heart pumps blood more efficiently, the kidneys are more able to cleanse it of wastes and toxins.

A wide range of cultures have used extracts of plants that contain cardiac glycosides. Ancient Egyptians employed dried, sliced scales of the bulb of the sea onion as a diuretic and heart stimulant. For hundreds, perhaps thousands, of years Chinese healers have used the dried skin of a common toad as a medicine for this same purpose. European folk medicine also used powdered toad skin.

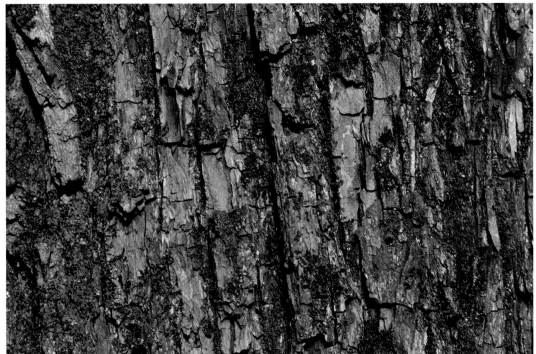

Bark of the willow tree contains salicylic acid, the active ingredient in aspirin. The full range of aspirin's effects is still not known. It cuts pain, reduces fever, can prevent strokes and heart attacks by inhibiting the clotting of blood, and may lower the risk of colon and rectal cancer.

Why do a plant chemical and a chemical in toad skin have such a similar effect? One possibility is that both the plant and the toad use the chemical for defense, presumably against some kind of microbes or fungi.

Some medical reference books use the word "digitalis" to denote the active glycosides in foxglove and other plants. Digitalis is now prescribed for congestive heart failure and for auricular fibrillation, irregular heart rhythm.

Digitalis's complex chemical formula is expensive to replicate, so modern pharmaceutical companies obtain the drug directly from plants by making a powder of their leaves and extracting the glycoside.

The success of digitalis has prompted the development of closely related drugs that act on the myocardium—the middle and thickest part of the heart wall—and treat heart problems. These drugs can be useful no matter what kind of problem—heart attack, infection, or leaky valves—has harmed the heart.

CINCHONA   Although cinchona bark, which the Spanish had obtained in the Andes in the mid-1600s, worked against malaria, most Europeans saw this remedy in terms of humors. They believed that what they called "spasms of the blood" caused the intermittent fevers of malaria and that cinchona bark fixed this malfunction by increasing the flow of the blood and the well-being of the muscles.

Problems with cinchona persisted. There are some 40 species, ranging in size from shrubby plants to tall, slender trees with symmetrical crowns, and leaves at least eight inches long. Bark adulterated with other ingredients was often sold, as was bark from one of the dozens of species of cinchona that contained fewer antimalarial properties. Given the variability in quality of cinchona, even the most skilled healers often had difficulty knowing what dosage of bark to prescribe. The bark, furthermore, was extremely bitter. Even when soaked in brandy or gin for a week, this bitterness was often too much for a patient to endure.

To make matters worse, cinchona was almost always expensive. The cinchona tree grew over wide areas—ranging from Colombia to Bolivia. Collecting cinchona bark was dangerous because the trees grew in rough terrain. Bark collectors had to climb into the mountains, braving insects, filthy water, fatal infections, and dangerous cliffs. They usually worked in groups so that if one or two died, the others could return with the bark. It was not unusual for them to encounter the bones of previous collectors.

One of the first acts of the U.S. Continental Congress was to appropriate 300 dollars for cinchona bark for George Washington's troops. Treating malaria, then the most common disease in America, was essential for the war effort.

Despite high costs, the potential demand for cinchona was extraordinary. Malaria was so common in the newly formed United States that many people took its fevers and chills for granted. They saw suffering from malaria symptoms as normal and did not even consider themselves sick.

When Thomas Jefferson, who had malaria, ordered Meriwether Lewis and William Clark to explore the recently acquired Louisiana Territory, Congress authorized expenditure of one-third of their medical budget for powder from cinchona bark.

The experience of Lewis and Clark demonstrates how the bark, despite its expense, was used for other purposes. Cinchona bark can reduce fever by dilating the small vessels of the skin, and it can give pain relief by suppressing some parts of the central nervous system. Someone on the expedition accidentally shot Lewis just below the hip joint. The explorer suffered great pain and a high fever. Treatment consisted of applying a heated cloth medicated with cinchona bark to the wound on the assumption that it combated all fevers no matter what the cause. Lewis spent a restless night. The next day he felt sore, but could move, and the fever was gone.

By the early 19th century, efforts were being made to locate antimalarial medicines from other plants. One candidate was lobelia, a flowering plant found in the eastern United States and Canada. Modern science has found it to have no antimalarial or anti-fever qualities. But it does stimulate the respiratory center of the brain stem, and from the 1920s to the 1950s Western doctors used it to restore breathing after shock. Because the

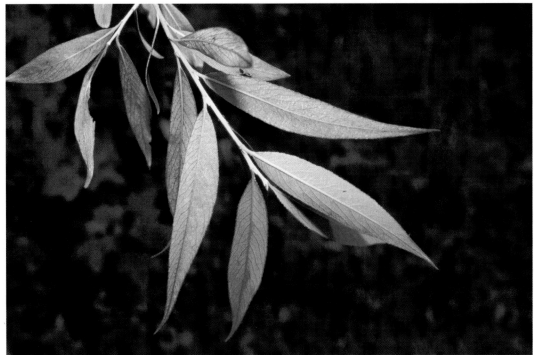

Ancient Sumerian, Assyrian, and Egyptian medical records mention the use of willow leaves for treating inflammatory rheumatic pain. Someone with an inflamed wound, advises a 3,500-year-old Egyptian medical papyrus found in a tomb at Thebes, should use leaves of willow to draw the heat out.

dried leaves and other parts of lobelia act like nicotine, some antismoking preparations include it.

Given the price of cinchona and the need to measure how effective any batch of bark would be, scientists kept looking for the active agent within it that reduces fever.

In 1820 French researchers isolated this agent and named it "quinine" after the Spanish word *quina* for cinchona. Quinine, which could be taken as a pill, was easier to administer than medications made from bark. It was also easy to establish and confirm dosage. When people bought quinine, unlike their purchase of bark, they could make sure they got what they were paying for.

Quinine probably kills malaria-causing parasites by preventing them from using glucose, but it kills only parasites in the red blood cells. When a person stops taking quinine, parasites elsewhere in the body bring back the disease.

Quinine, furthermore, can be slow acting—and it has major side effects: Among other things, it often causes rashes, dizziness, and ringing in the ears. And it can stimulate the pancreas to produce too much insulin. It can also bring about deafness and can cause miscarriages.

Although cinchona bark and quinine were effective and could be taken prophylactically to prevent malaria, knowledge about them did not spread as quickly as might be expected. Part of the reason was that many doctors, as well as patients, clung to the Galenic belief that for a cure to occur, the body had to expel a fluid. Further resistance to

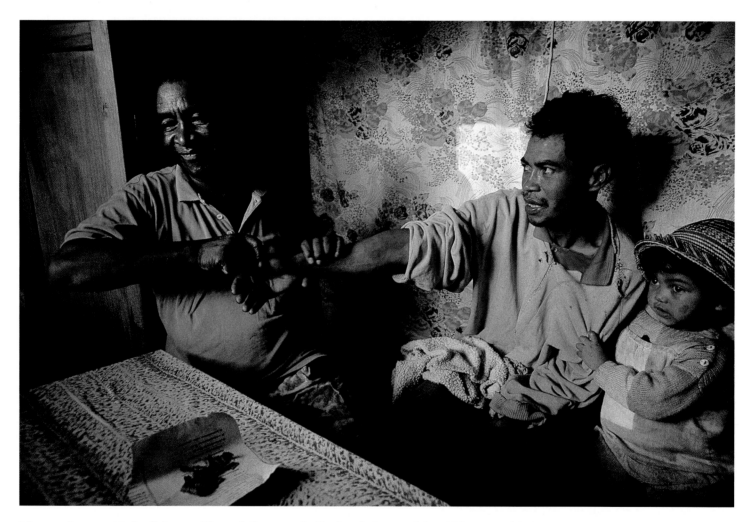

Like nearly two-thirds of the world's 6.1 billion people, Parfait Rakotomalala of Moranga, Madagascar, cannot seek help at expensive or inaccessible Western-style medical facilities. Sick with malaria, Rakotomalala sought help from a local healer, Pierre Rakotondramara, who prescribed seven plants to be boiled and drunk as a tea.

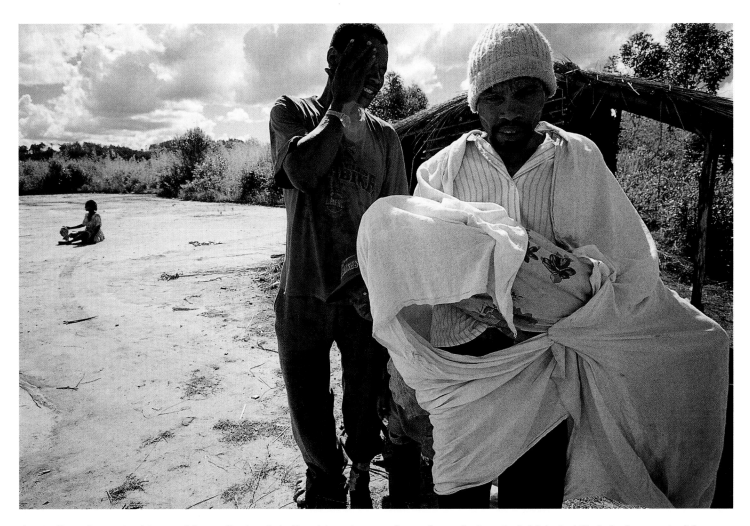

Justin Rapady carries his son, Mampolia Justilain Randriampionona, home from the hospital. Malaria killed the boy, as it did another of Rapady's children. Malaria deaths are common in developing countries, where people cannot purchase modern drugs. Most are synthetically derived from a compound first found in the cinchona tree; these drugs protect Westerners who travel to areas infested with mosquitoes that carry the malaria-causing protozoan.

their use came from continued ill feeling among Protestants toward the Jesuits. Price was also a factor. Cinchona bark lay unsold in some European ports in the late 17th century.

Many physicians in the United States did not routinely use cinchona until more than 150 years after its discovery. In the 1830s, according to the *New-Orleans Medical Journal*, malarial treatment primarily consisted of "thorough evacuation"—the giving of plants or chemicals that caused severe diarrhea—in the early stages of the fever, and then taking blood.

By the mid- and late 19th century, overharvesting of cinchona trees threatened the world supply. Repeated expeditions into the Amazon attempted to bring out species of cinchona trees that would grow well on plantations in other areas. These expeditions had to overcome obstacles. One aggressive Bolivian threatened to cut off the feet of anyone caught attempting to smuggle cinchona seeds from the country. Expeditions failed after leaving South America because seedlings died or because collectors had brought back seeds with a low yield of quinine. Then Charles Ledger, a British trader in alpacas, purchased 14 pounds of seeds from eastern slopes of the Andes in Bolivia. These seeds, he had been told, would produce trees that yielded high levels of quinine.

British authorities did not want to buy the seeds, but Dutch officials purchased one pound for 40 dollars. It produced trees of such extremely high quinine content that the Dutch bought the rest of the trader's seeds. Thirty years later, when Java's plantations dominated the world quinine market, the Dutch gave Ledger an annual pension. The person who told Ledger about the trees apparently received nothing.

Resistance to quinine became a problem of worldwide proportions by the late 19th century. Malaria then killed or crippled four million children under age ten each year in India alone. Epidemics occurred along the Thames River and persisted in areas of northern Europe. Malaria was prevalent throughout the southern portion of the United States. Well into the 20th century the disease was still the world's leading cause of illness and death.

The key to preventing and treating malaria was understanding how it is transmitted. Various cultures held a range of beliefs, including the correct observation that mosquitoes transmit malaria. In Swahili malaria is called *mbu*, the word for "mosquito." In some parts of Africa rural people associated malaria with the rainy—or mosquito—season, when they took herbs that provide protection against it. They used plants as natural insecticides and insect repellents.

Ancient Greeks associated malaria with swamps, but blamed the disease on night air. This thought was not far off target because mosquitoes fly mostly at night. But rather than notice mosquitoes, the Greeks blamed malaria on noxious miasma they believed was exuded by the ground. The word "malaria," derived from the Italian words *mala aria* or bad air, first appeared in writing in the mid-1700s describing a disease that seemed to emanate from swamps near Rome.

One researcher in Philadelphia in the early 1800s tested the theory that direct contact spread malaria. He inhaled vapors from vomit of people with malaria and injected their vomit into cats, dogs, and himself. None got malaria. This convinced him, scientifically, that the disease is not contagious.

In 1880 researchers realized that a protozoan causes malaria. They associated this protozoan with mosquitoes and suspected that drinking water in which mosquitoes had bred spread the disease. Scientists could not believe it possible for a parasite to live in a mosquito and then in a human. But by 1896, when researchers discovered that the malaria-causing protozoan could, indeed, live in mosquitoes and humans, researchers had confirmed that mosquito bites spread the disease to humans.

———

WHITE WILLOW   Ancient Sumerian, Assyrian, and Egyptian medical records mention use of willow leaves to treat inflammatory rheumatic pain. Someone with an inflamed wound, states an Egyptian medical papyrus, should use "leaves of willow" to "draw the heat out." Hippocrates recommended chewing willow bark to increase the flow of urine, and at least 15 Native American tribes used parts of the willow tree to relieve pain.

In the late 1750s Edmund Stone, a minister in Oxfordshire, England, knew that fevers were common in low, swampy, moist areas where willows grow. In keeping with the popular beliefs of the time, Stone thought that plants that grow in an area where a certain disease is prevalent can cure that illness. He decided to test the efficacy of white willow against fevers. Stone used dried, powdered bark to treat people suffering from fever, chills, and other symptoms. In 1763, after about a half decade of clinical observations, he wrote a letter to the president of the Royal Society reporting that willow bark was a good treatment for fevers.

"As this tree delights in a moist or wet soil, where agues [malarial fevers] chiefly abound," Stone wrote, his findings proved "the general maxim that many natural maladies carry their cures along with them or that their remedies lie not far from their causes...." The "intention of Providence" is clearly evident, Stone concluded.

Language like "intention of Providence" is not often found in scientific reportage today, but scientists' faith in this symmetry in nature— *(Continued on page 154)*

149

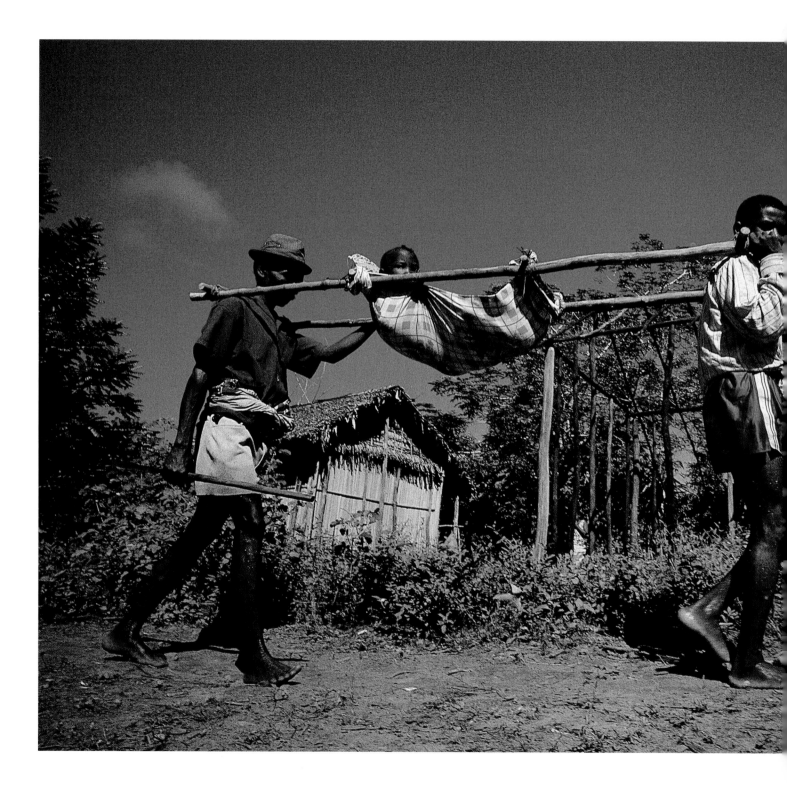

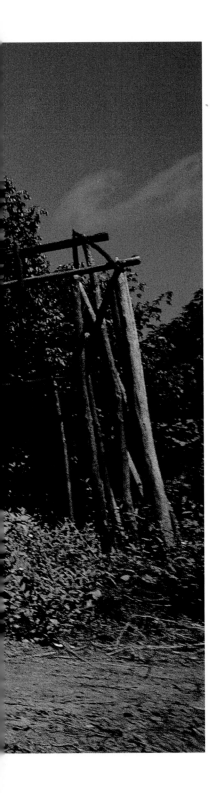

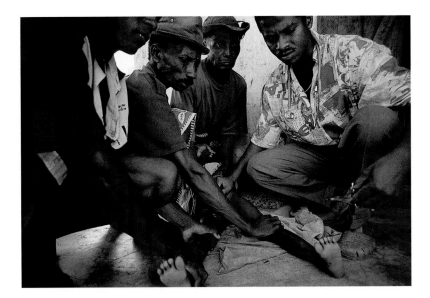

In northern Madagascar a child's father and uncle carry her, immobilized with a thorn in her groin (left). They will walk all day to reach a clinic in the remote village of Manongarivo that offers both Western and traditional medical care. As her father holds the girl down (above), medical doctor Jean Berthin Tida, in the blue shirt, uses a Western painkiller and forceps to remove the three-inch-long thorn. Traditional healer Ndronalahy, wearing a green shirt, then swabbed the area with an infection-fighting herbal solution. The men work side by side at the clinic. Most patients walk hours, even days, to benefit from their care.

At the Manongarivo clinic, Ndronalahy forces sap from a vine onto the burned belly of a patient named Natasha. Almost immediately, her crying and screams of pain stopped. Western-trained Jean Berthin Tida had little to help the girl, who suffered second- and third-degree burns from boiling water, but the traditional healer went into the forest and returned an hour later with a long piece of vine. One month later, after continued herbal treatment, Natasha's burn had completely healed.

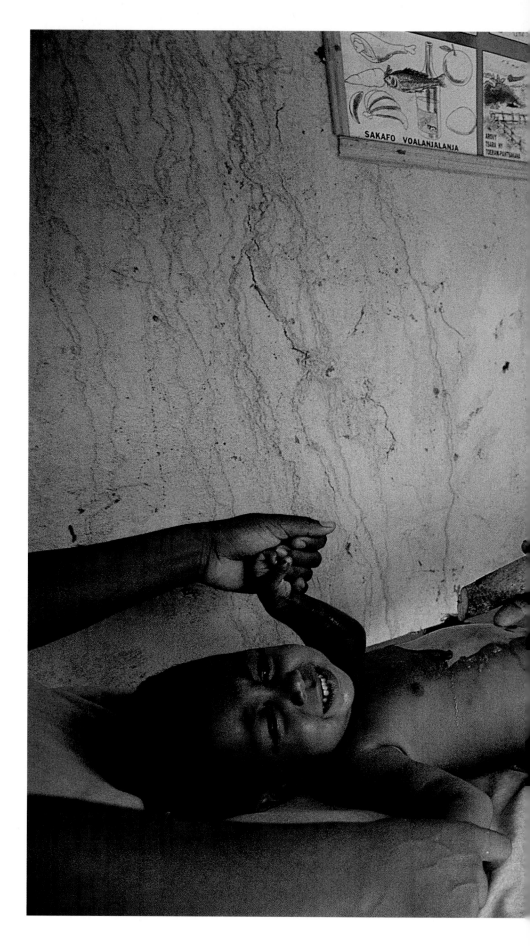

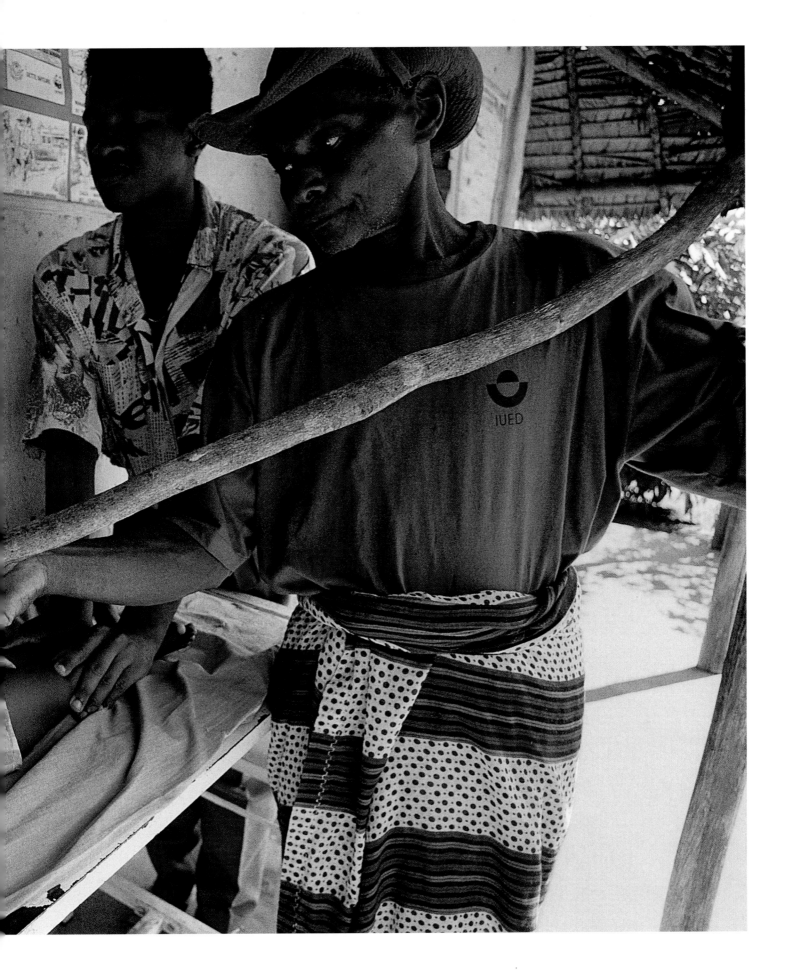

that plants cure diseases prevalent near the natural location of those plants—continued throughout the 19th century. In 1876, for example, an article in *The Lancet* reported on the effectiveness of willow bark as a treatment for rheumatism. The trees that grow in a "low-lying damp locality," it stated, work best because they are in areas where "rheumatic miasma seemed most to prevail." Stone hoped that willow bark would replace cinchona bark, which was expensive and hard to get. There is no evidence that he hoped to profit financially from use of willow bark, which was easily accessible to anyone.

The virtues of willow bark, however, were ignored for decades until a German scientist who knew nothing about Stone's work obtained the glycoside salicin from a sample of willow bark. In 1828 another scientist isolated salicylic acid, the active principle in the willow bark and leaves.

Other plants, researchers found, contain salicylic acid. Among them are meadowsweet flowers and oil found in the leaves of wintergreen, both traditional treatments for fevers. Salicylic acid was synthesized in 1859, and it is the active ingredient in all aspirin sold today. In 1874 a synthesized salicylic acid powder sold for one-tenth the price of willow-bark extracts. Salicylic acid was a bargain because much less of it performs the same function as willow bark. For example, to obtain relief from arthritis pain requires between 3 and 21 cups of willow-bark tea.

Use of salicylic acid, however, was negligible until 1899, when an employee of a pharmaceutical company gave it to his father, who was suffering from rheumatism. It worked so well that clinical tests were initiated. German, French, and British chemical and pharmaceutical industries were soon competing to improve extraction and synthesization techniques and to offer the best salicylic acid. Products eventually tried included aluminum aspirin, sodium salicylate, and chlorine salicylate.

In 1904 stamped tablets replaced powders on the marketplace in an effort to prevent adulteration. The Bayer company trademarked the name "Aspirin" in the U.S. and owned the name until 1921, when courts ruled that it had entered the public domain.

The full range of aspirin's effects and why they occur are still not known. Aspirin blocks the synthesis of prostaglandins, hormones that contribute to inflammation and pain. It disrupts interactions within cells, and it seems to interrupt the beginning stages of inflammation. Aspirin reduces fever by acting directly on a part of the brain called the hypothalamus. Low doses of the drug block excretion of uric acid by the kidneys; high doses stimulate excretion of uric acid. Aspirin may also cut the risk of colon and other cancers. But the drug can cause severe side effects that include stomach bleeding and the appearance of Reye's syndrome in children who have viral infections.

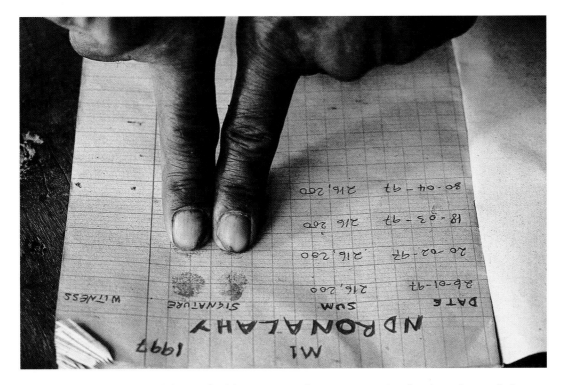

Traditional healer Ndronalahy at the Manongarivo clinic cannot write; he signs the pay ledger with his fingerprints. His vast knowledge of medicinal plants in the nearby rain forest is part of an oral tradition that possibly dates back to the arrival of humans on Madagascar thousands of years ago.

Some of the insights into aspirin have come about through epidemiology, patterns of disease in large populations. In the early 1950s a physician in California reported that none of 1,465 patients who had taken designated levels of aspirin for ten years had suffered from certain major heart problems. These findings sounded strange, and his cases presented a variety of unstudied variables. But his report provided one of the first strong clues about aspirin: It affects the aggregation of platelets, which is a leading contributor to heart attacks and strokes.

These effects are strong enough to earn aspirin regulation as a prescription drug (see Chapter 5). But the widespread use of aspirin—in 1950 it entered the *Guinness Book of Records* as the most popular painkiller in the world—has helped prevent government action.

———

THE ABOVE STORIES, modern science's first attempts to obtain medicines from plants, provide clues that are useful in today's search for new pharmaceutical drugs. All parts of plants—from flowers to roots—have yielded effective modern medicines. The plants came from a wide geographic range; information about traditional uses was available; and the efficacy of those uses had been proved before scientists began to focus on the sources.

The botanical medicines, furthermore, provided immediate, even dramatic, results. They sometimes addressed the cause of disease, but more often they worked on symptoms. Some medicines came from a single plant species; others (such as digitalis, aspirin, and antimalarial compounds) could be found in numerous species. But in each case a plant was used by itself, not in combination with others, which would have made isolation of an active compound very difficult.

Other circumstances seem essential to each medicine's eventual success. In every case, the active principle was discovered and could be standardized. The effect of a standard dose did not vary significantly between individuals. An adequate supply of the plants was available, and, when necessary, they traveled well and did not change chemically in transit. No specialized knowledge or techniques, furthermore, were required in collecting them.

All of the discoveries involved individual researchers, essentially working on their own. These researchers frequently experimented on themselves and on patients and friends. The experiments sometimes involved major risks, and they were often conducted without informed consent.

Whatever beliefs in Galenic medicine the researchers may have had, they recognized when their experiments provided clear, empirical proof of a plant's medicinal value. They reached correct conclusions, even though their analyses were often based on incorrect notions about how the human body functions and what causes disease.

Although desire for profit seemed to have motivated only a few of the researchers, they had no ownership rights to their findings, and they stopped playing a significant role as soon as large numbers of people were willing to pay high prices for the plant-based medicines.

Taking the lead in research, manufacturing, and the quest for profit were the large pharmaceutical companies that had started to emerge in the latter half of the 19th century. These companies were part of a larger phenomenon: Factories using techniques and equipment of mass production were replacing production by hand.

Economics of scale at these pharmaceutical companies encouraged, not further study of plants, but a focus on synthetic drugs that could be manufactured much more inexpensively than was possible when working with plants. That is a chief reason why the above list of modern medicines that were developed before the 20th century is so short.

Malagasy-born Jean Berthin Tida, a Western-trained medical doctor, consults with a patient and her mother. Working at a clinic in an isolated area of northern Madagascar, Tida sees local healers use freshly picked plants to provide treatments not possible with the modern medicines available at his disposal.

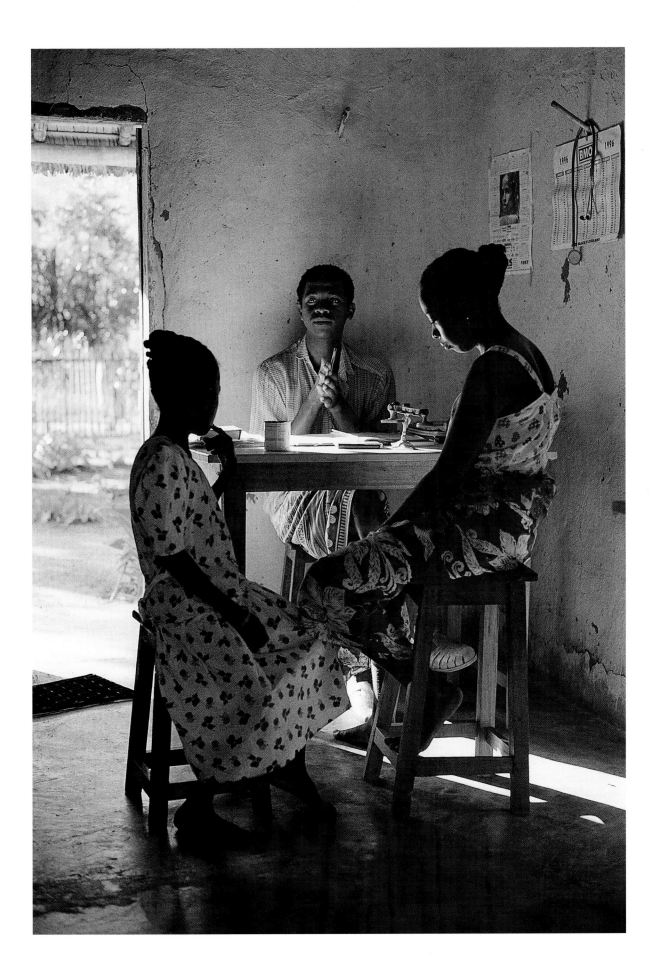

157

CHAPTER FIVE

Medicine Changes: Late 19th to Early 20th Century

In the early 20th century, as medicine began to adopt more scientific techniques, the American Medical Association published reports on nostrums, supposed cures it considered filled with "evil and quackery." Manufacturers of MacDonald's Atlas Compound Famous Specific No. 18, a typical nostrum, touted it as "The Greatest Remedy on Earth for Catarrh, Rheumatism, Blood, Stomach, Heart, Liver, Kidney and all Nervous Ailments." Laboratory tests showed that MacDonald's consisted primarily of sodium sulphate, sodium bicarbonate, and extracts from aloe and ginger. Another nostrum, Mexican Oil, contained red pepper and opium in a solution that was nearly 60 percent alcohol. Advertisements for Mexican Oil claimed that it cured gout, dysentery, cholera, sciatica, bronchitis, and rheumatism.

A traveling healer, who specializes in treatments for backaches, demonstrates his salve to a circle of villagers in Huasao, Peru. Hard labor on farms, poor nutrition, and cold temperatures contribute to many residents' back problems. Every culture, in every era, has had such itinerant healers.

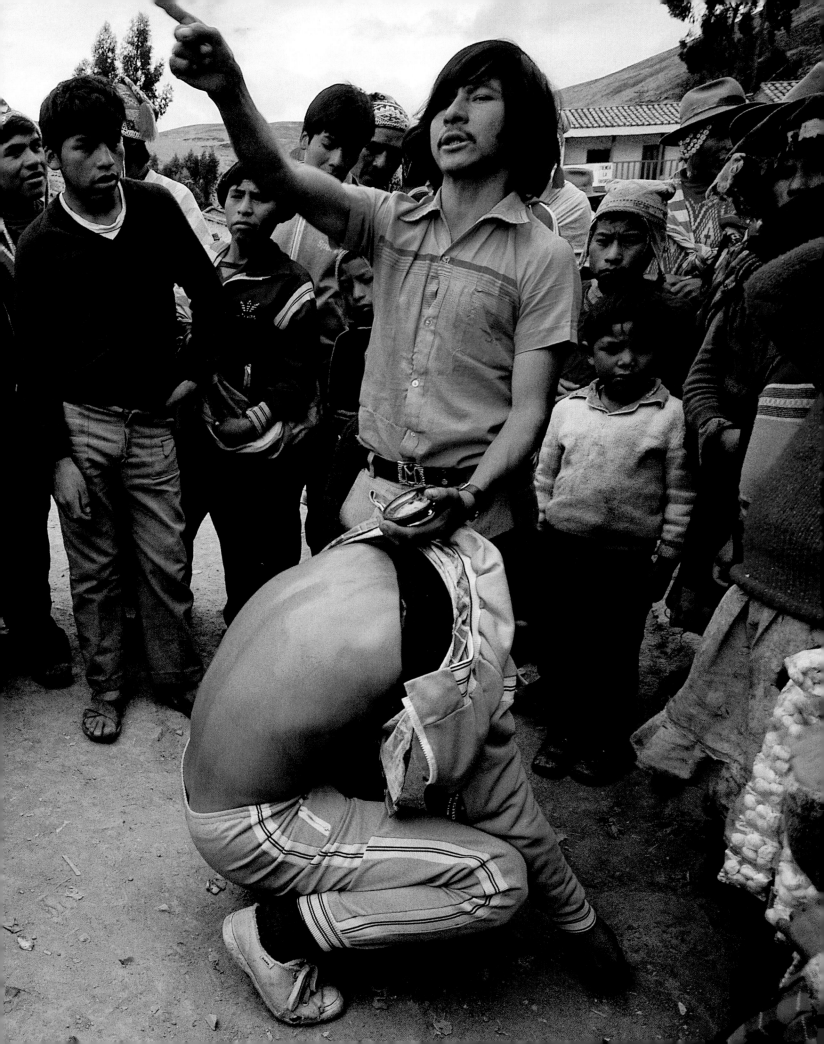

With the discovery that each natural alkaloid has a chemical formula and structure and that this structure can be reproduced using inorganic components, scientists attempted to create synthetic versions of alkaloids. Many early efforts centered on synthesizing quinine, whose prices were rising in the late 19th century due to dwindling Latin American supplies and an increasingly strong monopoly in the Dutch East Indies, present-day Indonesia.

But identifying the structure of an alkaloid and synthesizing it required large amounts of time and money. Scientists, therefore, began to work with chemicals not derived from plants, building drugs from their basic compounds. In 1883 came chemical synthesis of antipyrine, colorless crystals or white powder that combats pain and fever. Its use has been curtailed because it can produce a severe decrease in certain types of white cells.

Antipyrine's popularity stimulated development of other chemical drugs. One was carbolic acid, which was created by distilling coal tar and adding water, and was used to kill microbes. Other chemical drugs in use at the time included phenacetin, used to kill pain and reduce fever; iodoform, a greenish yellow powder, about 96 percent iodine, applied to the skin as a disinfectant; and chloral hydrate, colorless or white crystals used as a sedative. With these successes, drug developers began to understand that the effect of a drug—whether from a plant or other source—is related to its chemical composition. Thus, if quinine fought malaria, then chemicals resembling quinine could also have a beneficial effect. Before this insight, the best explanations of why a particular medicine worked had been the doctrine of signatures and the belief that plants grew where the diseases they cured were prevalent.

The pharmaceutical industry also continued searching for new drugs from plants and trying to find extracts in known plants. Companies protected their economic investment by taking out patents on characteristics found in certain plants.

Field agents acting on behalf of pharmaceutical companies collected material throughout the Western Hemisphere and as far afield as the Fiji Islands. Henry Rusby, who was born in 1855 and attended medical school, was a typical agent. In 1885 an American pharmaceutical company sent him to Bolivia.

Rusby's instructions were to investigate new sources of coca, to learn about the diseases common among the local people and how they cured themselves, and, if possible, to bring back any drugs frequently used by them. Another of Rusby's assignments was to collect specific plants that the pharmaceutical company wanted to investigate. One was cedron. This small tree had been brought to Europe in the 17th century, and people

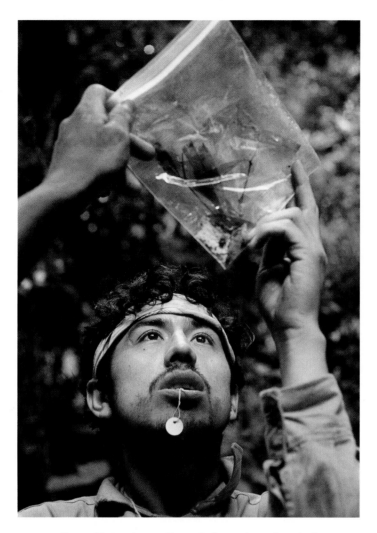

For more than ten years Percy Nuñez has collected plants from Peru's Amazonian rain forest for the Missouri Botanical Garden. Roughly a century ago modern pharmaceutical companies lost interest in such places as the Amazon as sources of medicine. Instead, the drug manufacturers focused their efforts on synthetic drugs. This trend continues into the 21st century.

treated fevers and digestive problems with it. South Americans used the plant to fight fever and to counteract the effects of snakebites.

Rusby struggled eastward from the Pacific coastal town of Arica, Chile, to the city of Belém on the Amazon Delta of Brazil. This journey covered 4,000 miles and took two years. On land, he traveled by foot and mule train. On the Beni, Mapiri, Madeira, and Amazon Rivers he used makeshift boats and rafts.

Along the way he encountered stinging ants, eight-foot-long poisonous snakes, waterfalls and impassable rapids, sunstroke, unfriendly tribes, and criminals fleeing from authorities. When he emerged from the jungle two years after leaving home, Rusby was so emaciated that his family, who had been told he was dead, did not recognize him. Many of the plants he brought back had been found by earlier expeditions. These included Jamaica dogwood, used in Western medicine as a painkiller and sedative; tonka, administered to combat muscle spasms and nerve *(Continued on page 166)*

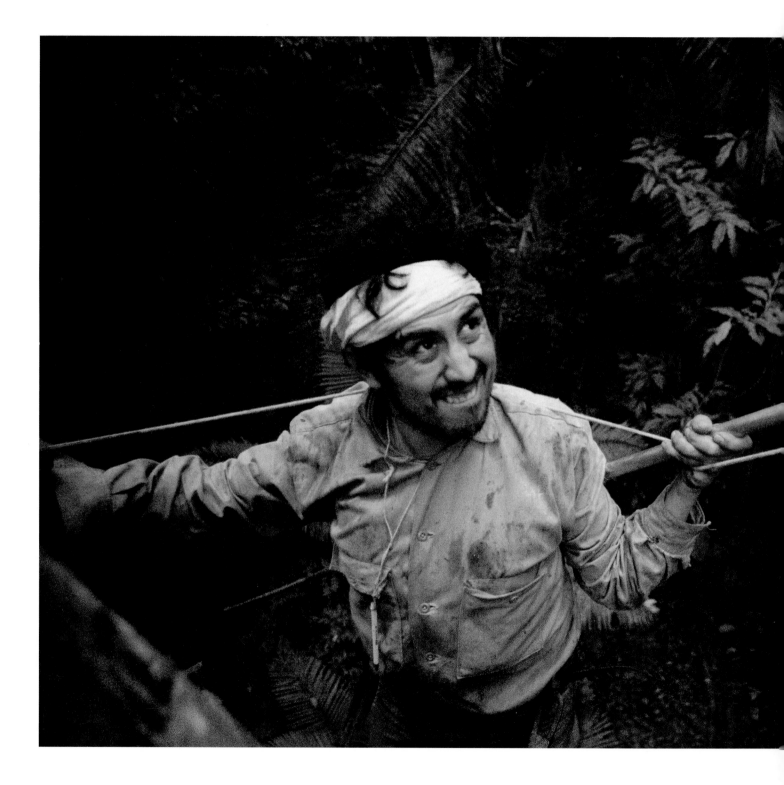

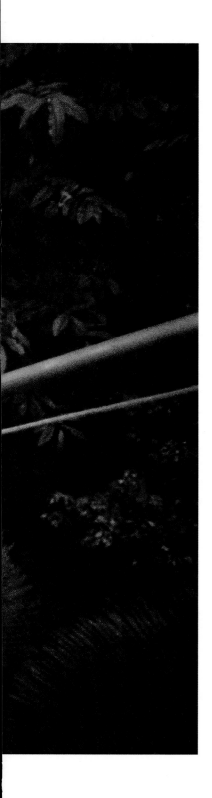

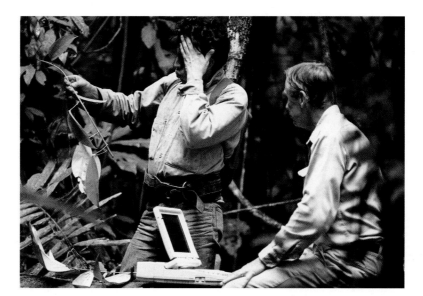

Plant collector Percy Nuñez works high in the canopy of the Amazon rain forest to gather plant samples using a long pole cutter (left). The National Cancer Institute will test these samples for anticancer activity. Heat, stinging fire ants, tree barbs, and loneliness are routine work conditions for such collectors—some of the reasons why by the late 19th century the focus of modern pharmaceutical research had turned to laboratory work. Nuñez and a colleague try to decide if they have seen a particular leaf before (above). Scientists have yet to compile and catalogue most plant species and subspecies in the Amazon.

FOLLOWING PAGES: On the Piches River in east-central Peru, papayas and other fruit rest at the bottom of a hand-hewn boat. In the late 19th century researchers discovered that papain, an enzyme in papaya juice, can yield drugs that dissolve blood clots and shrink ruptured or slipped discs.

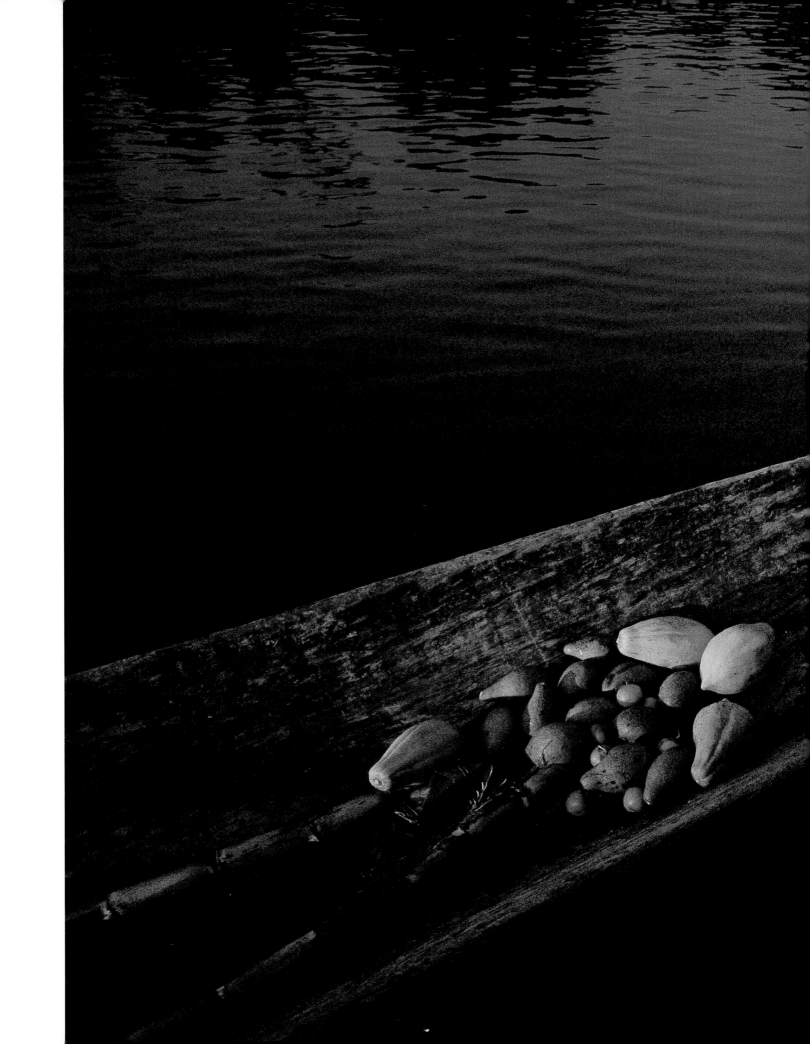

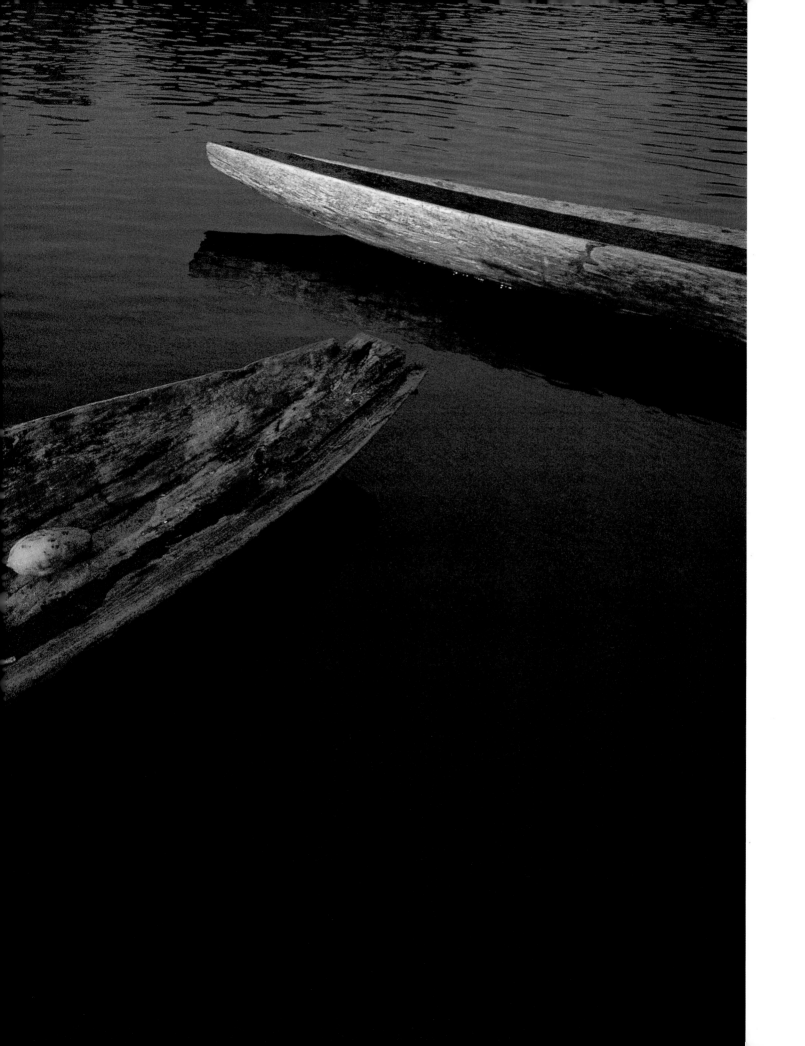

pain; and manaca, used to treat syphilis and rheumatism. Some of the plants Rusby collected were part of the transition to a reliance on alkaloids because chemists had already extracted a single active compound from them. Boldo, a Chilean evergreen that local people used for stomach and kidney problems, had yielded an alkaloid named boldine, which was injected hypodermically, paralyzing muscle fibers and motor and sensory nerves.

The way Rusby found drugs is instructive. He did not try to learn from local healers but seemed, instead, to have followed stories he heard. Arriving in the Bolivian tropics, he was told about an extremely powerful medicinal bark. The stories seemed too good to be true: The tree, called *cocillana,* was so strong that people who fell asleep beneath it never woke up. Rusby kept inquiring about the tree and was always told that it was "farther on." He began to believe it was only a myth, but in the small town of Guanay, Bolivia, a native showed him a plant about the size of an apple tree growing near a riverbank. Its fruit, his guide said, induced vomiting and diarrhea. Other townspeople had more complicated stories about its medicinal effects.

Rusby dried some bark from the tree, ground it into a powder, and gave it to one of the men traveling with him, who began sneezing and reported increased mucus in his mouth and throat. Rusby doubled the dose and gave it to two other companions, who developed runny noses and upper respiratory passages clogged with mucus. Rusby then quadrupled the original dose and took it himself. He became nauseated and pale and developed what he carefully described in his notes—reflecting what seems like a Galenic concern with body fluids—as "an abundance of thin, watery mucus, especially from the nose." The tree bark eventually became a cough syrup that sold well into the 20th century. The pharmaceutical company also sold it as a drug to induce vomiting. On a ship to Valparaiso, Chile, a fellow passenger told Rusby about *pichi,* a tree that yielded a drug local people used to dislodge small kidney and bladder stones. When he arrived in Chile, he asked for samples of the pichi tree. Rusby was not impressed with the branches that looked like cedar until he realized the pichi was related to the potato and could be useful. Then he shipped several hundred pounds of the branches home. It soon became a popular drug to counteract jaundice, urinary irritation, and stomach distress.

––––––––

AS MEDICINE BEGAN TO TURN away from plants and toward chemicals, expeditions like those of Rusby became outdated and unnecessary. In the decades following his Amazon trip, all of the plants that Rusby brought back were dropped by the *Pharmacopoeia of the United States.* The number of U.S. pharmacopoeia entries from plants, which had increased throughout most of the 19th century, peaked by 1890 at about 600—up from 425 in the first pharmacopoeia 70 years earlier. In 1890, 59 percent of the entries were from plants. In 1940, plant entries were 28 percent. The decline remained steady. In 1990 fewer than 2 percent of the entries were plant based. The European pharmacopoeias also dropped plants, but to a lesser degree.

Presumably the *Pharmacopoeia of the United States* dropped plants because their use by the public had declined and because experts considered them to be either useless or dangerous. But for the most part, no reasons were given, no studies were conducted, and no evidence was cited. Claims that no scientific evidence existed to support their use seem to have been enough to justify the exclusion of many plants. Those dropped included dandelion, black haw, cranesbill, pipsissewa, queen's root, and calamus. Some were replaced by their active principles, primarily alkaloids. A few new plants, however, were added. One was cascara sagrada, a powerful natural laxative, which entered the *Pharmacopoeia of the United States* in 1890 and is still there.

Movement away from plants reflected changes in Western society. With industrialization, the population of cities began to grow, a shift away from the land that continues today. In 1850 the vast majority of the American people lived on farms; by 1930 the figure had dropped to about 30 percent; it is now about 2 percent. Advances such as electricity further weakened peoples' connection to the rhythms of nature. Railroads, and then the automobile, increased mobility. Families became much more likely to move from place to place and much less likely to know—or care about—local medicinal plants. People no longer learned how to pick their own healing herbs and expected fewer of them to be recommended by their doctors. Europe and, to a lesser degree, Japan followed this same pattern.

With the growing distance from the land came a vague awareness, still present, that some primal connection to mankind's beginnings, some vital link to nature, was being lost in the name of progress. David Livingstone, a medical missionary and explorer who traveled through what was called "darkest" Africa in the mid-19th century, was amazed to discover what he considered to be the enduring power of the primitive. "We found some natives pounding the woody stems of a poisonous climbing-plant (*Dirca palustris*) called *busungu*, or poison, which grows abundantly in the swamps," Livingstone noted in his journals. The natives used this pulverized stem to kill fish. Later, he marveled at how the natives killed water buffalo using arrow poison from a plant called *kombi* (see Chapter 6). Livingstone could not imagine the presumably primitive Africans designing and conducting experiments that revealed the presence of such plant poisons.

How, Livingstone, asked himself, could Africans be better at recognizing plant poisons than English children, who would eat pretty, but poisonous, nightshade berries if left unattended. Somehow, he decided, the primitive people were more attuned to plants. "Probably the animal instincts, which have become so obtuse by civilization...," he noted, "were in the early uncivilised state much more keen."

———

GROWING RELIANCE ON IDENTIFIABLE chemicals from plants and toward synthetic chemicals fueled rebellion against modern medicine's reliance on the Galenic balance of humors. By the 19th century modern medicine routinely employed what came to be called, in Europe and the United States, heroic measures, assuming that the most extreme effects meant the most likely cure. The highest compliment of a medicine was often something like: "It works very violently both upwards and downwards," meaning that it caused violent vomiting and diarrhea—both highly desired effects. To choke on one's own mucus during treatment was not unusual.

Obeying what he believed to be Galen's edict to "destroy the fever at a blow," a prominent early 19th-century graduate of the Jefferson Medical College in Philadelphia routinely felt a patient's pulse. If the rate was too high, he made a hole in a vein in one of the patient's arms and took out 16 to 30 ounces of blood. If the patient fainted or vomited, the treatment was deemed to be a success. In the doctor's words, "the fever is vanquished." If it returned, the doctor resumed what he called the *coup sur coup* combat with the fever, bleeding the patient again. To facilitate bleeding, some doctors used the scarificator, a device with a triggered spring that made several small cuts in the patient at once.

Heroic medicine, which called the poisonous element mercury the "Sampson of the materia medica" and "a safe and nearly an universal medicine," emphasized the use of chemicals. Accepted medical advice dictated that travelers always carry calomel—mercury combined with chloride. Lead, antimony, and silver were also popular medicines.

In late 19th-century lectures to the Harvard Medical School, Oliver Wendell Holmes, Sr., one of the nation's most influential physicians, warned about such "alien substances," which he called "troublesome, painful, uncertain, or dangerous remedies."

———

THE DISCOVERY OF THE CAUSES of many diseases helped justify the rejection of the Galenic view that health is a function of the balance of fluids in the body. French scientist Louis Pasteur (1822-1895) discredited the concept of spontaneous generation—the belief that heat, moisture, and other conditions generate worms, insects, and other living things—a concept that had been in force since the time of Aristotle. Pasteur, Robert

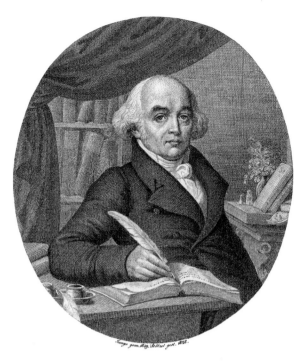

An early 19th-century portrait depicts Samuel Hahnemann, the German physician who founded homeopathy. After experimenting with cinchona bark and other plants, Hahnemann devised a medical approach based in large part on what he called the law of similars: "Like cures like." Make drugs, Hahnemann said, that produce in a healthy person symptoms similar to those of someone who has the disease. Many people worldwide use homeopathic remedies successfully.

Koch (1843-1910), and other scientists showed that various microorganisms cause numerous afflictions, including tuberculosis, diphtheria, typhoid, plague, tetanus, cholera, boils, malaria. The word "germ," which had been used since the early 19th century as a vague reference to the cause of a disease, began to denote a whole new world.

Suddenly, nothing was the same. "Wash your hands. You have millions of tiny organisms living on them," sounded strange to people who believed that if something looked clean it was clean. Florence Nightingale (1820-1910), whose reforms of hospitals and nursing emphasized cleanliness, rejected all contentions that bacteria are related to disease. Nightingale persisted in believing, as did most of her contemporaries, that miasmas—noxious gases emanating from the earth—cause illness.

Discovery of bacteria augmented the growing sense of reductionism—reducing human health to mechanical, cause-and-effect principles—that still dominates Western medical thinking. Just as the cause of many diseases could be pinpointed to alien entities, so, too, the belief went, functions of the human body are best understood as a series of finite operations. French mathematician and philosopher René Descartes (1596-1650) had set the tone for reductionism with his assertion that the human body is "an earthen machine" that operates according to mechanical principles.

By the end of the 19th century modern thinking began to see medical treatment as warfare—one-on-one combat between the medicine and whatever caused a particular

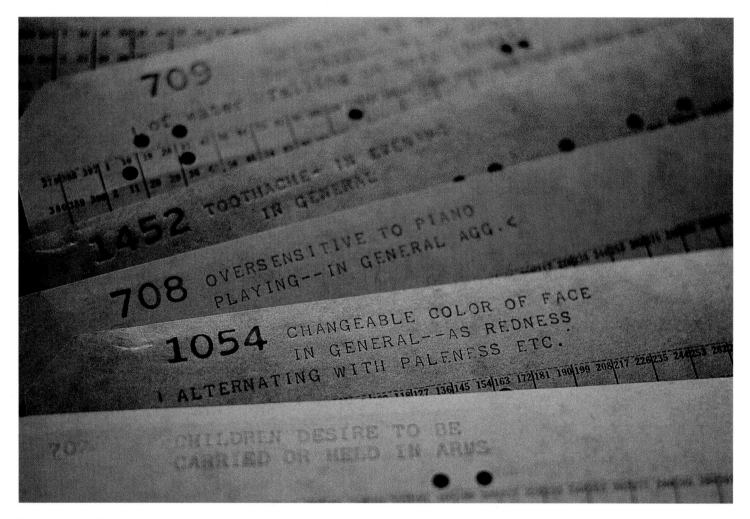

Diagnostic cards from 1922 listed personality traits and symptoms important to homeopathic doctors. To determine a remedy for a particular patient, homeopaths selected appropriate cards, then decoded the perforations to determine a treatment. In the middle of the 19th century, one out of every seven doctors in the United States prescribed remedies that followed homeopathic principles. Those included recommending treatments based on the individual and called for in-depth psychological knowledge of each patient.

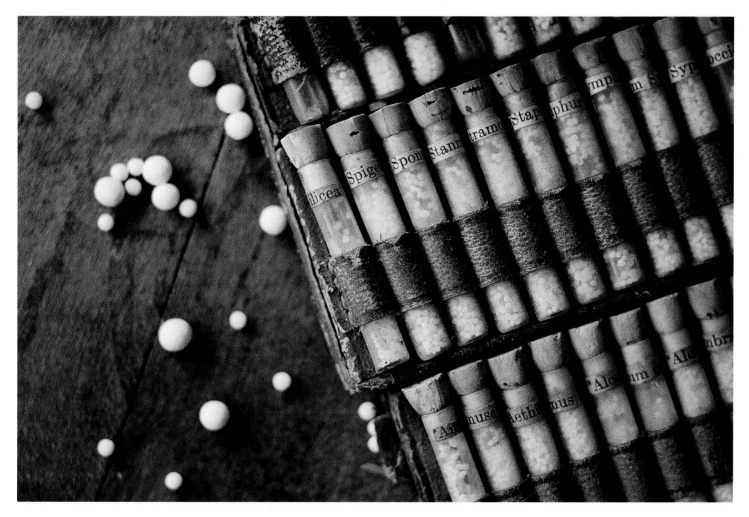

Homeopathic medicines, like those in a mid-19th-century travel kit, rely on infinitesimal doses of drugs, most of which are derived from plants. Many of the plants used in homeopathy—such as ignatius bean, bryony, aconite, and arnica—can be poisonous if taken at higher doses than the minute portions prescribed in homeopathic remedies.

disease. The resulting role of drugs—to kill the invader—fit well with the growing focus on developing drugs from single active agents found in either plants or chemicals. The reductionist mechanical model reflected the growing industrialization in Western society. Sir William Osler, an influential and progressive medical thinker during the late 19th and early 20th centuries, compared the human body to a steam engine. Previous cultures had found explanations for health and disease in the gods, luck, fate, and even the stars. Modern science discounted all of these as unrelated, misleading, and unprovable. It embraced an approach that still prevails: Look for the smallest piece possible because to get smaller and smaller is to get closer and closer to the truth.

———

THIS APPROACH WAS MOST successful in developing a cure for syphilis. In the early 20th century treatment for syphilis consisted primarily of spending time in a dry climate; exercising; eating a bland diet; bleeding and purging; taking mercury and herbs; and using ointments, often roots of daffodils, for syphilitic ulcers. Not much had changed since the Lewis and Clark expedition a century before, during which all of the men may have suffered from syphilis. Their prime treatment had been pills that consisted of calomel—a compound of mercury and chlorine—and extracts from the jalap plant. Americans then called these pills thunderclappers because they caused explosive vomiting and diarrhea. A variation of this treatment, introduced in 1834, combined mercury with potassium iodide. Mercury was the prime medicine for syphilis. Patients swallowed it, rubbed it on their skin, and had it injected into their veins. The lucky among them only lost weight, were disfigured, and had their teeth fall out.

In the late 1800s Paul Ehrlich, a German physician and pharmacological researcher, began to focus on chemical dyes as possible cures for diphtheria and sleeping sickness. Chemists had been using dyes, which were derived from coal tar, to help identify and observe bacteria under a microscope. If bacteria absorb synthetic dyes, Ehrlich reasoned, why not find a toxic dye that would kill disease-causing organisms? "We must learn to shoot microbes with magic bullets," he told colleagues. Such a bullet would kill microbes without harming human tissue.

Ehrlich said he relied on the "four G's," *Geduld, Geshick, Geld,* and *Glück*—patience, skill, money, and luck. He tried more than 600 chemicals on bacteria. The microbe responsible for syphilis had been isolated in 1905. In 1910 the 606th chemical Ehrlich had tried, arsphenamine, a synthetic compound derived from arsenic, worked against the syphilis bacterium. Arsphenamine was trademarked as Salvarsan. An indication of its potency was that manufacturing it generated vapors that could burst into flame. A shot of Salvarsan was no routine matter. One doctor advised "a day's previous rest in bed, securing the usual movement of the bowels, proper food, etc. so generally employed before any operation." One writer called Ehrlich's discovery "miraculous" and "Biblical." It accomplished what no herb had: Quick results, few side effects, and the disease was gone.

Although in the 1940s antibiotics replaced Salvarsan as the chief treatment for syphilis, the compound introduced a concept and an expectation that still defines much of modern medicine: Medicines should be magic bullets.

———————

EHRLICH'S MAGIC BULLET was only one of several ways scientists questioned Galenic medicine. In the late 18th century a German physician named Samuel Hahnemann (1755-1843) learned that cinchona bark caused people to sweat—just as the malaria it was treating did. He experimented on himself, drinking a remedy made of cinchona bark even though he did not have symptoms of malaria. "Briefly, all the symptoms usually associated with intermittent fever appeared," he noted in his journal.

Hahnemann coined the word "allopathy" to describe the medical system prescribing remedies that produced effects different from the symptoms of a disease it treated. He then began to outline the principles of a new approach to medicine. Its fundamental concept is the law of similars—*similia similibus curantur*, or "like cures like." Make drugs, Hahnemann said, that would produce in a healthy person symptoms similar to those of someone who has the disease. Thus Hahnemann's medical system—homeopathy, from the Greek roots *homeos* meaning "similar" and *pathos*, which means "disease"—uses extract of poison ivy to treat itches. The principle can be found in Ayurvedic writings and in the works of Hippocrates and Paracelsus.

Homeopathy has other prominent characteristics. Treatment is designed for the individual, based on the totality of a person's physical and emotional characteristics. Before advising a patient, a homeopathic doctor may question him for hours. Although the goal for all patients is to stimulate and guide the body's own healing mechanisms, different people with the same disease but dissimilar symptoms may receive different remedies—the homeopathic term for a medicine or combination of medicines. Most homeopathic remedies are tiny beads that are taken sublingually, or under the tongue.

Another fundamental homeopathic principle—the law of infinitesimals—is the use of exceedingly small doses that are designed not to kill whatever is causing the disease but, rather, to trigger the body's own immune responses. Reliance on infinitesimal doses roughly resembles the modern scientific observation that the human body needs minute amounts of trace elements and hormones for healthy functioning. Nonetheless, many scientists today dismiss homeopathic remedies, saying that the active components in them have been so diluted that none of their molecules can be located. Homeopaths respond that often the more diluted a remedy is, the more effective it is.

The *Homeopathic Pharmacopoeia of the United States*, first published in 1876, now consists of more than 1,300 remedies based on close examination of how various substances have affected people. A drug's impact on a statistically significant number of people is not studied. Before a remedy is recommended to homeopathic doctors, however, findings about its effects and side effects are confirmed via double-blind studies in which some subjects take a placebo. Some remedies in the *Homeopathic Pharmacopoeia* are minerals, but most are the same plants that were once used in non-homeopathic medicine. Many plants frequently used in homeopathy—such as ignatius bean, bryony, aconite, and arnica—were dropped by mainstream medicine and can be poisonous if taken internally at higher than the minute doses prescribed in homeopathy.

Such plants have a rich history, which most often suggests uses that differ from those found in homeopathy. Calling plants by their Latin names, homeopaths prescribe *Pulsatilla*—the anemone flower—as a treatment for colds, coughs, eye and ear infections, and other ailments. In ancient Egypt the anemone was the symbol of illness. Chinese called it the "flower of death." Greek mythology says that it arose from tears that Venus shed as she wandered through the forests, weeping over the death of Adonis. Traditional European herbal uses of anemone include treatment for headaches, malaria, rheumatism, leprosy, lethargy, inflammation of the eyes, and malignant ulcers. Another plant used differently in homeopathy is *Lycopodium*, or club moss. Ancient healers dried the entire plant and treated stomach and kidney complaints with it. After the 17th century physicians used its spores—which look like yellow powder—for a number of ailments, including dysentery, diarrhea, gout, wounds, and various skin diseases. Homeopathic medicine uses *Lycopodium* to treat, among other things, digestive problems and hepatitis.

One of the few plants commonly used in homeopathy and modern medicine is *Atropa belladonna*, which got its name because Italian women supposedly placed an extract in their eyes to dilate—and hence brighten—their pupils. Young women in Louisa May Alcott's 1870 novel *An Old Fashioned Girl* *(Continued on page 180)*

Calendula probably originated in Egypt, where healers relied on it as a rejuvenation herb. Some doctors during the U.S. Civil War used the leaves on wounds. Today, herbalists use calendula ointment for insect stings and calendula tea for fevers. Homeopathy prescribes the flower for numerous ailments, including headaches and head wounds.

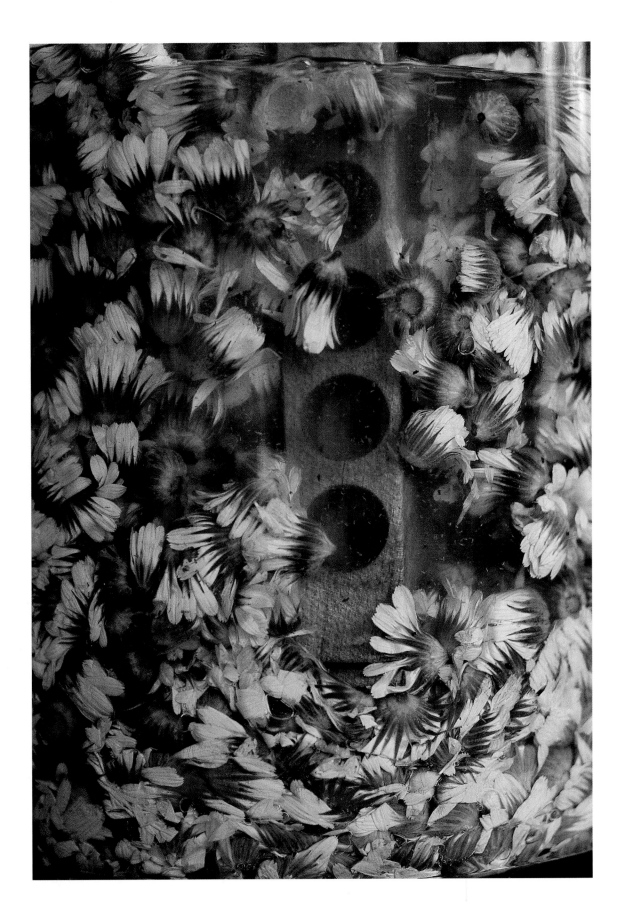

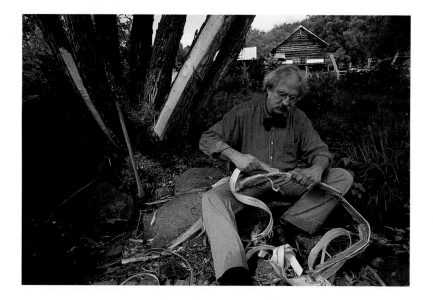

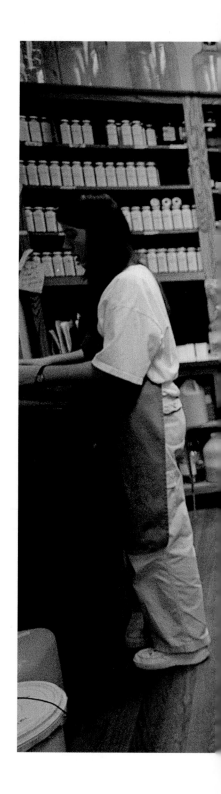

On his West Virginia farm Joe Lillard strips bark from the branch of a black willow tree. It will become part of a homeopathic remedy used primarily to treat menstrual pain. Joe and his wife, Linda, owners of Homeopathy Works in Berkeley Springs, West Virginia, have made homeopathic remedies for nearly a decade. Codi Parker and Belle Lillard prepare poison ivy pills at the shop. Instead of using medicines to attack invading bacteria, homeopathy uses remedies designed to stimulate the body's own health-promoting capabilities. The body has a natural tendency toward health, homeopathy contends, and only when it is run down or overwhelmed does it exhibit symptoms of disease.

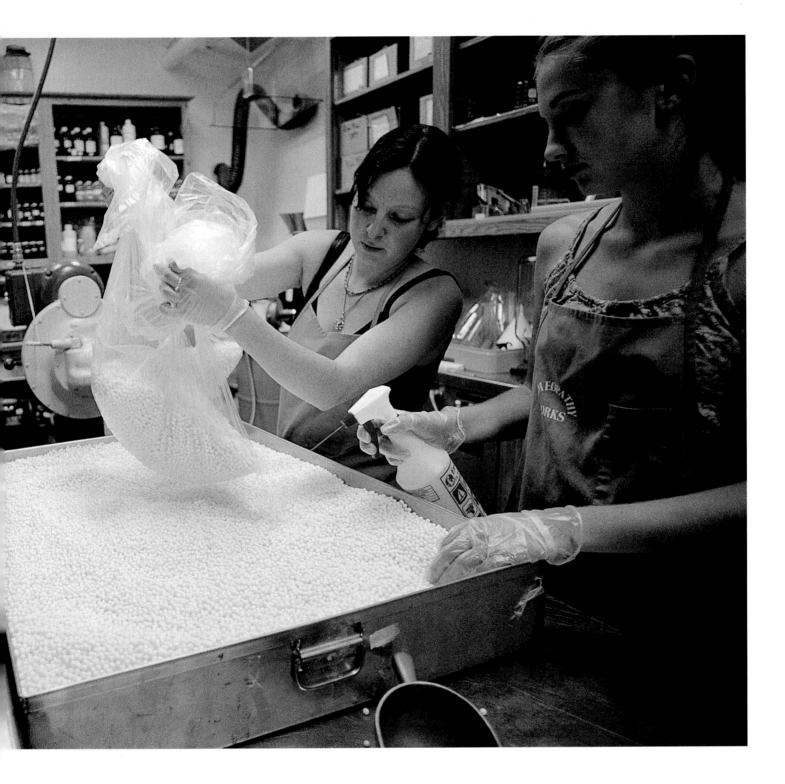

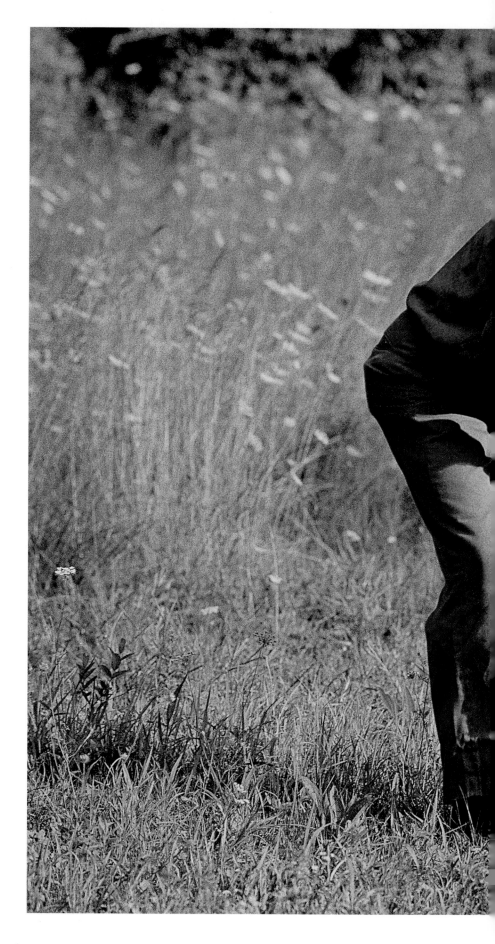

Enjoying the music of her father's fiddle, ten-year-old Emi Lillard represents a medical miracle. She has a rare genetic disorder that brought on septicemia, system-wide blood poisoning, when she was six months old. Her doctors announced she had hours to live, and hospital monitors attached to her body documented that she was dying. Her parents, Joe and Linda Lillard, credit homeopathic remedies with saving her life.

Did the homeopathic medicine really work a miracle, and if so, what does her story teach us about the power of plant chemicals and the need for a range of ways to use them? Or, did Emi live because, as her doctor said, she is "one tough kid"? Emi, who does not have normal speech and hearing, loves music. Her best smile comes when her father plays the fiddle: She enjoys touching it and feeling the vibrations.

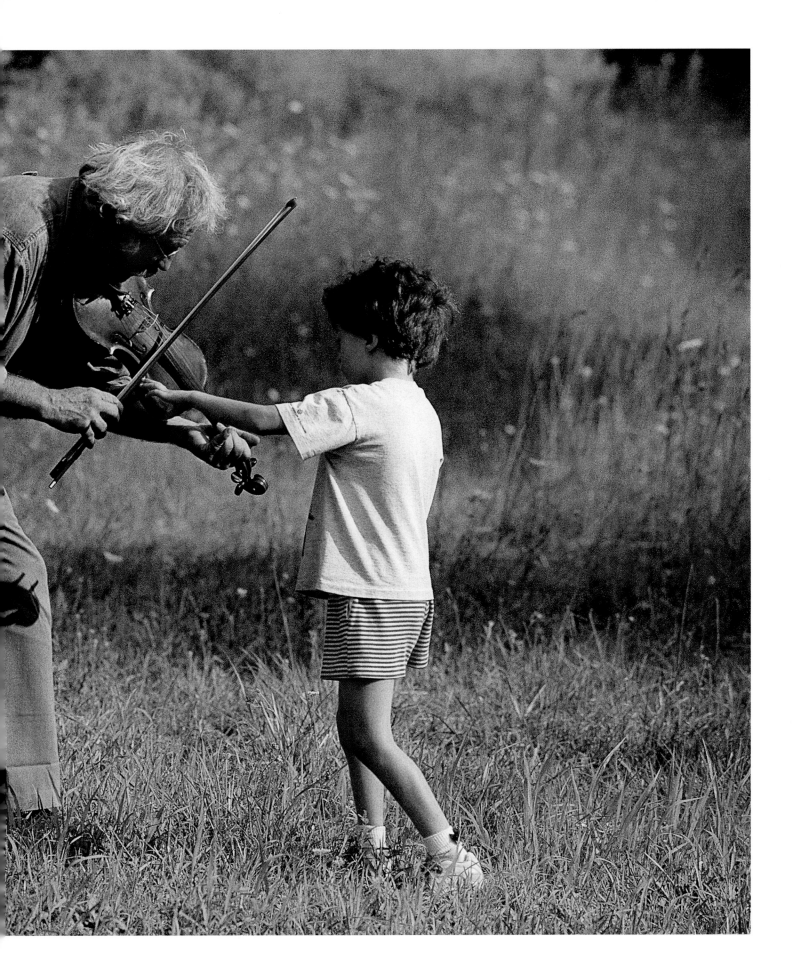

used it for this purpose. During the Roman Empire *Atropa belladonna* served as a poison, favored because it can be slow acting.

Belladonna attracted the attention of Western scientists in the early 19th century after British colonists in India noticed people burning jimsonweed, which is closely related to belladonna, and inhaling the smoke as treatment for asthma. Like belladonna, jimsonweed is a member of the nightshade family.

The alkaloid atropine was isolated from *Atropa belladonna* in 1831. The plant also contains the alkaloids scopolamine and hyoscyamine, whose functions in modern medicine, along with atropine, include dilating the pupils during eye exams, relaxing muscles during spasms caused by Parkinson's disease or stomach disorders, increasing heart rate, and acting as an antidote to toxins. Although all of these alkaloids can be produced synthetically, the primary source of hyoscyamine today is the Australian corkwood tree, another member of the nightshade family. This is part of a larger pattern in medicine—to use such natural sources when synthesizing a plant chemical is too expensive.

Homeopathic practice currently advises using belladonna for, in part, "Restless, red, and hot/Cold, flu, sore throat, cough, fever, headache, earache. Earaches, especially in the right ear, after getting the head cold or wet."

Homeopathy became popular in Europe and the United States; by the middle of the 19th century one out of every seven doctors in the U.S. was a homeopath. Competition between them and mainstream doctors continued into the 20th century. The battleground included accreditation of schools, government licensing, access to research money, and eligibility for insurance reimbursement. Newspapers often described this competition as mainstream medicine, or the Regulars, against the Irregulars. Many of the Irregulars were called Botanics, distinguished by their reliance primarily on plants—and, as is clear in the case of homeopathy, the way in which they use plants. Another major group that still relies on plant-based medicine is called the naturopaths, who draw upon Chinese, Greek, and other ancient systems. Founded in the early 20th century, naturopathy still focuses on diet, exercise, and other means to harness the body's own healing systems. For medicines, naturopaths rely on herbs and nontoxic chemicals.

By the post-World War I era the Regulars had won the battle in Europe and the U.S. To be licensed as a medical doctor meant training in an approach and in the use of medicines oriented toward chemicals. But homeopathy, naturopathy, and some of the other approaches did not die. As the 21st century begins, they are gaining in popularity and remain strong in many European countries, where the split between mainstream and plant-based medicine is not as pronounced as in the United States.

THROUGHOUT THE 19TH CENTURY doctors in the West relied on imports for many of their medicinal herbs. Often the herbs were contaminated, diluted, or counterfeit. This prompted action by the U.S. Congress in 1848, when charges that bad medicines were killing American troops in Mexico aroused the public. The Import Drugs Act of 1848 ordered inspections of medicines, including checks of their purity and potency. The act resulted, however, in little effective action, because the drug examiners had been appointed according to their political connections rather than competence.

The lack of regulations that focused on safety, honest labeling, and validity of claims led to extensive abuses. By the latter part of the 19th century, Oliver Wendell Holmes, Sr., was telling Harvard Medical School students that an end to all use of drugs would "be the death-blow to charlatanism, which depends for its success almost entirely on drugs, or at least on a nomenclature that suggests them." Holmes made it clear that he was discussing "charlatanism in and out of the [medical] profession...all the inconceivable abominations"—from noxious plant growths, cankering minerals, the entrails of animals, and the poison bags of reptiles—being "thrust down the throats" of patients. He called profiteers from such sales "toadstool millionaires."

Medicine sold throughout Europe and the U.S. in the late 19th century was often high in alcohol and opium. Many marketers promised that they could renovate the liver and kidneys, cure cancer, and strengthen weak hearts—and that their medicines were "absolutely harmless." Posters promoting drugs often featured bare-breasted women pointing the way to plants. Offerings in the U.S. included Warner's Safe Cure for Diabetes and Brown's Iron Bitters, "a certain cure for diseases requiring a complete tonic, indigestion, dyspepsia, intermittent fevers, want of appetite, loss of strength, lack of energy, malaria and malarial fevers, & removes all symptoms of decay in liver, kidneys and bowels, assisting to healthy action all functions of these great organs of life."

Traveling medicine shows are part of the minstrel tradition, common to virtually all cultures, that provides rural entertainment. Hucksters in the United States augmented this tradition by using Native Americans to appeal to the popularity of the supposedly primitive. While massacres of Native Americans were still taking place in the West, traveling medicine shows with natives in full regalia vouching for "Indian Compounds" crisscrossed the East.

Not all abuses came from so-called patent medicines. Large pharmaceutical companies also were selling drugs with high opium and heroin content. In the early 20th century, muckrakers, who were focusing on abuses by the meat-packing, petroleum, chemical, and other industries, turned their attention to medicine. A cartoon in *Collier's*

Weekly that ran a series of articles entitled "The Great American Fraud" shows a huge, hollow-eyed skull. On its forehead is written "The Patent Medicine Trust, Palatable Poison for the Poor." The skull's teeth are bottles labeled "slow poison for little children," which are connected by tubes to the eyes. One eye is labeled "Laudanum," a compound made with opium, and the other is marked "Cheap Poisoning Alcohol."

The Food and Drugs Act of 1906, passed in response to such publicity, was intended to protect public safety. But the act forced the government to prove a drug-maker's claims were fraudulent. To avoid legal repercussions, manufacturers simply had to say that they believed their medicines' claims were true. Enforcement was left to the Bureau of Chemistry. It had originated in the mid-19th century as part of the Department of Agriculture and by 1931 had evolved into the Food and Drug Administration.

Abuses persisted. The phrase "snake oil," now synonymous with fraudulent medicine, entered the language because so many salesmen passed off products with names like snake oil as miracle cures. Another popular word was "quackery," derived from the term "quacksalver," someone who quacked like a duck while praising his salves.

But problems with pharmaceutical, not herbal, drugs prompted the next major government actions. In the 1930s German pathologist Gerhard Domagk, inspired by Paul Ehrlich's work, discovered sulfanilamide, which was extremely successful in treating streptococcal infections such as meningitis. To make one sulfanilamide product, a syrup called Elixir Sulfanilamide, easier to swallow, one manufacturer had added diethylene glycol, an antifreeze additive whose toxicity was well documented. In 1937, 105 people, 34 of them children, died after taking the syrup. If all the elixir had been consumed, the number of deaths could have exceeded 4,000. The sulfanilamide deaths prompted passage of the Federal Food, Drug, and Cosmetic Act of 1938. This act required drug manufacturers to provide scientific proof of a product's safety. Until then, drug manufacturers did not have to test their products for toxicity. An FDA official later described the policy of the company that had manufactured Elixir Sulfanilamide as throwing "drugs together, and if they don't explode they are placed on sale."

One unintended consequence of the 1938 law was that it encouraged pharmaceutical companies to drop or to stop pursuing plant-based products. To receive the newly required FDA approval for a product required an investment of millions of dollars in laboratory work and tests, a huge amount at the time. Companies were unwilling to invest such large sums in plant products that could be difficult or impossible to patent because they had been created by nature, not by human ingenuity. The 1938 law led to FDA regulations, transformed into law by Congress in 1951, requiring that certain

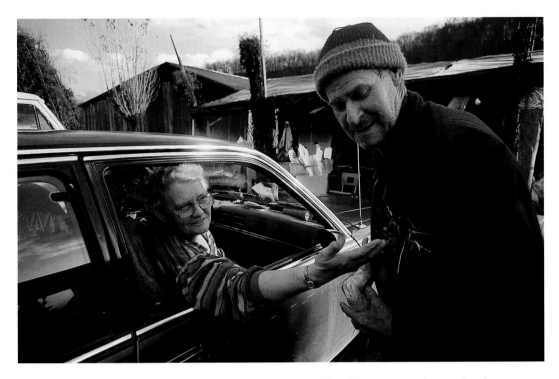

People drive for hundreds of miles to buy herbs from a West Virginia man known for forgotten reasons as "Catfish-Man of the Woods." Guided by local Appalachian traditions, he picks herbs that grow wild in the countryside. Due perhaps to Appalachia's lower-than-national-average per capita income level and the fierce individualism of its people, herbal healing traditions have remained particularly strong in this part of the United States.

drugs be available only on the instructions of a doctor. This distinction between prescription and over-the-counter drugs still defines American medicine.

The prescription, or bill, had become common in England as early as the 1500s as a written instruction from a physician to an apothecary. "The Physician cannot always be present at the making or the delivery of such medicines," explained a book published in 1548. "He may be twenty or forty miles from the Apothecary, when sending the Bill to him." Prescriptions that served only this purpose had continued in the United States until 1914, when Congress regulated the sale of narcotics such as opium. Thus, before 1938, any drug that did not contain narcotics could be purchased in the U.S. without a prescription.

———

PATENT MEDICINES, PHARMACEUTICAL COMPANIES, and government regulations had little effect on a common practice that continued throughout the 19th century and forms the core of much of today's herbalism. American families, especially those moving westward, relied on home treatments, and on what were called the root and herb doctors of their community. Treatments were an evolving and inventive mixture of traditions settlers brought with them, learned along the way, and absorbed from Native American practices and folklore. Problems addressed by home remedies ranged from the serious to the annoying, including cuts and scrapes, itches, burns, indigestion, colds, coughs, ringworm, rheumatism, venereal disease, dysentery, and cancer.

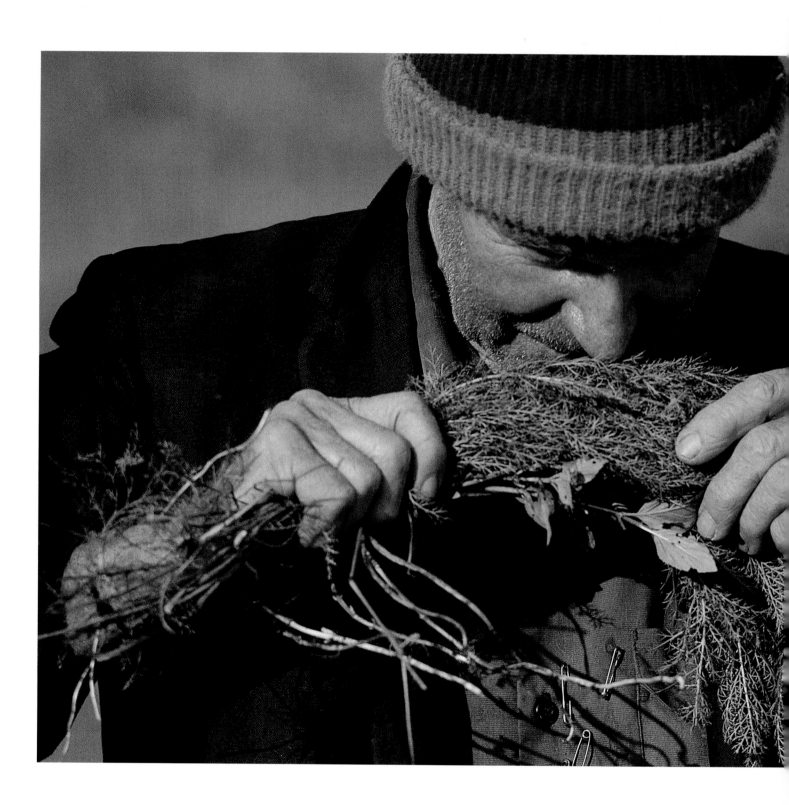

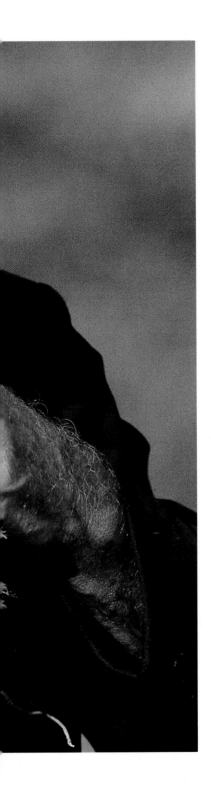

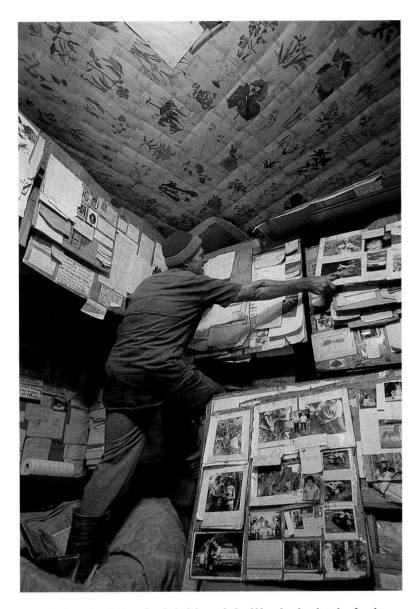

Appalachian herbalist Catfish-Man of the Woods checks the freshness of a handful of wild asparagus (left). People use it as a diuretic, to help eliminate kidney stones, to treat urinary tract infections, and to fight insomnia. When taking such herbs, it is essential to learn about correct doses and possible interactions with pharmaceutical drugs. Although he learned from other herbalists and has no formal degree, Catfish-Man surrounds himself with pages from herbal books. He attracts a stream of clients, many from faraway cities.

To find the possible virtue in some of these treatments strains the imagination. In the pre-Civil War American South, for example, men with bald spots were told to "rub the part morning and evening with onions until it is red, and rub it afterwards with honey." The herbal tradition was particularly strong in the South, in large part because it was predominantly rural and because slaves there had brought with them from Africa an appreciation of herbal remedies. One author catalogued nearly 800 Zulu words for plants, for example, and noted that 225 of them had some medicinal use or property.

It was not unusual for Southerners, particularly those fearful of heroic medicine, to turn to their slaves for help. A Louisiana planter wrote to his brother, "Your Doctors are rather a rough set—they give too much medicine. We Doctor upon the old woman slave and have first-rate luck." Another observer wrote about a female slave who served as a healer on a plantation, "I was sorry not to ascertain what leaves she had applied to her ear. These simple remedies resorted to by savages, and people as ignorant, are generally approved by experience, and sometimes condescendingly adopted by science."

Slave knowledge and traditions helped the South during the Civil War when a naval blockade imposed by the North impeded the import of drugs. Southerners also turned to old family herbals. Women traveling with Sherman's army through Georgia picked herbs to help treat the soldiers. Blackberries were used for diarrhea, jimsonweed as a painkiller, and wild cherry and bloodroot to stimulate the heart.

————

IN JULY 1924, people throughout America began to wait tensely for the next newspaper headline and radio bulletin. Calvin Coolidge, Jr., the 16-year-old son of the President, was very ill. Coolidge had stopped all but essential work. He and Mrs. Coolidge were at their son's bedside. Calvin Jr., who had a high temperature, was near delirium and in great pain. At first White House doctors thought he might have appendicitis. But the situation was graver than that. The teenager had septicemia, or blood poisoning. Toxins were in his blood and spreading rapidly throughout his body. The toxins came from a blister that had developed on the big toe of his right foot while Calvin Jr. was playing tennis at the White House with his brother. The blister had been "treated locally" but had become infected.

Since it was too late to amputate the infected part of the foot, early the next evening surgeons at Walter Reed Army Hospital sliced the boy's leg open to the bone and inserted drains to extract the poison. The next day they injected white blood cells into him. He was on sedatives, semiconscious, and unresponsive to all these efforts. Less than a week after playing tennis, the President's son died.

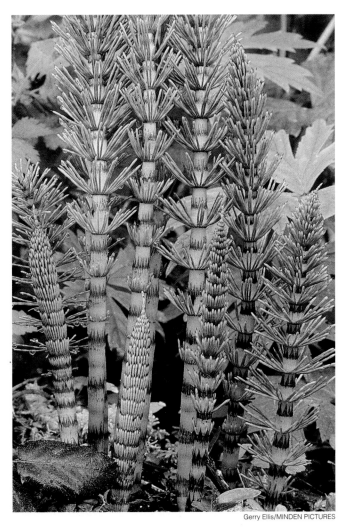

Horsetail, sometimes used to polish metal because its high silica content makes it abrasive, has been used to help clot bleeding from wounds, to treat urinary problems, and to promote healing of eczema and other skin diseases.

Four years later, in 1928, a British bacteriologist named Alexander Fleming was studying variations of staphylococcus bacteria as part of his interest in influenza. He entered his laboratory one morning and found that mold had grown on staphylococcus culture dishes he had absentmindedly left exposed to air. The area around this mold was free of bacteria. Pursuing this clue, Fleming published his results: *Penicillium notatum,* a type of fungus, kills certain bacteria.

Fleming saw little potential for *Penicillium.* He thought that this newly discovered substance could help grow cultures for laboratory experiments and might be used as an antiseptic to place on wounds. But he was not hopeful. "The trouble of making it," he explained, "seemed not worth while."

In 1939 a team led by scientists Howard Florey and Ernst Chain at Oxford University focused on *Penicillium* as a possible antibacterial drug. In 1941, thanks in large part to financing and technical support in the United States—which was assuming leadership in the research and production of pharmaceuticals—Florey and Chain

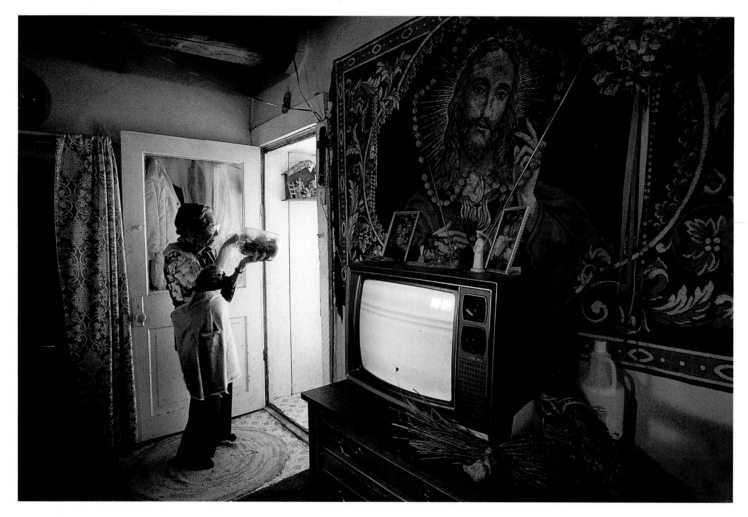

Failing eyesight brings Doña Gabrielita Pino to the strong mountain light in her doorway in Las Vegas, in northern New Mexico. A *curandera,* a healer who melds Spanish and Native American traditions, Doña Pino combines a vast knowledge of medicinal plants and massage with an intense and abiding faith in God. The light helps her find the proper herb for each remedy.

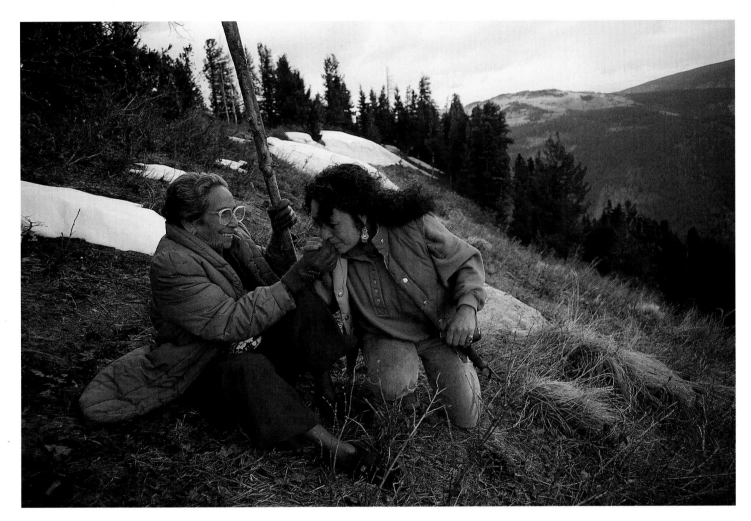

Youth honors age as herbalist Doña Pino and her student, Virginia Alaniz, collect plants on a mountain slope. None of Doña Pino's 17 children, 76 grandchildren, or 83 great-grandchildren has shown more than a passing interest in learning her herbal skills. But an attentive Virginia Alaniz, who has been interested in herbal healing for two decades, has assumed responsibility for seeing that the herbal knowledge does not die.

introduced a new drug called penicillin. It was the first antibiotic, a drug based on a fungus that is able to kill other microorganisms.

Penicillin was scarce and expensive. Throughout World War II it was rationed, with soldiers receiving priority and strictly monitored amounts allocated to the civilian population. This rationing ended in the late 1940s with the development of synthetic penicillin.

Shortly afterward came the discovery of many more antibiotics such as chloramphenicol, streptomycin, and bacitracin, all of which were called wonder drugs because of their miraculous effects.

These wonder drugs largely superseded the chemical sulfonamides—antibacterial drugs devised from chemical dyes—that had reached the market in the late 1930s. Antibiotics were developed from bacteria, fungi, and microbes. What these sources had in common was that the organisms are all biologically simple. They are one-celled, not multicellular as are plants, and thus relatively easy to master, modify, duplicate, synthesize—and patent.

———————

APPARENTLY NONE OF THE RESEARCHERS who discovered and developed penicillin knew that an old wives' tale in Europe and the U.S. had advised that placing bread mold on open wounds could prevent infections. Likewise, Chinese healers for thousands of years had covered wounds with fermented soy to prevent and treat infections.

As wonder drugs dominated newspaper headlines, people wrote letters to medical journals about such folk remedies that cured infections. "It was during a visit through Central Europe in 1908 that I came across the fact that almost every farm house followed the practice of keeping a moldy rye loaf on one of the beams in the kitchen," one man reported. "When I asked the reason for this I was told that it was an old custom and that when any member of the family received an injury such as a cut or bruise, a thin slice from the outside of the loaf was cut off, mixed into a paste with water and applied to the wound with a bandage. I was assured that no infection would then result from such a cut."

Such letters came from all over the world. "There exists in Brazil," one physician wrote, "a belief in the curative action of a field mould when applied in natural condition to cuts and wounds. This mould is found in the fields, chiefly in pastures, and its appearance is that of a ball more or less the size of a lemon…. It is a home remedy and very much employed….according to the popular belief the wounds thus treated do not require further care and heal without any complication."

None of these folk practices, as was typical of medicine's century-long movement away from such influences, ever led to the discovery or development of a new antibiotic.

By World War II memories of the role that plants had already played and the willingness to learn more about plants were fading. American surgeon Gordon S. Seagrave earned worldwide fame from the 1930s to the 1950s for running a hospital in Namkham, in the mountainous jungles on the Burma-China border. Seagrave lived and worked with people from more than a half-dozen cultures, including Chinese and Burmese—all of which had long medical traditions and a ready supply of medicinal plants. The traditions and plants never interested Seagrave. During his decades on the Burma-China border Seagrave took great pride in saving lives using Western pharmaceuticals. Among those he frequently cited were digitalis and quinine, both of which were derived directly from folk medicines. Yet Seagrave derided native botanical remedies as "quackery."

Seagrave described an experiment with one such "quack" remedy, which was called "umckaloabo" and came from Africa. Three doses of the drug a day were supposed to be highly effective against tuberculosis. During the middle of the war, when he had no other medicine to offer, Seagrave let a doctor on his staff give umckaloabo—*Pelargonium reniforme*, a type of geranium—to some patients on a trial basis. "We had all been skeptical but we were so no longer," Seagrave wrote about the results. Umckaloabo immediately improved the patients' appetites and cut their fever. Then, he reported, it cleared "the tubercle bacilli from the sputum and cause[d] the disappearance of all physical signs…." Only one patient taking the herbal drug died of tuberculosis, and many people were cured. Even with these impressive results, Seagrave refused to treat American or British soldiers with umckaloabo. He tried it only on a German prisoner of war and on Chinese patients.

When the end of World War II initiated an era of mid-century prosperity, chemicals and synthetics accounted for more and more of the drugs listed in the *Pharmacopoeia of the United States*. Pharmaceutical companies had essentially stopped looking for plants. Botanical expeditions continued, but their prime purpose was to discover and catalogue new species of plants for general scientific knowledge, not medicines. In the 1950s, to cite a typical example of the new attitude that had taken hold, one team from a major American university met a woman in a remote area of Peru who took them to what local people called Cerro Botica, Apothecary Mountain. She referred to each plant by a special name that described how local people used it as a medicine. The American researchers were not particularly interested.

CHAPTER SIX

The 20th Century: A Limited Role for Plants

In the 1920s farmers in Wisconsin panicked when some of their cows started to hemorrhage. The cause of the bleeding, which seemed to begin spontaneously, was found to be sweet clover, part of their usual fodder, that had been stored in overly dry conditions. The dryness facilitated development of a mold that produced dicumarol, a chemical that keeps the blood from clotting. In 1948 a synthetic version, warfarin, was introduced as a rat poison. Experts assumed it was unsafe for humans until 1951, when an Army inductee attempted suicide by taking warfarin—and lived. Today, extracts of dicumarol and similar substances from sweet clover and other plants—as well as synthetic versions of plant extracts—yield anticoagulants commonly used to treat a variety of vascular and cardiac conditions.

At the central marketplace in Antananarivo, the capital of Madagascar, a vendor arranges for sale finely ground herbs high in iron and other elements. Of the hundreds of medicinal plants sold in this African market that are indigenous only to Madagascar, only one—the Madagascar rosy periwinkle—has yielded a modern pharmaceutical drug.

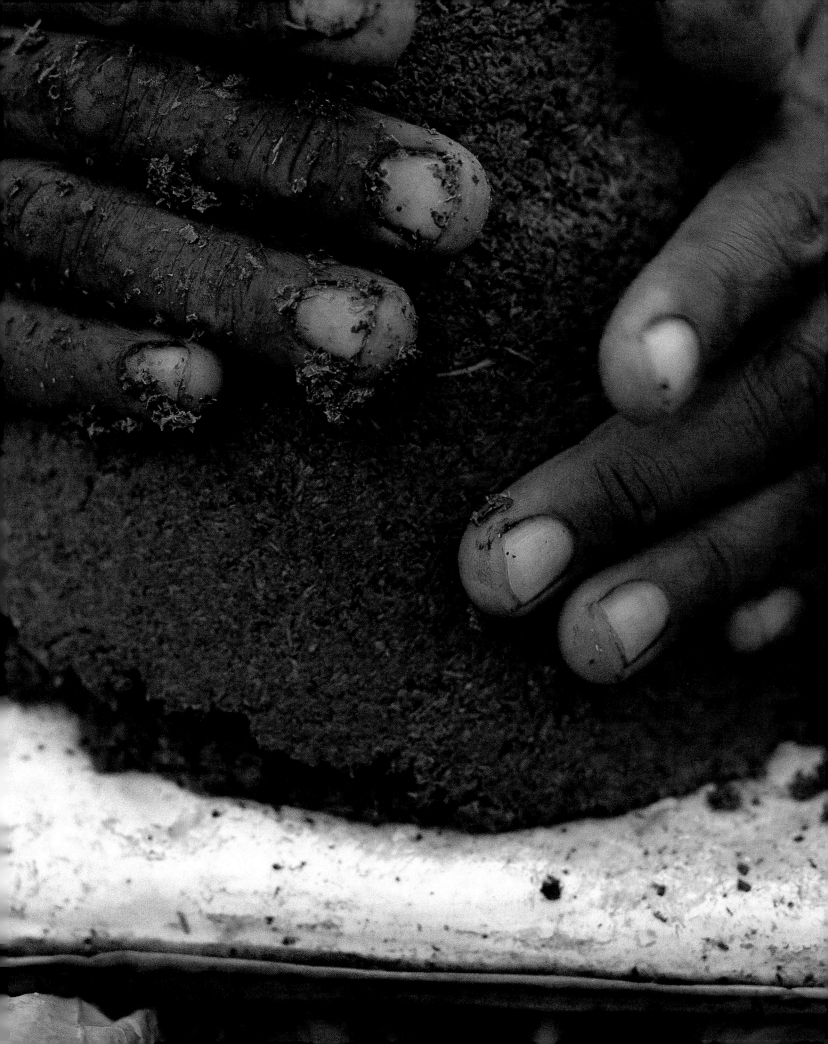

ery few new major drugs based on plants have their origins in the 20th century. The stories of these drugs are fascinating for the insights they provide into medicinal plants and into the process by which modern medicine makes discoveries about them. All of these stories are essentially links in the evolving relationship between medicine and plants, and they raise fundamental and provocative questions—such as the distinction between the words "natural" and "synthetic"—that demand answers. At the same time, the stories are deceptive because they create the impression that many such successes occurred.

The first of these stories involves a plant—chaulmoogra—that for hundreds of years provided the only known treatment effective against leprosy, one of the diseases that has most tormented mankind.

CHAULMOOGRA   Leprosy is a disease that, in its most extreme form, erodes the bones, causing deformities, particularly of the fingers and toes. It dates back to antiquity, and signs of it have been found in Egyptian mummies. "To drive away leprous spots on the skin," a medical papyrus suggests, a person "cooked some onions in a mixture of sea-salt and urine and applied it to the spots." Vedic texts mention leprosy, as does the Bible, which includes elaborate purification rituals and sacrifices. In the New Testament Jesus touches a leper and, in the Gospel according to Matthew, "immediately the man's leprosy disappeared."

There are two basic types of leprosy. The milder form, in which the human body's immune response encases the disease-causing bacteria, is not contagious. The more serious form, in which the bacteria move more freely throughout the body, can be spread through the air and via skin-to-skin contact. But until fairly recently, perhaps in response to the grotesque deformities they sometimes saw, people had an exaggerated sense of how contagious leprosy was. Most societies have myths about how families, including royalty, took loved ones to a forest, placed provisions in a cave, and left them. Until modern times, leper colonies for those suffering from this "living death" existed throughout Europe. Funeral services were held for living lepers, who often had to ring a bell as they walked near other people. If lepers came to church to pray, they frequently had to view services through a special leper's slot.

A 20th-century cure for leprosy came from traditional Chinese medicine, whose other remedies might involve such ingredients as arsenic, snakes, and scorpions. The Chinese cure derived from the chaulmoogra tree, which is native to Thailand and is also found in Cambodia, Malaysia, Vietnam, and eastern India. The tree grows from 50 to

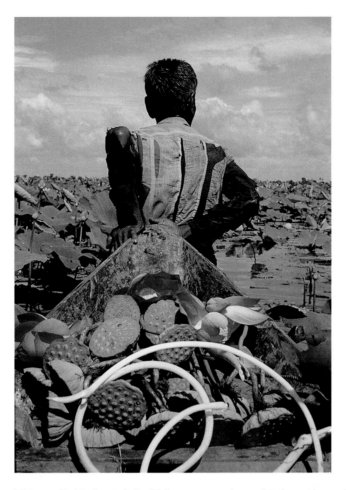

Lotus farmer Chen Nhim pulls his boat full of blossoms, pods, and tubers through a pond clogged with the plants near the village of Day Eth, Cambodia. People in Asia use lotus seeds to treat digestive problems, the flowers to stop bleeding, and the tubers to treat a range of ailments. Modern scientists have derived no pharmaceutical drugs from the lotus.

65 feet high and has a thick trunk, drooping branches, and long leaves that turn yellow. Animals eat the fruit of the chaulmoogra, but it can be toxic to humans.

According to one legend that describes the discovery of chaulmoogra's antileprosy powers, the King of Burma suffered from the disease. Because his doctors could do nothing for him, he turned his throne over to his son and retreated into the jungle, where he lived like a hermit. There, the gods advised him to eat the leaves and fruit of a tall tree with yellow leaves. Cured, he returned to his family. An alternative version of this myth says that the hermit king ate the leaves and fruit on his own, without specific instructions from the gods.

The remedy that comes from the chaulmoogra tree is its oil, which probably arrived in China sometime in the 14th century along with the knowledge of how to use

FOLLOWING PAGES: People in some parts of Nigeria, like this woman, lick the leaf of the "headache plant" and hold it against their skin to cure headaches. They use the plant for skin sores, also. Chemicals from the leaf may enter the body transdermally, or through the skin.

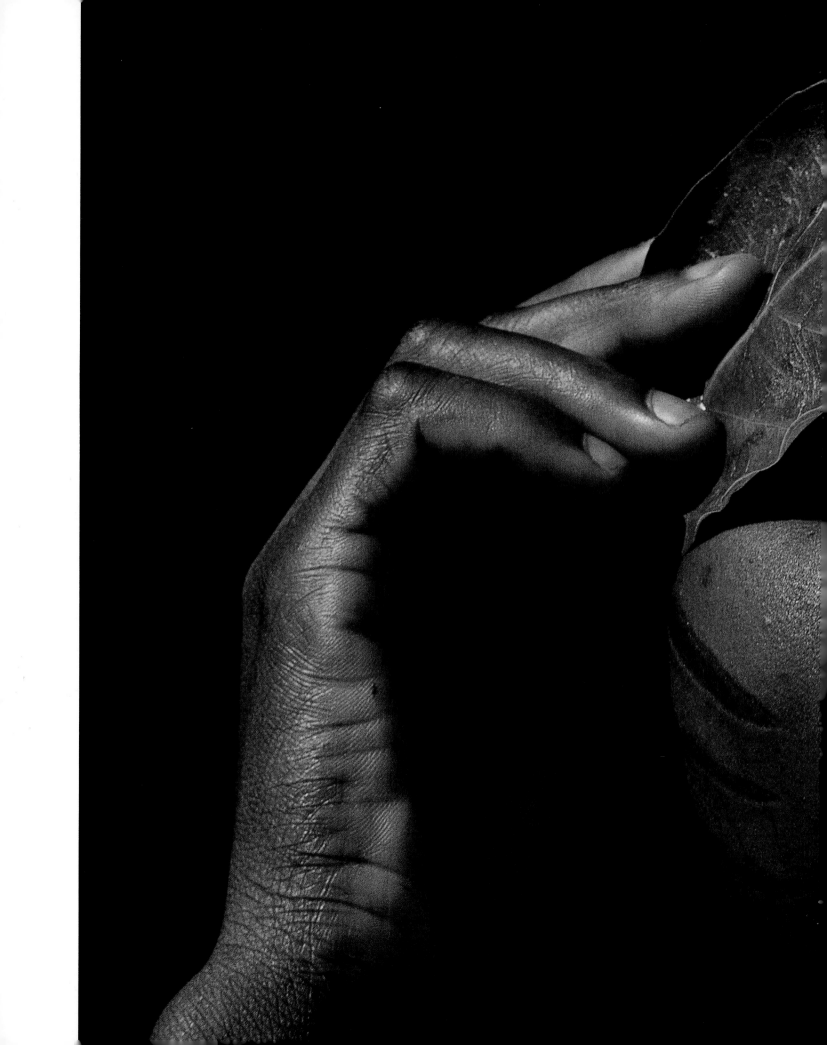

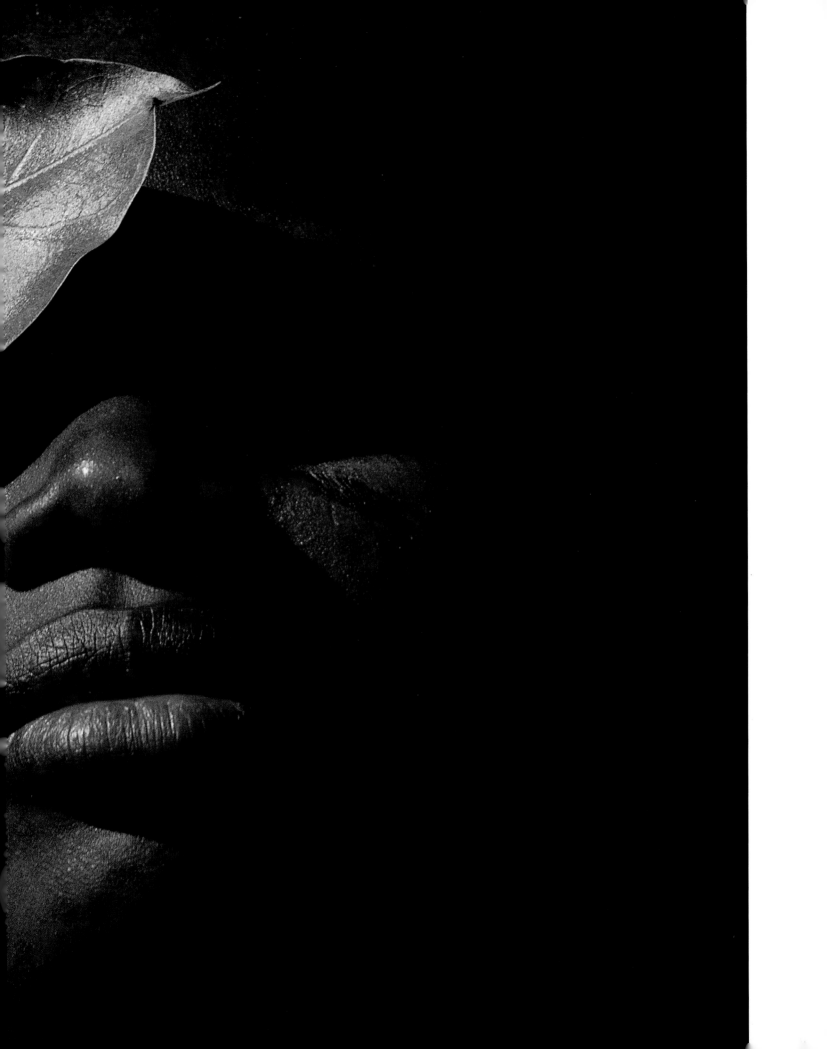

it. Purchasing chaulmoogra oil had been one of the tasks assigned to the 15th-century treasure ships (see Chapter 1).

According to traditional Chinese teachings, chaulmoogra oil was most effective in the early stages of the disease. This could make scientific sense. The bacterium that causes leprosy has a long incubation period and can lie dormant for three to five years before major symptoms appear. The bacteria may have been most susceptible to chemicals in the oil during this dormant period.

Chaulmoogra oil also had a reputation in Asia for working on wounds, ulcers, early stages of tuberculosis, and rheumatism and other causes of pain. In 1853 a physician in the British Indian Medical Service came upon Hindu and Chinese writings that discussed this treatment: Take 10 to 20 chaulmoogra drops after meals, and apply the oil directly to skin sores; continue this procedure for three months. The doctor tried this procedure on leprosy patients, found the results encouraging, and by the late 19th century Europeans had adopted chaulmoogra-oil treatment. It was taken orally or injected.

The oil did not cure advanced leprosy. It provided great relief from the symptoms and often seemed to be a cure, but the disease returned 80 percent of the time. Taking the oil, furthermore, was such a hardship that many people decided to forgo treatment. When taken orally, it can cause great nausea and stomach irritation. Injection is very painful because the oil is so thick. Large abscesses can form where the needle enters.

In 1873 a Norwegian researcher, Armauer Hansen, isolated the bacterium that causes leprosy. (In the 1940s some people began calling the illness Hansen's disease to avoid the stigma associated with the word "leper.") This discovery did little to change treatment, which continued to rely on chaulmoogra oil. But the oil was often unavailable because chaulmoogra seeds were difficult to cultivate outside the plant's natural habitat. In the 1930s chaulmoogra trees were grown around leper colonies to obtain oils of constant strength and quality. The plant was also cultivated in Africa.

No alkaloid or other active element has ever been found in chaulmoogra oil, which is 49 percent hydnocarpic acid. This acid is probably what kills the leprosy-causing bacteria, although about a half dozen other acids are also present. Use of chaulmoogra oil was discontinued in the 1940s, when the antibacterial chemical drug dapsone proved effective against leprosy.

Dapsone kept leprosy-causing bacteria from growing but did not kill them. It continues to be used in combination with rifampin and other antibiotics. Today, multidrug therapy is used against leprosy. Such reliance on more than one drug is becoming much more common (see Chapter 8) as disease-causing organisms develop resistance to modern drugs built around a single active agent. Chaulmoogra trees, once threatened when valued for their oil, still grow in the wild.

————————

EPHEDRA   This evergreen plant grows mostly in desert regions and produces yellow flowers and masses of red berries. It can be found worldwide, although some species, including most native to North America, seem to lack pharmacological effects. For more than 4,000 years Chinese healers have used *Ephedra sinica*, which they call *ma huang*, to treat coughs, asthma, bronchitis, and other respiratory problems. Plants are collected in autumn, sun dried, and sectioned. The sections are boiled, often in a mixture of honey and water, and then roasted until all the water evaporates. Many Chinese tie the stems of the plant in bunches and use them as a tea to treat fevers, cough, and postpartum problems. They use the roots and joints to cause sweating.

Ancient Greeks used a species of ephedra to stop bleeding and cure coughs. Native Americans in Texas and Mexico used it to treat kidney diseases. Teas made with ephedra have been used to treat numerous ailments. The Mormons in Utah used it as the basis for Mormon, or desert, tea, a treatment for venereal disease.

Nagayoshi Nagai (1844-1929), a Japanese organic chemist who had studied in Germany, worked with ephedra because he knew that it had been used as "a drug which for thousands of years had been appreciated" for fighting fevers. Japanese—or Kampo—medicine, whose roots are in Chinese healing, uses ephedra to treat headaches and chills as well as fever. Kampo healers also prescribe ephedra to help maintain the flow of energy—or qi—to the lungs, thus fighting coughs and wheezing.

In 1887 Nagai isolated ephedrine, an alkaloid in ephedra, but his work—although published in scientific journals—was quickly forgotten. In the early 1920s two young American researchers working at the Peking Union Medical College were looking for plants with bioactive qualities. They injected extract of ephedra into dogs and found that it raised their blood pressure, which led to the researchers' discovery that ephedrine and other alkaloids in ephedra stimulate the central nervous system.

Some of ephedrine's effects on the central nervous system resemble those of amphetamines, addictive chemical drugs that were synthesized in 1887. Although ephedrine is weaker than amphetamines, its similar effects create the possibility for abusive and dangerous use.

Ephedrine's most important effects are to relax the smooth muscles of the bronchial tree, dilate the bronchial passages, decrease congestion in mucous tissue, improve air exchange, increase capacity, and relieve mild spasms of the bronchial tubes.

All these effects are extremely important to those suffering from bronchitis or asthma. Injections of ephedrine can also help during acute bronchial or asthmatic attacks.

Ephedrine quickly entered clinical use. By 1925 and 1926 it was a leading treatment for asthma, and since then has led to the development of at least a half dozen other pharmaceutical drugs, many of which have been made by modifying the chemical formula for ephedrine. The alkaloid is also used to stimulate the central nervous system in cases of narcolepsy (recurrent, brief, uncontrollable episodes of sleep), to counteract poisoning by a central nervous system depressant, to prevent low blood pressure during spinal anesthesia, and to dilate the pupils.

Pseudoephedrine, another chemical found naturally in ephedra, has effects that are milder than those of ephedrine and is used as a nasal decongestant.

———————

INDIAN SNAKEROOT   *Rauwolfia serpentina*, commonly known as Indian snakeroot, is a shrub that grows throughout much of southern Asia. Ancient Ayurvedic medicine used it to treat diarrhea, dysentery, and snake and insect bites; to fight fever; and to cause contractions of the uterus. Villagers today give it to their children to help them sleep. The part of the plant most used is the root, which is made into a powder.

Knowledge of Indian snakeroot may have reached Europe in the mid-16th century with publication of writings by Garcia da Orta, a Portuguese doctor living in India. Da Orta's work on Indian medicinal plants, however, did not become widely read in Europe or available to scientists until the late 19th century.

A myth associated with Indian snakeroot is that the mongoose, a small, short-legged mammal, eats snakeroot leaves to protect itself from poison before fighting a cobra. If bitten, according to this myth, the mongoose eats more leaves, rests, and returns to the fight. The myth does not say what the snake does while the mongoose rests. The only true part of the myth is that mongooses and snakes fight. A mongoose often attacks, relying on speed and agility to avoid the snake's fangs. The mongoose bites the snake's skull, breaking it. Mongooses eat no herb to attain immunity from snake venom and often die from it, as do other small mammals.

In the 1930s Indian physicians trained in Western medicine were using snakeroot to treat hypertension and psychoses. At the same time, Mohandas K. Gandhi (1869-1948), the leader of India's independence movement, reportedly chewed on snakeroot while meditating and drank a tea made with snakeroot before going to bed. These acts had symbolic importance for Indians because Gandhi represented an appreciation of India's ancient wisdom in the face of pressures to emulate the modern, industrial world.

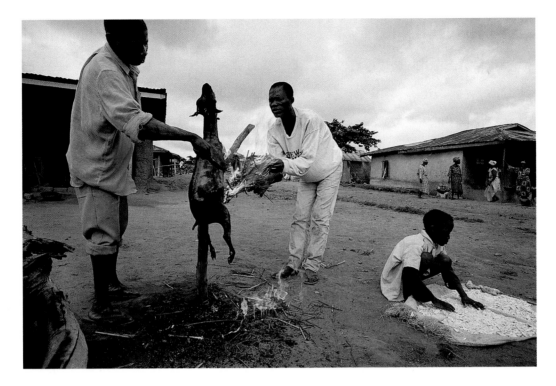

Villagers in central Nigeria prepare for a feast day. The boy dries cassava, a shrub whose roots provide a staple of their diet. Traditional healers around the world use cassava to treat a range of ailments including skin problems, diarrhea, and scabies. In most cultures the use of a plant as a food as well as a medicine is not unusual.

In 1952 researchers isolated the alkaloid reserpine in the root of the snakeroot. This root has at least 50 known alkaloids, of which modern medicine uses only reserpine. It interferes with the sympathetic nervous system, something no previous drug had accomplished. Western doctors began to use reserpine to treat some emotional and mental problems, including mania and schizophrenia, and physicians felt optimistic about its unique ability to affect certain chemical processes in the brain. But reliance on reserpine was curtailed because it can trigger severe depression and nightmares and affects blood pressure. Synthetic drugs that act in a similar manner on the brain have been developed. These drugs lack reserpine's power but do not provoke its negative side effects. Reserpine is still used, however, to treat high blood pressure and as a tranquilizer.

Although researchers synthesized reserpine in 1956, the process is expensive and time-consuming, and medicine is still obtained from the actual plant. Because cultivation of snakeroot has proved difficult, most plants are still harvested from the wild.

———

PAREIRA   In the 1540s Spanish and Portuguese explorers in South America reported seeing animals killed by darts and arrows dipped in a gummy substance. The poison did not affect the edibility of the animals, but it completely immobilized them

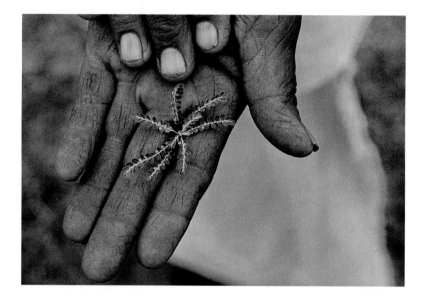

In the village of Jodagette, near Bangalore, India, a man holds a plant that local people use to treat fevers (above). Fifty miles to the north, an area with similar vegetation, villagers use a different plant with equally effective fever-fighting properties. Such a wide range of available plants has made it difficult for modern pharmacological researchers to identify which ones are the most likely candidates to provide drugs. Water hyssop yields its medicinal juices as Minashi and Shanda Vishalagi prepare a medicine at the Poonkutil Mana Hospital, an Ayurvedic treatment center in Karala, India (right). The medicine will be used to relieve anxiety in mentally ill patients.

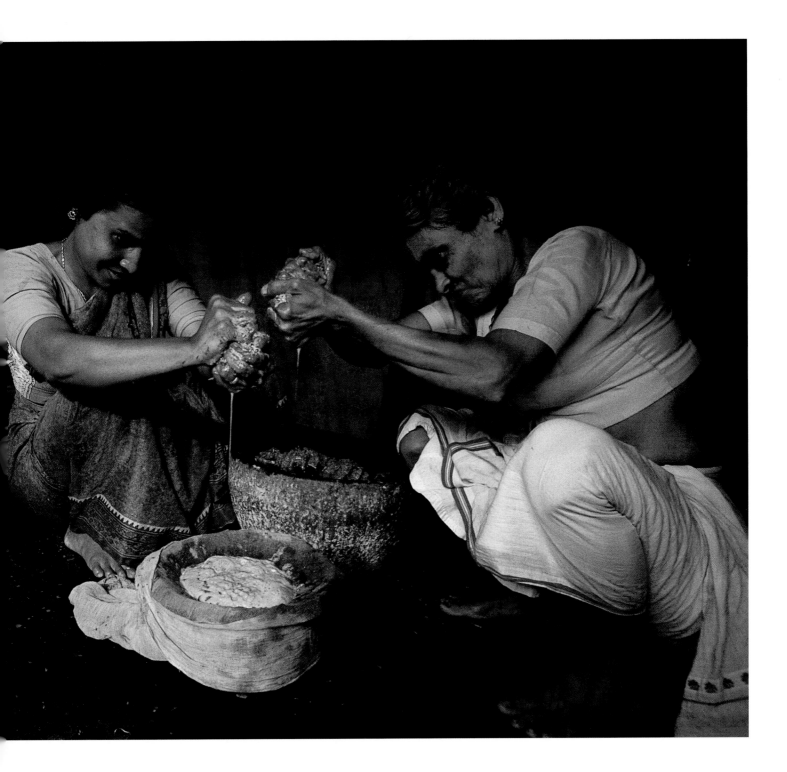

before they died. One observer noted that they had seemed at peace, not distressed about their impending death.

The poisons frightened the Europeans, who saw that one nick of an arrow could kill a man instantly. Proposed antidotes included garlic juice, salt or human urine, and sugar. One suggestion made in 1600 was to use a razor to slice off all skin and flesh that had been in contact with the poison.

Natives throughout South America used such dart and arrow poisons, which can also be found in cultures on other continents. The word "curare," which may come from *urari*, one of the many native words for poison, refers to plant-derived poisons of Central and South America.

Not all these poisons are equally effective or constituted the same way. Curare from the Amazon relies on plants with neuromuscular-blocking alkaloids, while poisons from Asia and Africa come from plants whose alkaloids block the central nervous system. Amazonian curare is almost always derived from plants, and, like dart and arrow poisons from other areas, can include snake, scorpion, frog, and centipede venom in addition to plants.

Sensational stories in Europe attributed curare to snakes, boiled ants, spiders, bat wings, toads, and a combination of snake blood and ant heads. According to one widely believed myth, curare was made by old women locked in huts. If they tried to escape, according to the myth, the women were beaten. And if they breathed fumes from their concoction, they died slowly, over three days—and the men of the tribe knew the poison was good.

In South America scores of tribes used dozens of formulas to make curare. All the makers were secretive about their poisons, which made sense. Natives used curare for hunting and to protect themselves against intruders, especially the Spanish and Portuguese—who were, after all, not teaching them how to make guns or swords.

By the late 16th century the Spanish and Portuguese had brought some curare back to Europe for study. The price they paid for it was often an amount of silver equal in weight to the weight of the curare, but they never got the formula for making it.

In 1769 an American doctor provided the first written recipe for curare, a dark brown-to-black sticky mass with a tarry odor: "Take of the Bark of the Root of Woorara, six parts; Of the bark of Warracobba coura, two parts; Of the Bark of the Roots of Couranapi, Baketi, and Hatchybaly, of each one part." It is impossible now to know what woorara, warracobba coura, couranapi, baketi, and hatchybaly are. Even people in the 18th century probably had no idea.

Over the centuries finding curare was one of the primary goals of jungle expeditions to South and Central America. Many of these explorers died; at least one was eaten by natives. Written stories from those who survived, however, describe how natives made curare: Work was done, not by old women locked in huts, but by skilled craftsmen. These artisans followed strict rules and conducted empirical tests to ensure that their poison was at the correct strength. One such test was to prick a lizard on the toe, put some poison on the cut, and see what happened. The poison-makers knew that lizards are cold-blooded. The time for the poison to act would therefore be about twice that required in a warm-blooded animal.

The poison, Europeans learned, retained its strength for about two years. To renew the potency, natives added juice from the root of the cassava, an edible plant whose tubers are used to make flour and tapioca. They then buried the poison in the ground for two days.

We now know that curare is a complicated combination of roots, stems, tubers, leaves, fruits, seeds, bulbs, latex, resin, and other elements from numerous species of plants. Recipes can be extremely complicated. Most seem to include the stem of the climbing vine pareira, and some types of curare use tubers from at least eight plants.

Curare-makers claim to recognize signs of an extremely potent plant, such as yellow rather than red sap color when the stem is cut, that professional taxonomists do not see. Traditional plant-hunters also insist that they can look at a plant and see if it has many or few toxic products.

Native healers knew that curare can harm humans only if it enters the bloodstream, and that it can have considerable medicinal value. It was applied directly to bacterial or fungal infections of the skin, and it was employed as a contraceptive by both sexes. Healers still use it to kill worms and parasites, to help with stomach problems, and to cauterize wounds.

Europeans in the 16th and 17th centuries began to employ some of curare's constituent parts for their own medicine. Among these plants were *Strychnos nux vomica* and ignatius bean. Some of the initial European experiments on curare were a bit crude. In 1838 researchers wounded a donkey in the shoulder and exposed it to curare poison. Ten minutes later, the animal seemed to be dead. They then cut into the donkey's windpipe and used a pair of bellows to keep its lungs working. After two hours the donkey could breathe on its own. Not surprisingly, the researchers reported that, "she looked lean and sickly" for more than a year. From this they concluded that curare somehow stopped its victim's breathing.

In 1844 French physiologist Claude Bernard began experiments with frogs and curare. He found that curare blocked nerve impulses from the brain to the muscles. When their lung muscles were affected, the frogs stopped breathing. Ironically, Bernard supported research with money from his wife, who was active in the antivivisection movement. Allying himself with those who opposed animal experiments, Alfred Lord Tennyson (1809-1892) wrote a poem about a children's doctor so insensitive he could "mangle the living dog that had loved him and fawn'd at his knee—Drench'd with the hellish oorali [curare]."

The chemistry of curare is not yet understood. One of its most lethal ingredients seems to be pareira, whose principal alkaloid, tubocurarine, was isolated from the bark and stems of this woody vine in 1895. No medicinal use was found for it until 1932, when physicians began to use it to treat spastic disorders and symptoms of tetanus, a bacterial infection that causes rigidity and spasms of the voluntary muscles.

Tubocurarine came into modern medicine by way of psychiatry. In the late 1930s doctors who were conducting convulsive therapy—administering chemicals that caused a psychiatric patient to experience strong convulsions—decided to curarize patients so that their muscles would relax and they could absorb stronger shocks. At the time some shock therapy caused convulsions that fractured the spines of more than 40 percent of all patients. Curare acted, in the words of one doctor, as a "shock absorber." Curare derivatives still serve as treatments for spasms associated with tetanus and convulsive therapy.

In the early 1940s tubocurarine's capacity to relax muscles made it a welcome addition to anesthesia. It prevents nerve impulses from activating voluntary muscles, accomplishing this by affecting the actions of acetylcholine, a compound released by the nerves and received at receptor sites on the muscles. Acetylcholine stimulates muscular contractions, so less effective acetylcholine means fewer and weaker contractions.

Tubocurarine is now used as an auxiliary in general anesthesia. It usually allows patients to need less anesthesia and effectively relaxes muscles during throat, rectal, and abdominal surgery, as well as during orthopedic procedures for broken bones.

Shortly after World War II more than 70 curare alkaloids were found. Many were synthesized by the late 1950s. Next came the manipulation of these synthetic compounds to produce medicines with fewer side effects. One such synthetic derivative, metocurine, doubles or triples the effect of tubocurarine in humans.

WILD YAM　　　In the first century B.C., the Roman poet Gaius Valerius Cattulus wrote to his lover Lesbia that he would like to share kisses: "As many as there are grains

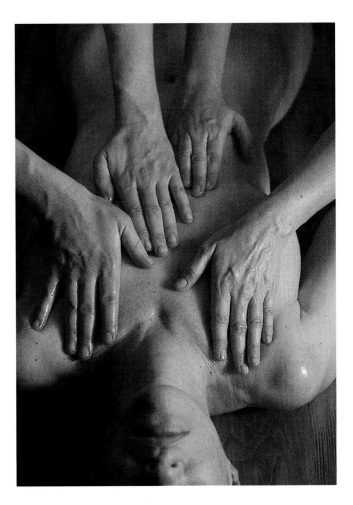

A woman in New York City undergoes a traditional Ayurvedic massage using herbal oils. It is part of a lengthy treatment process called *panchakarma* that cleans, purifies, and balances the mind, body, and spirit. This and other Ayurvedic practices are gaining in popularity throughout the developed world.

of sand on Cyrene's silphium shore." Cyrene was a Greek city on the coast of North Africa in present-day Libya. Its people became wealthy and famous because of silphium, a plant they found growing wild on the area's dry mountainsides when they arrived in the seventh century B.C.

Silphium is today called giant fennel. Ancient people used the sap of silphium roots and stems to treat coughs, but written sources report that it was used throughout the Mediterranean for a more important purpose: birth control.

Numerous attempts to cultivate silphium in other areas failed, and for reasons now lost to history, the plant grew only within a 30-mile area *(Continued on page 212)*

FOLLOWING PAGES: Many Asian cultures revere the lotus as a symbol that beauty and truth can arise from pain and ignorance. Every morning, at the botanical gardens in Singapore, people of all ages practice *tai chi chuan*, an ancient Chinese discipline that combines body movements and mental concentration to promote well-being.

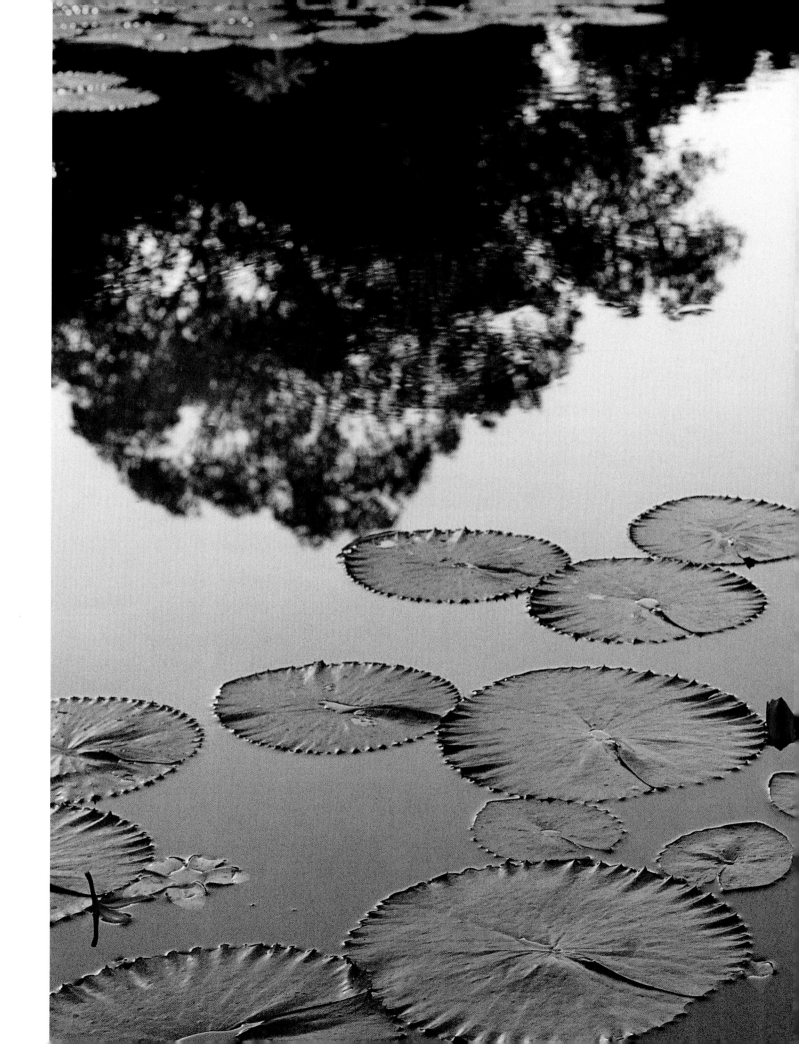

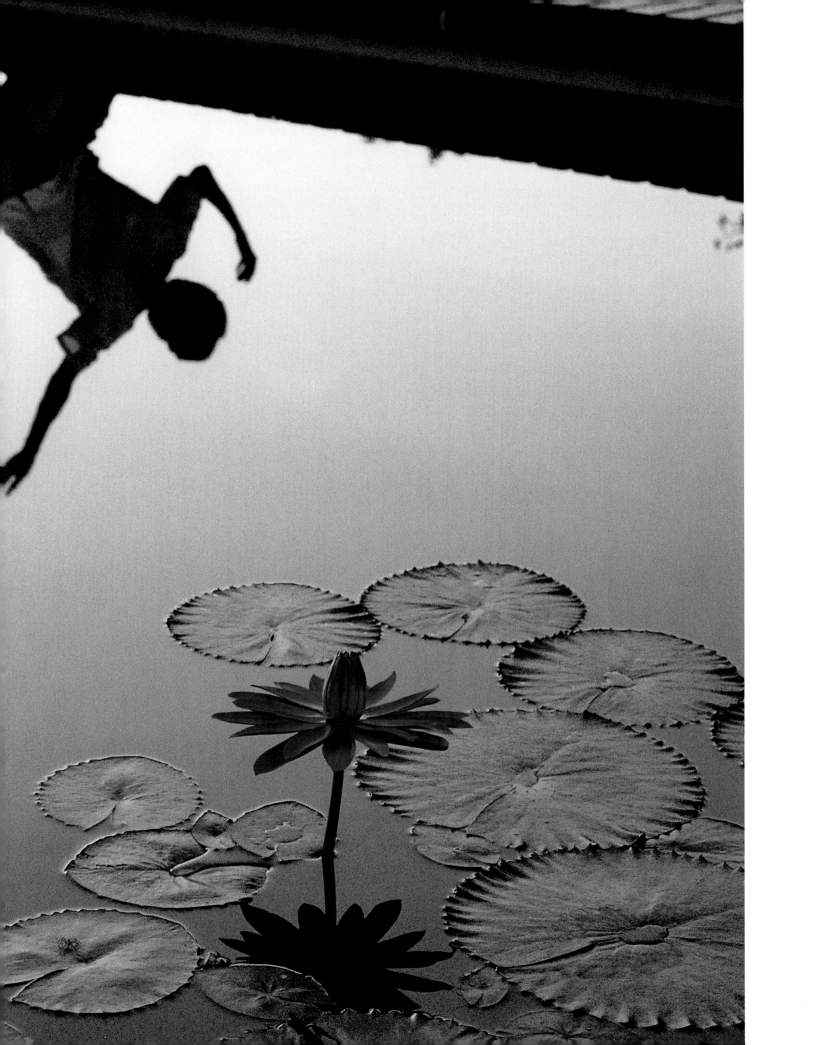

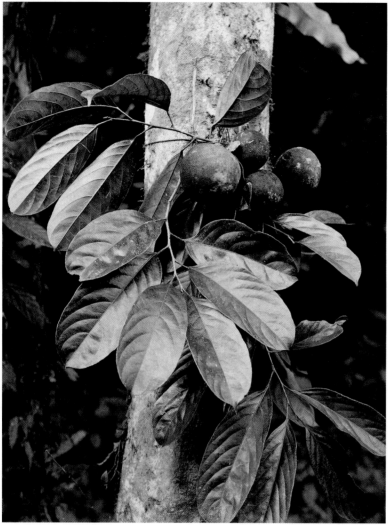

Joseph F. Rock

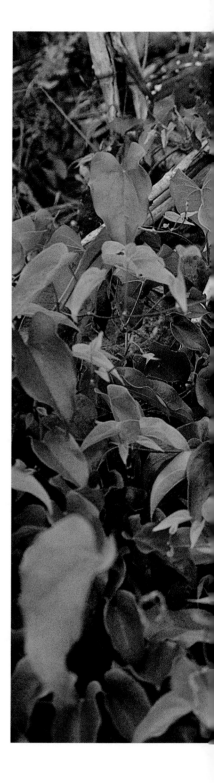

Botanist Joseph F. Rock pinned a fruiting branch to the trunk of a
chaulmoogra tree in a photograph taken about 1920 (above). From its
discovery in the jungles of Southeast Asia thousands of years ago
until the development of modern antibiotics, oil from the seeds of the
chaulmoogra provided the best known treatment for leprosy, which
can be contagious and disfiguring. Lepers often lived in colonies that
cultivated chaulmoogras. A Nigerian plants soybeans to help feed
people at an informal leper colony (right). Before the mid-20th
century, when antibiotics became the most effective treatment for
the disease, the use of chaulmoogra oil caused severe side effects.

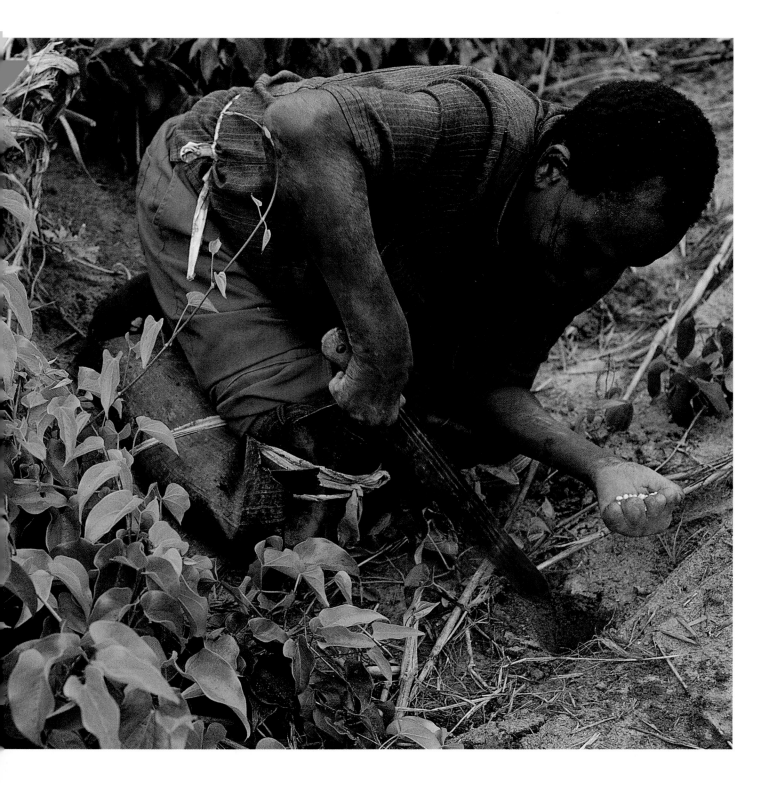

around Cyrene. By the first century A.D., overharvesting had made it scarce, and silphium was worth more than its weight in silver. By the third or fourth century A.D., the plant was extinct.

While silphium cannot be studied, it may have been one of a group of plants that contain ferujol, a chemical that studies have shown to be extremely effective at preventing pregnancy in rats.

Ancient cultures and native tribes used a wide range of plants as contraceptives. Egyptians, for example, employed a combination of acacia gum, dates, honey, and an unidentified plant. Contraceptives used in other countries included components taken from Queen Anne's lace, pennyroyal, artemisia, myrrh, and myrtle, as well as cedar and balsam trees. No one knows with any certainty how well any of these methods worked. Studies demonstrate, however, that many of them have chemicals that block or disrupt other processes that are essential to the beginning and continuation of a pregnancy. Modern analysis shows they could also poison the liver.

For reasons not understood, by the beginning of the Renaissance, doctors and medical texts no longer discussed contraceptives. They had disappeared from the medical literature.

Modern research into plants as sources of contraceptives came in the 1940s, with the study of chemicals in the Mexican wild yam, which grows in the southwestern United States and in northern Mexico. The wild yam is inedible, but traditional healers have used it for a range of purposes, including treatment for cancer, diarrhea, rheumatoid arthritis, colic, and muscle spasms. The yam's principal use, however, is to help with menstrual disorders and with the fatigue, inflammation, and pain associated with menstruation. Native women also use it for birth control.

The roots of the wild yam, researchers discovered, contain large amounts of a chemical called diosgenin. They devised a way to transform this diosgenin into progesterone, a hormone that in humans prepares the uterus to receive and develop a fertilized egg. Modern medicine had understood the role of ovarian hormones such as progesterone since the early 20th century.

Progesterone until that time could be obtained only from human placentas or the ovaries of pregnant sows—and it cost more than 38,000 dollars a pound. With wild yam's contribution, the price of progesterone fell to several dollars a pound, and birth control pills could be mass-produced.

Birth control pills combine the hormone estrogen with progesterone to inhibit the secretion of follicle-stimulating hormone (FSH), a necessary hormone for ovulation to occur. Until the early 1970s manufacturers used wild yam in making birth control pills, but the estrogen and progesterone used in birth control now are synthetic.

————————

CINCHONA   Reliance on the quinine derived from cinchona bark grew throughout the first half of the 20th century. Standard malaria treatment specified daily doses of quinine pills. Many people resisted treatment because of the side effects, which could become so serious that it had to be stopped.

Researchers made extensive efforts to find an alternative to quinine. They tried to derive an antimalarial serum from animals and from people with malaria. All those tested failed to provide any benefit. Mepacrine and amodiaqine, synthetics derived from coal tar, showed action against malaria, but many people were allergic to them. The Western world remained dependent on cinchona trees grown in Dutch-controlled Java, now part of Indonesia. The capture of Java by the Japanese in early 1942, shortly after World War II began in the Pacific, robbed the Allies of antimalarial medicine. This triggered the rationing of quinine, as well as increased efforts to develop man-made forms of the drug. Research efforts resulted in the introduction of the synthetic antimalarial drug chloroquine during the war. When it was over, the Allies learned that German had created the same drug as early as 1934.

Scientists are still not exactly sure how chloroquine kills the protozoan parasite that causes malaria. Like other synthetic drugs that followed, it seems to pursue the same principle as quinine. All seem to raise the acidic level within the parasite, thus interfering with its interaction with human hemoglobin and causing it to suffer structural abnormalities.

After World War II proguanil, pyrimethamine, and other synthetic drugs came into use. In the 1950s strongly drug-resistant malaria was becoming more prevalent. Drug-resistant parasites were often associated with cerebral malaria, the most serious and most frequently fatal strain of the disease. Doctors began to use quinine again because parasites were less resistant to it than some other drugs, as well as mefloquine and other new synthetic drugs.

Resistance to antimalarial drugs, however, continues to increase. Malaria has been resurging even in such remote areas as the mountainous regions of Peru and Ecuador, where cinchona bark first came to the attention of Europeans. Today, malaria affects at least 300 million of the world's 6.1 billion people and kills more than a million every year. Most of the victims live in poor countries, but global warming has brought the spread of disease-carrying mosquitoes into areas that have been malaria-free for generations. In the 1990s Texas, Florida, and even New York City had cases of malaria carried not by travelers returning from the tropics but by local mosquitoes.

Rapidly spreading resistance has raised the possibility that malaria-infested areas where the disease resists every known drug may become a growing international problem. Already, such zones may be emerging in western Thailand at its border with Burma and to the east, where it shares jungles with Cambodia. Parasitic resistance has triggered investment in plant-based antimalarial drugs. Much of the investment has come from the U.S. Army, which wants to ensure that its soldiers can operate safely and effectively everywhere. The only new drug so far has come from China.

Chinese pharmaceutical books dating to about A.D. 340 mention a malaria remedy named *qinghao* that fought fevers. Its principal ingredient was one of the *Artemisia*, a genus of about 180 species of plants now known to grow throughout the world, including the sagebrush that covers large areas of the North American plains. The plant usually tastes bitter, so animals do not eat it. *Artemisia* is named after the Greek goddess Artemis, who was associated in mythology with wild animals, the hunt, vegetation, chastity, and childbirth. Its common name in Europe, where it has been used to treat intestinal worms and various liver and kidney problems, is wormwood. It also was used, until the 1920s in the preparation of absinthe, an alcoholic beverage.

Chinese healers use artemisia plants to treat, among other things, faintness, headache, rheumatism, leukemia, dysentery, jaundice, tuberculosis, and fevers.

During the Chinese Cultural Revolution of the 1960s and early 1970s, dictator Mao Zedong was eager to widen the split between his country and the West. As part of this effort, he ordered that researchers thoroughly examine Chinese traditional medicine to find plants that could serve as the basis for modern drugs. Chinese researchers discovered that qinghao can be effective against malaria, and in 1972 they isolated *qinghaosu*, or artemisinin, its active principle.

Artemisinin and its derivatives, whose mode of antiparasitic action seems to be generally the same as quinine's, have demonstrated effectiveness against malarial strains resistant to chloroquine and other pharmaceutical drugs. In one test of Bangkok patients with severe, drug-resistant malaria, of 50 treated with quinine 18 died; of 47 treated with artemesia-based drugs 6 died. At least 70 other species of *Artemisia* have failed to yield evidence of antimalarial activity.

GOAT'S RUE   Diabetes is a disorder in the metabolization of carbohydrates and is caused by having either insufficient insulin, the hormone that regulates the burning of blood sugar—glucose—or by having insulin that does not work well. Insulin is produced by the pancreas. Diabetics accumulate too much insulin and too much glucose in their blood.

Descriptions of diabetes go back to Chinese, Indian, and Egyptian texts that are at least 2,000 years old. Sanskrit manuscripts talk about a disease of "honey-tasting urine," and Galen likened fluid passing through a diabetic person to the condition of the bowel during diarrhea.

Two types of diabetes have been identified. In diabetes I, the pancreas does not produce enough insulin. Before the 1920s, when scientists discovered the existence of insulin and developed ways to inject cow- and pig-generated insulin into humans, a diagnosis of diabetes I often meant death would soon occur. Insulin injections are required because the stomach would break down any insulin taken orally. Human insulin, made via recombinant DNA technology—the splicing together of DNA fragments from several different species—replaced animal-based insulin in the 1980s.

In diabetes II, non-insulin-dependent diabetes, the production of insulin is sluggish. This condition may be treated by exercise, changes in diet, and oral drugs that lower the levels of blood sugar. Oral medicines work in various ways, including decreasing the release of glucose that is stored in the liver, stimulating the pancreas to produce more insulin, and increasing the use of glucose. Many of these drugs cause negative side effects, however, such as extreme fatigue.

Traditional medicines have used approximately one thousand plants to help treat diabetes II and its symptoms. These include garlic, onions, turmeric, cloves, and cinnamon. In the body they can act like insulin and affect the burning of glucose. No plant, however, has provided any indication that it could serve as a substitute for insulin, and only one—goat's rue—has affected the development of a modern pharmaceutical drug used in treating diabetes II.

Goat's rue, usually considered a weed, is a legume with a leafy stalk and white or purplish flower. Traditional medicine uses it to make people sweat, and to treat fevers, plague, intestinal worms, and snakebites. In the 1870s French scientists documented that cows eating goat's rue produced more milk.

Research has isolated numerous alkaloids, glycosides, and other active elements from goat's rue. In the late 1920s French scientists realized that guanidine—one of the alkaloids in goat's rue—lowers blood sugar. Although it is too toxic for human use, in the late 1950s two pharmaceutical drugs based on a synthetic modification of guanidine were on the market in France. The drugs reduce the glucose stored in the liver; they also

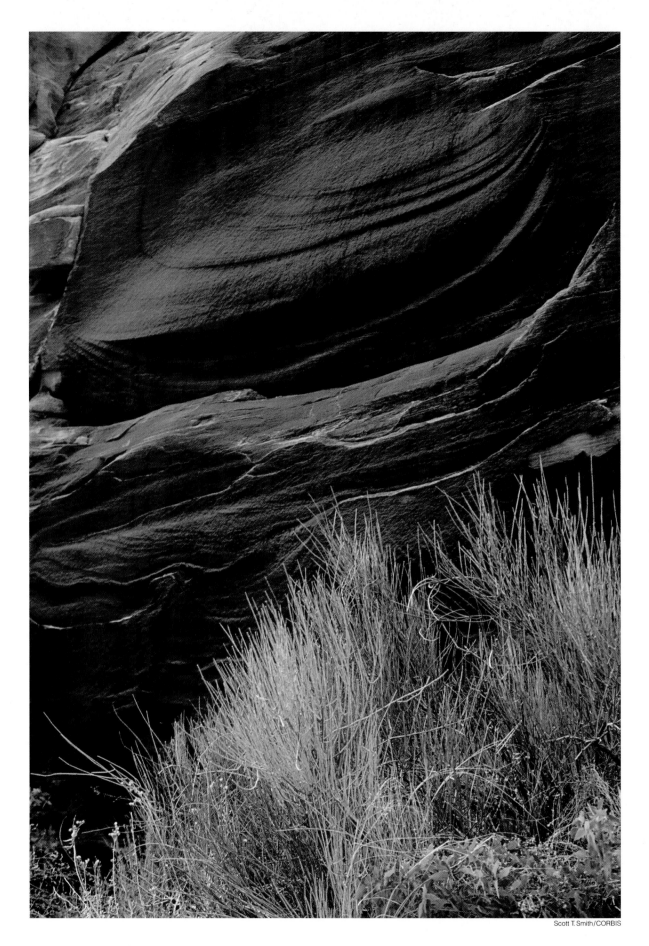

Scott T. Smith/CORBIS

216

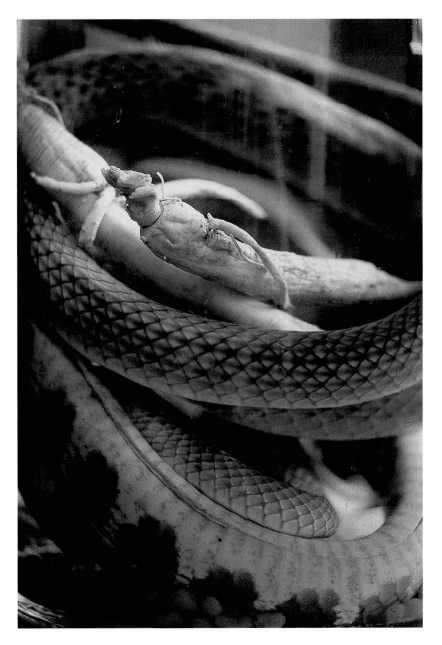

Ephedra, which has led to the development of several major modern pharmaceutical drugs that treat bronchial and respiratory problems, grows wild in Utah's canyon country (opposite). Many people use this plant as a ground cover or in rock gardens. Snake, ginseng, and other ingredients of an ancient Chinese health-promoting potion remain on display in a museum in Beijing, China (above). Such combinations of plant and animal material, not uncommon in the Asian pharmacopoeia, make it difficult for modern science to document remedies' effects.

reduce the intestine's absorption of glucose. In 1995 the FDA approved one of the synthetics for sale in the United States.

————

ROSY PERIWINKLE   The pink flowers of the Madagascar rosy periwinkle are often on posters for "save the rain forest" educational and fund-raising campaigns. Pictures of the plant pop out of mass mailings along with letters filled with arguments about how we must not destroy the Earth's biodiversity. Scientists at scholarly conferences discuss its virtues.

Such attention is deserved. Drugs made from the periwinkle help cure most cases of acute lymphocytic leukemia and Hodgkin's disease and treat testicular cancer.

This success has generated mythological tales about the wisdom and generosity of traditional healers. A 1996 book on alternative medicine, for example, praises the "spirit and expertise" of the shaman from Madagascar who—although never acknowledged or compensated— "revealed" the rosy periwinkle's usefulness. The true story is far more complicated.

In Madagascar traditional healers use the rosy periwinkle to treat a huge range of ailments. Throughout the island the plant is conspicuous in markets and gardens and along roadways. Although it is native to Madagascar, the rosy periwinkle's beauty has prompted people to transplant it throughout the world. In warmer climates it flowers most of the year. It requires sunlight, but is hardy. Wherever it grows, people develop their own medicinal uses for it. By the early 20th century healers in Brazil prescribed it to control hemorrhages and scurvy and to heal chronic wounds; in the British West Indies it helped treat diabetic ulcers; and in southern Europe, the Philippines, and South Africa it was an oral hypoglycemic, an agent that lowers blood sugar. In England during the 1920s, pharmacies sold a diabetic treatment called Vin-q-lin made from rosy periwinkle. In the early 1950s a team of Canadian medical researchers with a special interest in the use of plants by what they called "primitive people" received a letter from a patient who was visiting Jamaica. She told them that local people made a tea from a plant known as the Madagascar periwinkle, and that this tea helped with what they called blood problems. These tea drinkers were people with diabetes who could not afford insulin treatment.

The Canadian woman enclosed with her letter some leaves from the plant, as well as the endorsement of a Canadian doctor practicing in Jamaica who felt that the herbal tea helped his diabetic patients. After their tests of the leaves showed positive results, the researchers in Canada sent two colleagues to Jamaica.

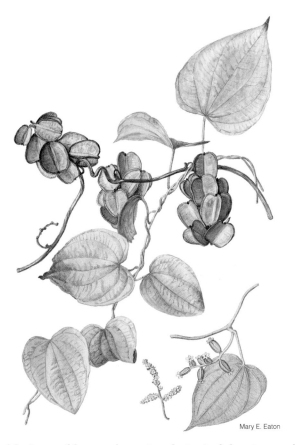

Mary E. Eaton

Native women use the Mexican wild yam, shown in a botanical drawing made before the advent of color photography, for menstrual problems and as a contraceptive. The plant contains chemicals that contributed to the development of modern birth control pills. Traditional cultures have used a wide range of plants as contraceptives.

The Canadian doctors examined diabetic patients who were drinking periwinkle tea but taking no insulin. The patients seemed fine. Skeptical about the power of periwinkle, the researchers at first thought that they had encountered a previously unidentified type of diabetes. In their judgment the patients should have been dead because they were not taking insulin.

Back in Canada the researchers tried the periwinkle tea on a few patients who volunteered and could find no significant impact. They then ground up the entire plant, soaked it in alcohol, and injected it into laboratory rats. The rats' white cell counts plummeted. The scientists made an extract of the plant and injected it into more laboratory rats. Three days later all the rats were dead. Weakening the extract by diluting it, the researchers injected it into a new group of rats. Three days later all these rats were dead, too. Diluting the extract once again before injecting it led to the same result.

The researchers cut open the dead rats and tested to see what had killed them. No poison from the plant was at fault. The rats had all died of a particular bacterial infection that was common to the feces of laboratory animals. This finding indicated that their white cells, which normally combat such bacteria, were not acting effectively. After injecting a new group of rats with the periwinkle extract, the researchers checked the rats' white cell count. It was again down significantly.

The next step was logical. The periwinkle was killing white blood cells. What disease generates too many white cells and calls for a medicine to kill them? Leukemia.

The researchers introduced leukemia into rats, then injected them with the plant extract and watched to see what would happen. The periwinkle extract showed some antileukemic action, but work proceeded slowly because the researchers focused most of their efforts on other projects. To understand the periwinkle was a slow and costly process. More than a year of looking was required before the scientists isolated the active alkaloid that cut the rats' white cell count. It was a novel structure that had been encountered nowhere else.

Obtaining an adequate supply of rosy periwinkle was a constant problem. The doctor in Jamaica continued to send dried leaves. When drought in Jamaica created difficulties, the researchers tried to grow periwinkle in southern Ontario. It died every winter. Plants grown in the northern climate, furthermore, produced fewer alkaloids.

In 1958 the Canadians published a paper, "Role Of Chance Observation In Chemotherapy: *Vinca Rosea*." Scientists at an American pharmaceutical company noticed this paper at an academic conference. These American scientists knew that during World War II people in the Philippines had used rosy periwinkle when insulin became unavailable. This had prompted the Americans to look at rosy periwinkle as a diabetes treatment. Like the Canadian researchers, they had failed to substantiate the plant's hypoglycemic claims and had noted the plant's antitumor qualities.

In 1959, after licensing use of the alkaloid—called vinblastine—from the Canadians, the American pharmaceutical company began clinical trials. The drug received approval from the Food and Drug Administration in 1961, and in 1963 the company received permission to sell drugs based on vincristine, another alkaloid from the periwinkle.

These alkaloids are highly toxic and have harsh side effects. To be tolerated and effective they must be given along with a careful regime of other drugs. But the treatment resulted in high cure rates for some of the most fearsome cancers.

A difference in only one element accounts for the distinction between these two periwinkle alkaloids. Vinblastine has methyl, and vincristine contains formyl. Although the periwinkle plant has a thousand times more vincristine than vinblastine, obtaining a supply of either alkaloid remained difficult. Fifteen tons of dried leaves were required to produce one ounce of vinblastine.

Both alkaloids are too complicated to synthesize economically, but periwinkle plants with a high yield in alkaloids can be cultivated. For several decades vincristine and vinblastine sold in the United States came from periwinkles grown in Texas. Now they come from plants grown in India that have a higher alkaloid content.

Why do vincristine and vinblastine work on one kind of leukemia and not another? Why on Hodgkin's disease and testicular cancer, and not on other cancers?

All cancers are basically the same. What makes them different is the type of cells that become cancerous and the reasons these cells grow uncontrollably. There is to date no explanation for why a plant alkaloid—or a synthetic chemical—works better on one type of cancer than another.

Other chemotherapeutic drugs, which are mostly derived from chemicals, kill cancer cells by interfering with their DNA or by directly disrupting the process by which they multiply. Vinblastine and vincristine work in a way that differs from all of them. These two plant alkaloids are antimicrotubules. They destroy elements that give structure to the cancer cells. This, in turn, keeps the cancer cells from multiplying. The process by which the two plant alkaloids work is so complex that no synthetic anti-microtubules exist.

PACIFIC YEW Ancient Greeks and Romans used the sap of the yew tree as a deadly poison. In his war memoirs Julius Caesar notes that Cativolcus, a chief of the Gauls, killed himself by drinking yew-bark tea. Pliny, a first century Roman writer, called it a "cursed tree" that is "unpleasant and fearful to look upon...." A few decades later Greek historian Plutarch warned that if you fall asleep under its shade, you will die. The witches' brew in William Shakespeare's *Macbeth* contains "gall of goat, and slips of yew sliver'd in the moon's eclipse."

In Britain yews were planted in graveyards: According to a folktale, yew roots grow around the throats of the dead, so yew branches would whisper their secrets. In the mid-20th century, poet T. S. Eliot wrote about wind that shakes "a thousand whispers from the yew."

Various species of yew range across the Northern Hemisphere. The tree is usually found in moist, dark areas and can grow more than 80 feet tall. Its needlelike leaves stay on the yew tree no matter how cold or windy the weather. When a branch breaks off and falls to the ground, it can sprout a new tree.

Chinese healers use yew to treat arthritis; people in India employ it against rheumatism; and the Japanese treat diabetes and induce abortions with it. Native Americans of the Pacific Northwest use it as a disinfectant and as a treatment for tuberculosis, digestive problems, and skin cancer.

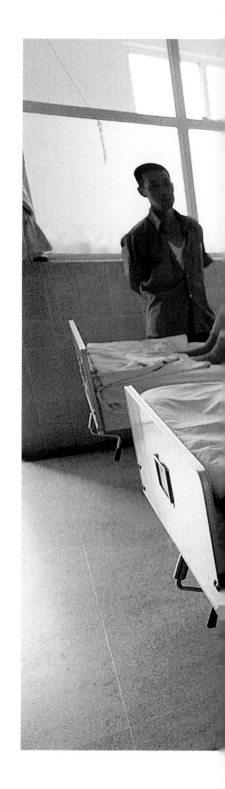

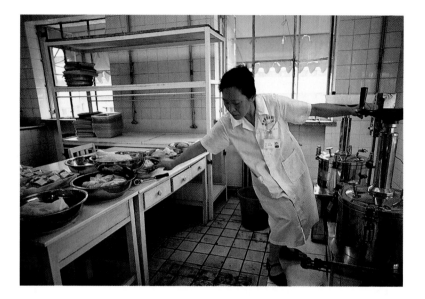

In the Xi Yuan Traditional Chinese Medicine Hospital in Beijing, China, a worker prepares individualized herbal treatments for patients (above). Combined in the hospital pharmacy, the complicated herbal recipes are then steamed in large pressure vats. The oncology ward of the hospital fights cancer four ways. One patient takes Western-style chemotherapy while the pads on her legs deliver sound therapy. She combines these with special nutritional supplements—she is drinking a cup of watermelon juice—and herbal remedies.

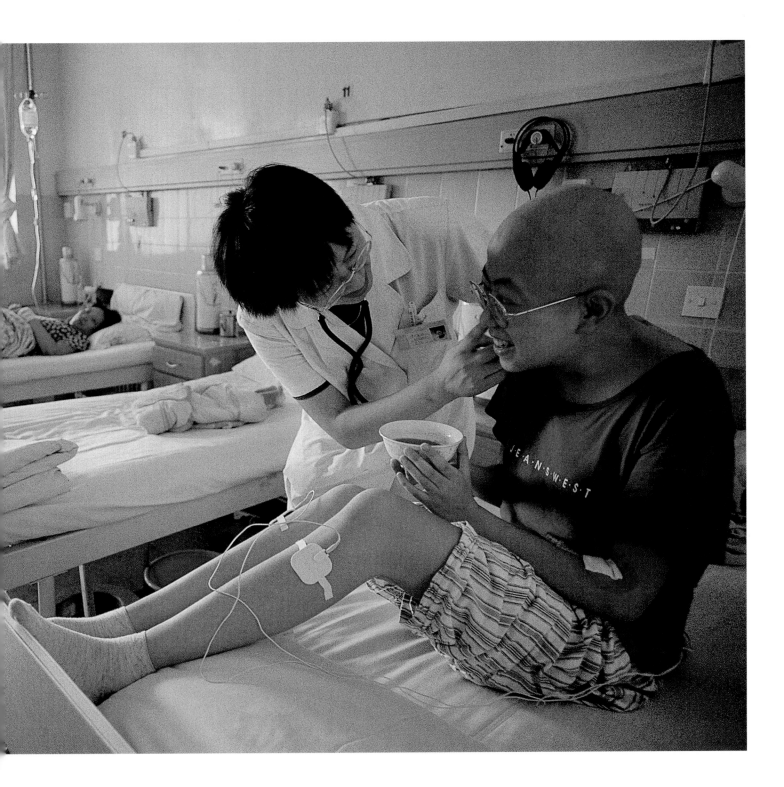

Traditional uses of the yew played no role in its development as the source of a modern medicine. Nor did its unique qualities. In the late 1950s and 1960s the National Cancer Institute began to collect samples of natural products from all over the world. In 1962, as part of this effort, a 22-year-old part-time U.S. government worker collected samples at random from forests in the Northwest. Red, berrylike seeds hanging from a branch of what looked like a creeping shrub caught his attention. Red seemed out of place amid the thick forest greens and browns. He took some berries, twigs, roots, and bark.

The red seeds belonged to the Pacific yew, which foresters and loggers treated as a trash tree. Logging companies sometimes sold it as fence posts, but they regarded it mostly as a nuisance. They burned yews to gain better access to spruce and fir trees.

Tests revealed that the Pacific yew seeds and the fleshy fruits surrounding them contained taxines, deadly alkaloid poisons. The bark, researchers discovered, has even stronger poisons that show greater anticancer activity. By the late 1960s researchers had isolated the responsible alkaloid, paclitaxel. (Its more common name, Taxol, has been trademarked.) But alkaloids from other natural products were more promising, and yew findings were filed away.

In 1979 researchers discovered that paclitaxel works against cancer because it binds to a cancer cell's microtubules, part of the cell's skeletal structure, and keeps it from dismantling. Microtubules must disintegrate for the cell to divide, so paclitaxel, in effect, freezes the cancer cell in place until it dies. No other known substance did. The action was so unusual that researchers at first thought that their sample had been contaminated. Since then researchers have discovered other substances, natural and synthetic, that work the same way.

Paclitaxel has proved effective against ovarian and advanced breast cancers, malignant melanoma, and small-cell lung cancers. It became available for clinical use in the early 1980s, about 20 years after the young government employee first put it in his collection bag. After paclitaxel received FDA approval in 1992, supply became a major problem. Logging the yew was difficult. Its usual growth pattern is scattered, and forests were sometimes closed due to fire danger. A Pacific yew tree grows slowly, and each tree yields about ten pounds of bark. Collecting bark, furthermore, can kill the tree. A 1991 study estimated that it would take 625,000 pounds of dried bark from 62,480 trees, yielding 55 pounds of pure paclitaxel, to treat 12,000 patients—the number of American women who died from ovarian cancer each year. That comes to three trees per person. Another study estimated that it would take six trees to treat one patient.

Attempts to harvest paclitaxel-like compounds from a fungus that grows on Pacific yew trees, and from the needles of related species of yews—all yews produce paclitaxel—did not yield enough of the necessary alkaloid. Expeditions to collect rare species of yews also generated nothing useful.

Paclitaxel is too complex to be synthesized in the necessary quantities. One factor contributing to this complexity is that yews belong to the Taxaceae, a family of plants that has survived since the early Jurassic, nearly 200 million years ago. To help survive that long, they have devised some complicated chemicals. As one indication of such age-related complexity, cycads, which have survived even longer, produce some of the strangest and most bioactive compounds yet discovered. Some of these compounds induce liver and colon cancer in humans. Others have been linked to neurological disorders such as Guam dementia, a neurodegenerative disease that people in the western Pacific may get from eating *fadang*—a food that is made from cycad cones and looks like thick corn chips.

Paclitaxel and other related cancer-killing substances are now produced by chemical manipulation of a compound taken from Pacific yew needles, thus not harming the tree.

————

ALTHOUGH THE ABOVE STORIES are typical, other less famous plant-based drugs have been developed during the 20th century. Mayapple, a white flowering plant indigenous to northeast North America, has yielded semisynthetic drugs called etoposide and teniposide. Ouabain from squill, the dried bulb of the sea onion, is used, like digitalis, as a heart stimulant. An enzyme from the papaya, chymopapain, helps shrink or dissolve ruptured discs. Quinidine, derived from quinine, helps control irregular heartbeats. Pilocarpine, from South American shrubs of the genus *Pilocarpus*, is a topical treatment for glaucoma. Similar treatments for glaucoma come from the alkaloid muscarine found in the *Amanita muscaria* mushroom and the alkaloid arecoline from the betel nut. Calabar beans yield the alkaloid physostigmine, which led to a drug that also treats glaucoma. Capsaicin, derived from cayenne, is used to treat pain caused by arthritis and by herpes zoster infections. Drugs based on the alkaloids caffeine, theophylline, and theobromine—and found in coffee, tea, kola, and numerous other plants—can help treat a wide range of conditions that involve smooth muscles, the central nervous system, cardiac muscles, and the kidney. They are sometimes helpful in cases of asthma and in stimulating preterm infants who have stopped breathing.

The discovery of such plant-based drugs in the 19th *(Continued on page 230)*

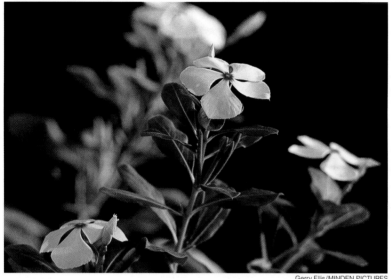

Time together remains especially precious for Audra Shapiro and her mother, Mara Bershad, as they share a hug outside their home in Chevy Chase, Maryland (right). The Madagascar rosy periwinkle plant (above) contains a chemical called vinblastine, which was central to the chemotherapy that cured nine-year-old Audra of leukemia. She endured more than two years of treatment that often kept her out of school, but without vinblastine her illness probably would have been fatal. A talented musician and singer, Audra now appears often with professional companies and has represented the United States at an international children's music festival in Finland.

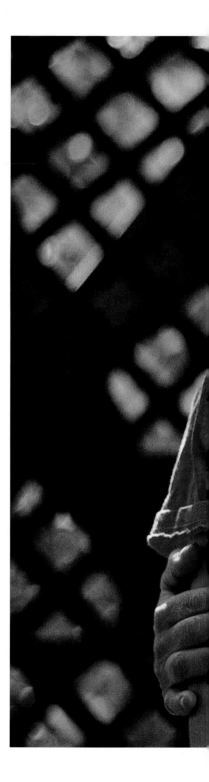

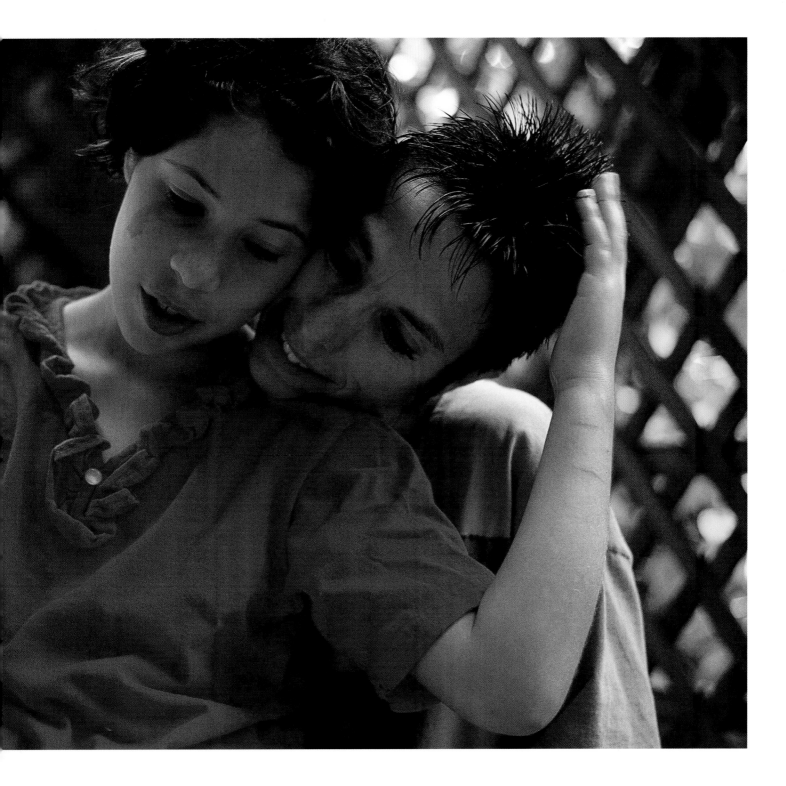

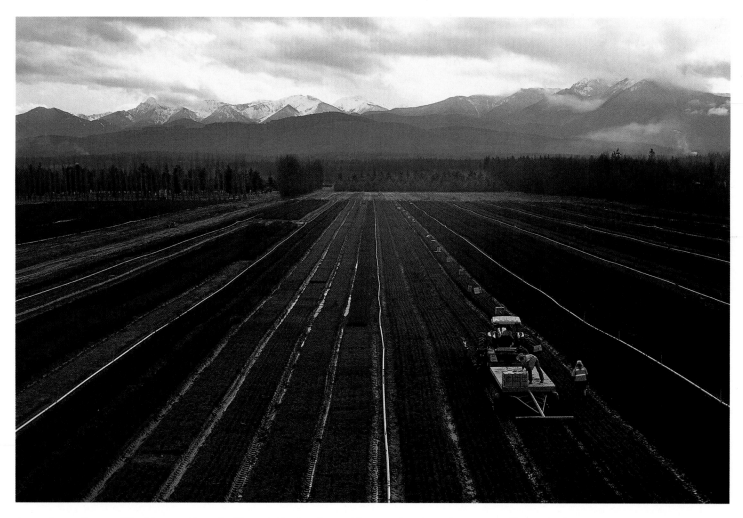

At a plantation on Washington State's Olympic Peninsula, employees plant Pacific yew seedlings. A chemical in these trees kills cancer cells by binding to their skeletal structure. The yews will contribute to the production of the chemical paclitaxel—trademarked as Taxol—which has proved effective against ovarian cancer, advanced breast cancer, and malignant melanoma.

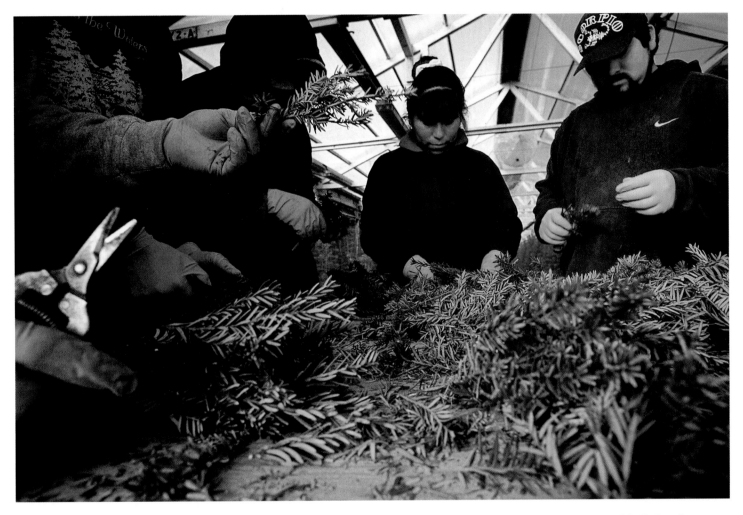

Workers trim Pacific yew branches before shipping them to a pharmaceutical company for further processing. Of all the plants native to North America only a few, such as the Pacific yew, have yielded modern drugs.

and 20th centuries shared many of the same dynamics. Hard work, luck, and perseverance were crucial; the discovery and development of any of these drugs was not inevitable. The flow of knowledge, from traditional societies to science and within the scientific community itself, was often rough. All types of plant parts were involved, and some medicines came from groups of plants as opposed to one specific plant. Plants that yielded medicines came from a wide range of cultures and geographic areas.

Significant changes, however, did occur between the 19th and 20th centuries. With exceptions such as scientists seeking antimalarial drugs, researchers no longer had direct contact with people actually taking plants as medicine. Reflecting changes in what society would allow, 20th-century scientists also conducted fewer experiments on human subjects. Finally, increasingly sophisticated science and technology in the 20th century brought experimentation at the cellular and the subcellular levels. Largely because of the great investment in equipment required, this work was conducted by teams of researchers and funded by large organizations—in contrast to the 19th-century scientists who usually worked alone in their laboratories. Advances in science and technology also contributed to the most dramatic change: more emphasis, at an earlier stage, on developing synthetic versions of natural substances. These drugs used chemicals derived from a plant, or they used a chemical formula taken from a plant. In either case, the drugs transformed a plant-based medicine into something beyond what nature had created.

Plant-based drugs discovered in the 19th and 20th centuries raise five interrelated questions that are important for today's use of medicinal plants both as pharmaceutical drugs and as herbal remedies (see Chapters 7 and 8).

(1) How useful is traditional knowledge?

All plant-based drugs discovered and developed in the 19th century relied on traditional uses of the plants. This mostly held true in the 20th century, when only one major drug—paclitaxel derived from the Pacific yew—was found without the use of traditional knowledge. But when paclitaxel became famous, some native tribes in the Pacific Northwest began to complain that it had been taken from them. Their healers had been using the yew, they said, for hundreds and perhaps thousands of years to treat, among other things, cancer. This claim may have been true, but had it nothing to do with the discovery of the new drug.

Such claims probably could be made about any drug derived from plants. For virtually any plant, there is a traditional society somewhere that uses it for a range of medicinal purposes.

Traditional societies often have difficulty documenting their claims because most did not have a system of writing until outsiders—whether Europeans, Chinese, or Arab traders—arrived. The traditional societies accumulated knowledge about medicinal plants and passed it orally from one generation to the next. To them, plants and knowledge were gifts from the gods, even though village healers may have guarded this information to protect their livelihoods or positions of power. In the stories cited above, traditional people resisted sharing their knowledge only in the case of curare, which they used as a weapon. Today, in an era concerned about ownership, profits, and what is called biopiracy, drug discovery will be able to rely less and less upon such openness (see Chapter 7).

(2) What are the advantages and disadvantages of pursuing the single active compound or molecule?

This search is at the core of pharmaceutical drugs based on plants. With the exception of chaulmoogra oil, which was replaced by an antibiotic, plants in each of the preceding instances yielded an active compound that, in turn, formed the basis for the modern medicine.

Relying on the single active compound can have definite disadvantages. In a process straight out of Charles Darwin's theory of evolution, disease-causing organisms have proved adept at resisting drugs based on one active element. Quinine, for example, kills a huge percentage of malaria-causing parasites. But those parasites it does not kill become increasingly plentiful as other parasites die. Such resistance has become a major issue in medicine, most notably with microbes that develop resistance to antibiotics.

Side effects are another major variable. In some cases it is impossible to know whether use of the single active compound generates side effects that are harsher than those that would come from a whole plant or plant part. Rosy periwinkle and the Pacific yew, for example, yield highly toxic drugs that can be extremely harsh. Yet these drugs achieve something—killing cancer—that the periwinkle and the yew are unable to offer without the intervention of modern science. There seems to be the trade-off: more punishing side effects in exchange for a benefit otherwise unattainable.

An additional advantage of isolating the single active compound is that it can make it much easier for people to absorb enough plant chemicals to get a therapeutic effect. To take enough willow bark to achieve the benefits aspirin provides or to take enough foxglove to achieve the full lifesaving effects of digitalis is much more easily accomplished via a pill than by eating natural substances. To ingest other plants, such as the

Mexican wild yam, in sufficient amounts to achieve a therapeutic effect might be physically impossible, especially on a regular basis.

Using the single active compound, however, means losing whatever medical power may be embodied in the plant parts, or whole plants, or multi-plant medicines. It also defines medicines as a weapon against disease, diverting attention from the use of plants to maintain health and prevent disease (see Chapter 8).

The lost opportunities, and enticing possibilities, for finding new plant-based medicines seem endless. Each plant discussed above has dozens of bioactive compounds that modern medicine ignores. Many of these compounds offer promising leads that are yet to be successfully pursued. Tea made from rosy periwinkle, for example, does seem to have helped people with diabetes. Yet the periwinkle plant is not used today as a modern medicine to treat diabetes.

If such significant drugs can come from one active agent in each plant discussed in Chapters 4 and 6, how many extraordinary drugs could come from combining two or three compounds? What about modifying those two or three to produce even better drugs? We cannot, or do not, pursue the answers to such questions for many reasons. Prime among them are the limitations of our technology, the methods we use to document the safety and efficacy of drugs, and the economic structures we have imposed on drug development (see Chapters 7 and 8).

The wildflower valerian provides a typical example of what modern medicine misses. For uncounted centuries people in China and India have used a wildflower from a related species—not an isolated active ingredient, but extracts from the flower itself—as a sedative and to combat, among other things, muscle spasms, leprosy, hysteria, eye disease, itches, boils, heart palpitations, bruises, and sores. Galen specified the use of valerian as a sedative. Medieval Europeans used it against pestilence, coughs, shortness of breath, sores, and menstrual and vision problems. Medical authorities during both World War I and II used it to treat shell shock: "Given in hysterical and neurotic conditions as a sedative," medical instructions in 1941 dictated.

Much of valerian's effects come from its volatile oils, which generate a distinctive smell. This has contributed to romantic myths. A young woman with a small branch of valerian always has enthusiastic lovers, according to one folk belief.

In the early 19th century, scientists began to investigate valerian's chemical composition. They made little progress for a hundred years, but by the mid-20th century dozens of terpenoids and other bioactive compounds had been identified. Since then much information about their structure, and the processes that give valerian its volatile

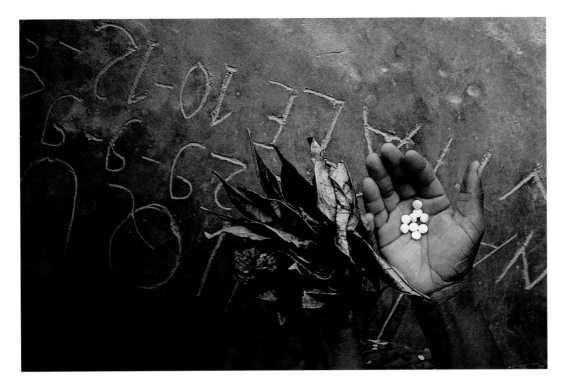

Pills or Plants—Western medicines or traditional herbs? A clinic in remote Manongarivo, Madagascar offers both. The concrete cornerstone of the building bears proud inscriptions from the innovative doctors and traditional healers who founded it.

oils, has been accumulated. Researchers have also documented how valerian affects glucose consumption in various parts of the brain.

None of this, however, has led to development of a drug with anything near the medical strength of valerian itself—which people continue to take as an herb and not as a modern pharmaceutical drug (see Chapter 8) because it relaxes smooth muscles, acts as a sedative and antidepressant, and induces sleep.

No one knows why isolation of active elements within valerian has been a medicinal dead end. Maybe plants whose active compounds do yield drugs are the rare exceptions. Or maybe the failure to develop a valerian-based pharmaceutical drug reflects something about valerian itself. A possible clue is that its bioactive compounds are far more unstable and decompose far more easily than those in most plants. Once isolated from each other, these compounds may therefore lose their pharmacological potency.

(3) Is it necessary to know how a drug actually works in order to combat a particular disease?

Only recently, probably since the 1950s, have scientists known enough about the workings of medicine and the workings of the human body to benefit from that knowledge in the development of drugs. Such knowledge is increasingly important to modern drug development because it allows researchers to focus on chemical processes within the human body that they know to be associated with disease (see Chapter 7). But does it limit our ability to benefit from plant-produced chemicals?

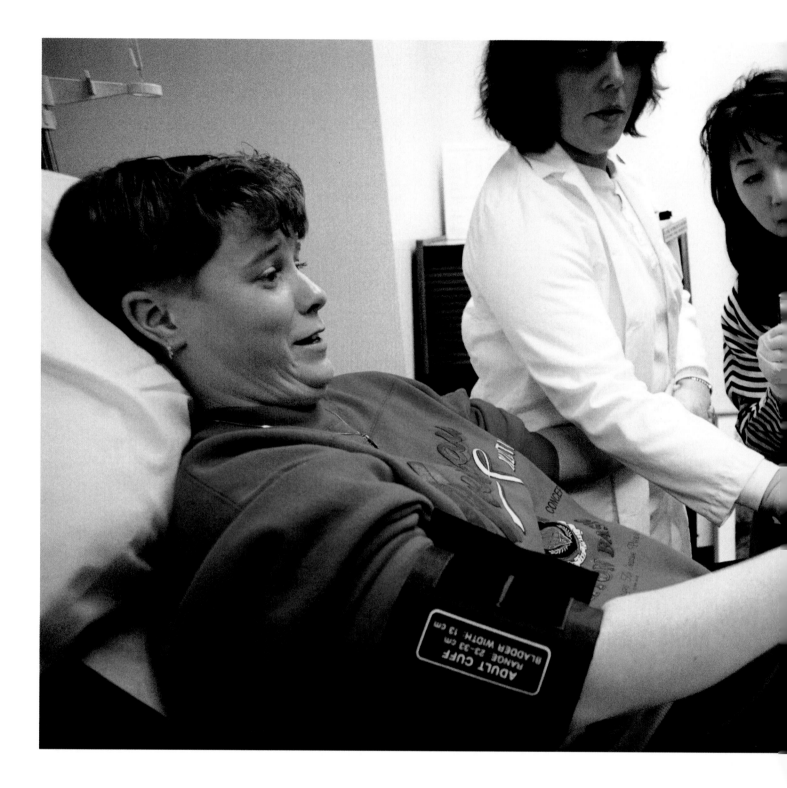

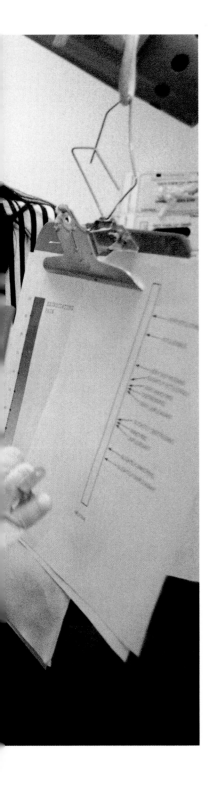

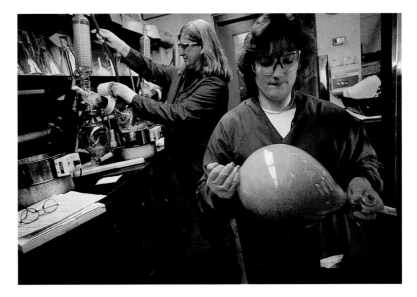

At the National Institutes of Health in Bethesda, Maryland, researchers test the power of capsaicin, a chemical derived from red pepper (left); a volunteer subject charts the extent of her discomfort. Modern doctors often prescribe capsaicin to treat pain caused by herpes zoster infections (also know as shingles) and by arthritis. Traditional cultures use different types of peppers to treat arthritis, colic, skin inflammation due to exposure to cold, and other ailments. "Grind and find" is a motto of workers at the Natural Products Division of the National Cancer Institute (above). Natural substances from across the globe yield thousands of bioactive agents. Often the journey from laboratory to drug has proved difficult, and very few products have become modern drugs.

Traditional medicine has not known, and has not seemed concerned about, the mechanics of how a plant works within the body. For thousands of years books on herbal medicine have not mentioned this topic. They have been concerned with the preparation of drugs, and with the drugs' effects—not with the hows and whys of what happens because of them.

All the stories cited in this chapter prove that it is possible to discover and develop significant drugs based only on the knowledge of effects. In this regard it is noteworthy that the drugs discussed in Chapters 4 and 6 have a documented and powerful impact on almost all of the human body's basic systems. Examples include the nervous system (opium, coca, Indian snakeroot) and circulatory (digitalis), respiratory (ephedra), reproductive (wild yam), musculoskeletal (pareira), endocrine (goat's rue), urinary (digitalis), and digestive (ipecac, papaya). Some plant-based drugs, like those that yield the salicylic acid found in aspirin, seem to work upon several systems.

The only human body system unaffected by any current pharmaceutical plant-based drug is the immune system. Logically a close link should exist between alkaloids and other secondary metabolites, which play a defensive role in plants, and the human immune system, whose prime purpose is also defensive. Plants do affect the human immune system (see Chapter 8), but scientists are still developing the sophisticated technologies and techniques necessary to distinguish and measure these effects.

(4) Is natural or synthetic better?

With few exceptions, such as digitalis, vincristine, and vinblastine, all the drugs discussed in Chapters 4 and 6 have been synthesized. There is no known difference between how natural and synthetic drugs work in the body. Both are made from the same elements combined in the same manner. Synthetic paclitaxel and paclitaxel derived directly from a Pacific yew tree have the same effect, at least as far as it has been measured, on cancer. All drugs, moreover, are organic molecules. Whether synthetic or natural, they combine carbon, hydrogen, nitrogen, oxygen, chloride, sulfur, phosphorus, and sometimes fluoride or iodine into chains, rings, and other formations that interact with receptors inside the human body.

This similarity raises the question of what the word "natural" means. Humans are part of nature. If we combine certain natural elements in a laboratory, is the result by definition different from what a plant creates when it combines those exact same elements in the exact same way? It can be argued that humans have, philosophically and practically, set themselves apart from nature. Our intelligence and the technology we have developed based on that intelligence certainly have given us a unique capacity to change nature. But are all such changes by definition "unnatural?"

Bias enters this discussion from both sides. Some people regard natural as automatically better than synthetic. Others, reflecting a view that took hold in the West sometime in the early to mid-20th century, prefer synthetic drugs because only they are so-called wonder drugs.

Whatever one's opinion, synthesizing plant-based drugs offers numerous advantages. It helps solve supply problems and can prevent destruction of a plant through overharvesting. It allows researchers to take full advantage of their ability to find interesting compounds in plants, and to use their modern technology to do what it increasingly does well—manipulate elements at the cellular and subcellular levels—to create drugs that would not otherwise exist. Synthesization also makes patents possible (see Chapter 7), and without patents pharmaceutical research would be a much less attractive investment.

To synthesize does have disadvantages beyond those imposed by relying on the single active molecule. One clear example can be seen by traveling through rural areas of virtually any developing country. People are extremely poor. Growing urbanization, disruption of traditional village cultures, and other variables have left huge areas of farmland abandoned or irrevocably changed. Medicinal plants are one of the primary natural resources of these countries, particularly those in the tropics. If Western pharmaceutical companies relied more on actual plants and plant parts, then it is reasonable to believe that huge numbers of people could be employed in growing and harvesting them. These people, and their families, would make a vital contribution to the world economy, which would, by definition, contribute to the stability and well-being of their own countries.

Of course, such scenarios would never become real unless it was in the economic interest of pharmaceutical companies to make them real.

(5) What is the role of the profit motive?

While desire for profit did not seem to play a role in the early 19th-century drug-related discoveries, it clearly has played a huge role in all of the stories in this chapter. Indeed, the profit motive provided the incentive to find, develop, and bring to market all the drugs discussed.

Difficulty in patenting plant compounds may be the single most important explanation of why the list of plant-based medicines is so short. It is possible to patent extraction techniques or changes to a natural compound, but if a pharmaceutical company cannot patent a plant, why would it invest the hundreds of millions of dollars necessary to discover an active element and bring a medicine to market?

———————

COUNTS OF PLANT-BASED medicines, especially tallies that have entered accepted popular wisdom, tend to exaggerate the importance of plant-based medicine. Claims are usually that modern societies get anywhere from 25 to 75 percent of their medicines from plants. It is necessary to examine what is being counted.

Some of the higher counts result from regulators in other countries having approved numerous plant-based drugs that the U.S. Food and Drug Administration has not approved. Typical examples are ajmalicine, which comes from Indian snakeroot and is used as a vascular dilator to treat circulatory disorders, and gossypol, which is extracted from the cotton plant and is used as a male contraceptive.

The number of plant-based pharmaceutical drugs approved for use in countries—industrial and non-industrial—other than the U.S., however, is not high. While no scholar has conducted an exact count, it is no more than a small percentage of the pharmaceutical drugs in use throughout the world. Most analysis, moreover, continues to focus on the U.S. because it is the wealthiest market for pharmaceutical drugs, and because the FDA maintains what are by far the strictest standards for drug approval.

Also often counted in some studies are drugs that have been derived from chemical formulas found in plants. In some of these instances the plant may have played no role other than as, in essence, a textbook providing researchers with a formula to manipulate. Thus, one recent study concludes that "at least 119 compounds from 90 plant species can be considered as important drugs currently in use in one or more countries." Another study reports that 30 alkaloids and 19 non-alkaloids from higher plants have led to usable drugs in the United States.

Another variable that leads to misunderstandings is the phrase "natural sources." In addition to plants, natural sources include animal parts and hormones; venom from snakes and other reptiles and amphibians; fungi; bacteria; and marine animals.

Typical examples of non-plant natural sources are the ergot alkaloids produced by a fungus that grows on grains, especially rye. Insects and the wind carry spores of this fungus, which often infects entire crops. When ingested by humans, infected grain can cause strange and terrifying symptoms such as gangrene of the feet and arms. Tissue can become mummified and fall off without loss of blood. Limbs blacken, and victims feel a terrible burning sensation. Medieval Europeans hit by such plagues called them St. Anthony's fire, after a shrine where they sought relief.

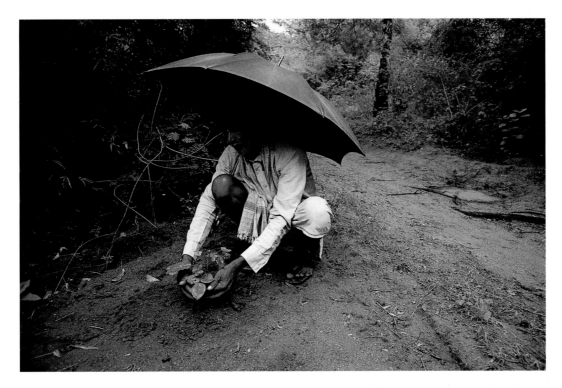

At the edge of a village near Bangalore, India, the caretaker coddles herbs on a special medicinal preserve. Over-collection, destruction of habitat due to population growth, migration to cities, and overgrazing by animals now threaten an uncounted number of medicinal plants. Many will probably disappear before modern scientists can study them.

Healers and midwives used ergot to induce labor, a practice European doctors adopted in the early 19th century. Physicians today have learned that ergot can kill fetuses, but ergot alkaloids are sometimes used to stimulate uterine contractions and stop postpartum hemorrhages after delivery. Some of the alkaloids, of which there are dozens, have proved effective as treatments for migraine headaches and to improve certain behaviors in cases of senile dementia.

COUNTING SOURCES such as ergot alkaloids, 45 percent of the 99 most prescribed drugs in the United States in 1993 came from natural sources or were made based on chemical formulas taken from natural sources. Of these 99 drugs only 6 came from plants, and another 13 were synthetically derived from plant material. According to a 1967 study of more than a billion prescriptions, 25 percent contained "principles from higher plants."

The studies reveal clear trends: The percentage of prescription drugs that come from natural sources, and from plants, is shrinking. Most of these drugs have their origins in centuries-old knowledge, not in current research. And, while some plant-based drugs have supplemented synthetics, few have ever replaced a synthetic pharmaceutical drug as the preferred treatment for a medical problem.

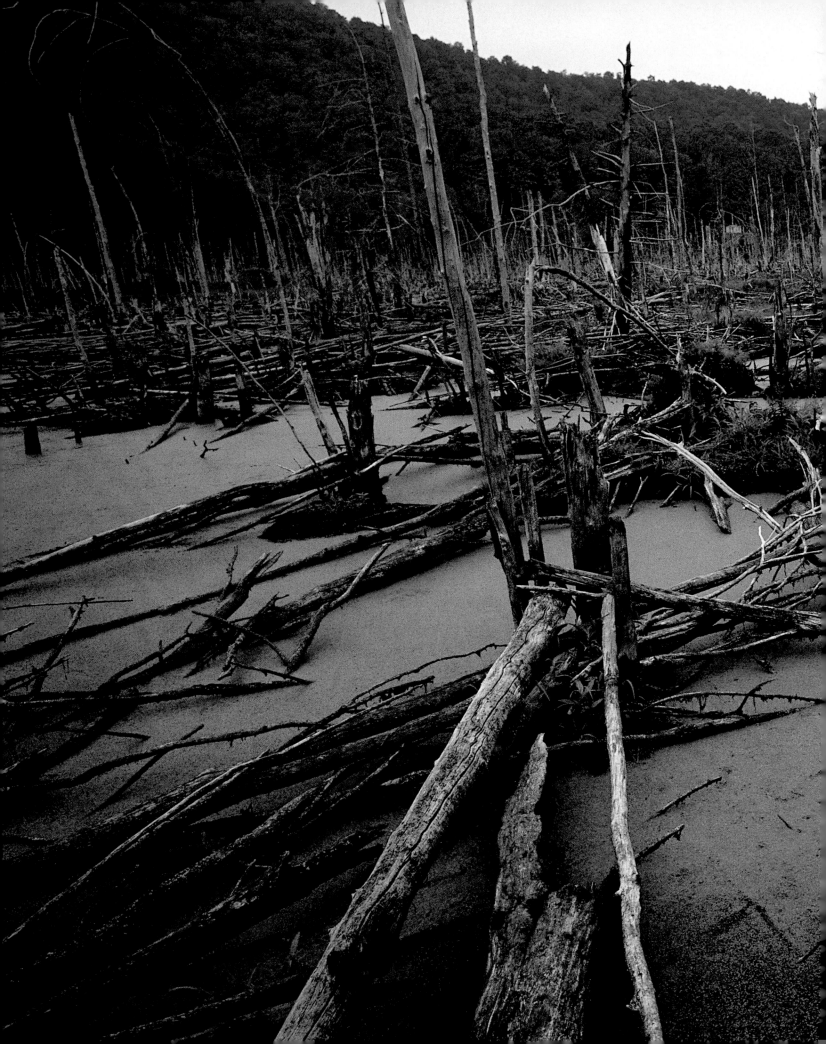

SHAPING
THE FUTURE OF
PLANT-BASED
MEDICINE

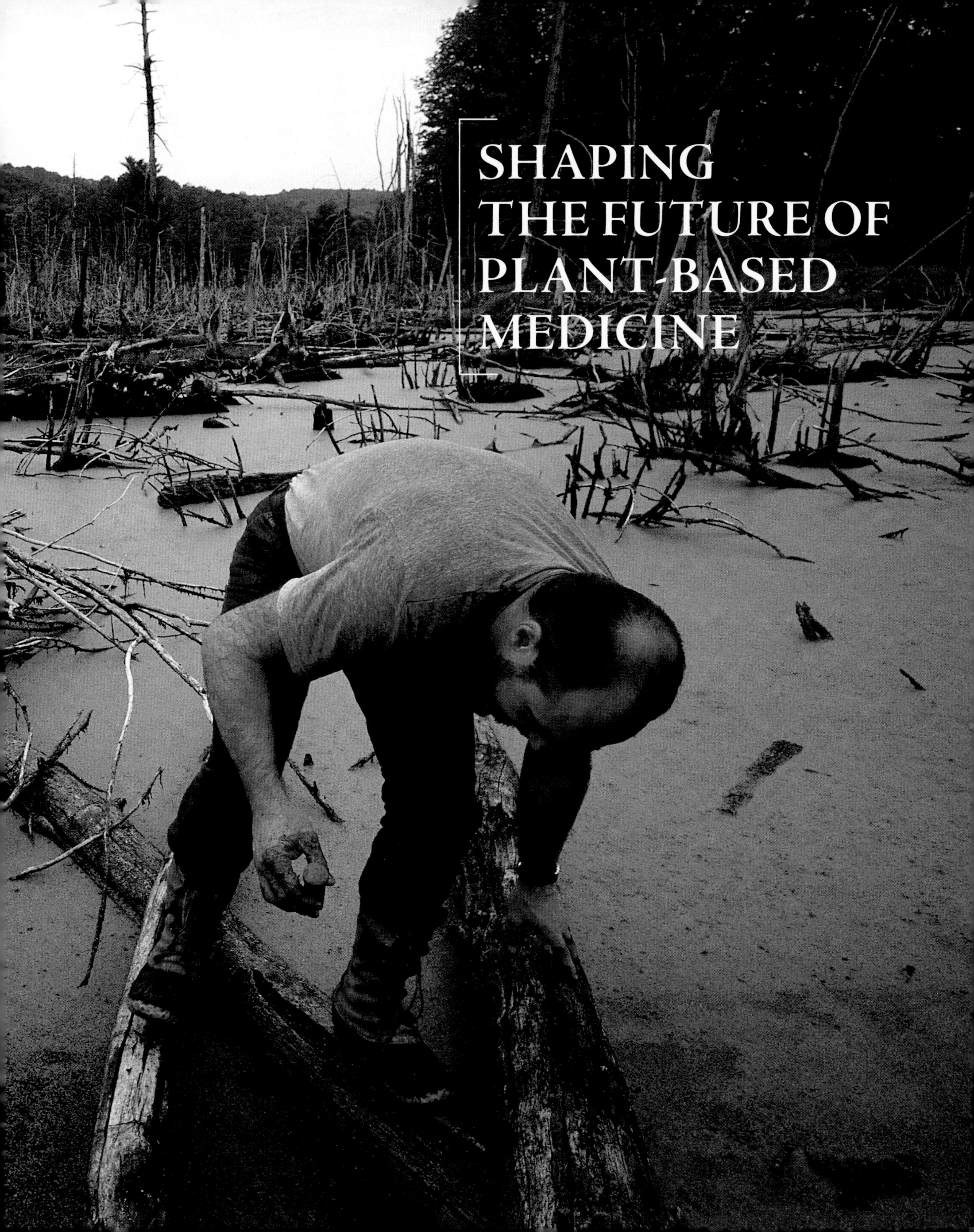

CHAPTER SEVEN

Modern Medicine Keeps Trying to Use Plants

In 1997 nine Madagascar rosy periwinkle plants were included in the cargo of two National Aeronautics and Space Administration shuttles. This periwinkle is the only source of two cancer-fighting alkaloids, vincristine and vinblastine, and scientists wanted to see if weightless conditions increased the plant's production of them. The periwinkles, whose longest period in space was 16 days, did appear to have higher levels of lifesaving chemicals. Whether this resulted from overall stress or as a direct effect of weightlessness remains unknown. Also unknown is whether weightlessness changes the intensity or bioactivity of such plant-produced chemicals. Future flights may take periwinkles into space for months, part of the continuing efforts to use technology to maximize medicinal benefits derived from plants.

Botanist Stefano Padulosi and a local farmer use a loupe to examine a plant in Nigeria. Modern science has yet to identify what may be the majority of plant species, and not all of those are deep in rain forests.

PRECEDING PAGES: In an upstate New York forest, newly protected to preserve existing biodiversity, James Babcock of Cornell University collects samples.

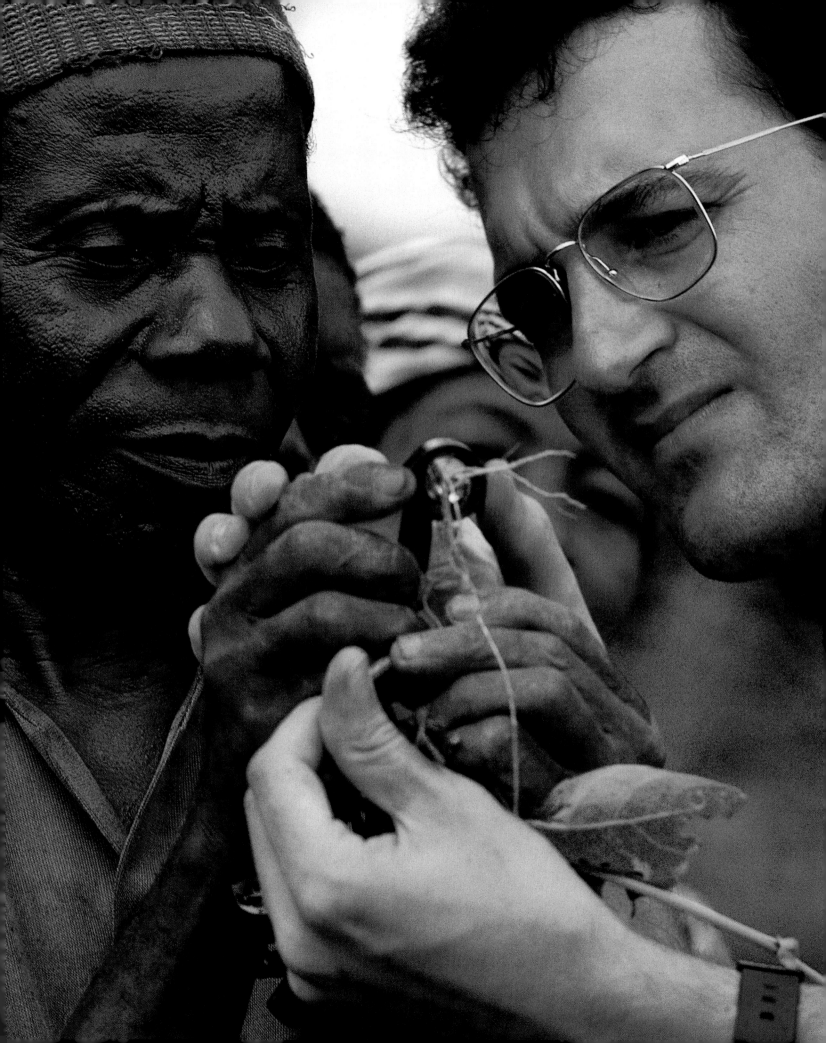

THE PREVIOUS FEW CHAPTERS have outlined two basic facts that make sense individually but that together are contradictory. The first: Given the power of plants, the extraordinary pharmaceutical drugs that they have yielded, and the thousands of years of experience available from other cultures, modern science has found surprisingly few drugs from them. Indeed, the more sophisticated science has become, the more complete has been its failure in this effort. Paclitaxel is one of the few FDA-approved plant-based drugs to emerge in the last third of the 20th century. This fact is painful to admit, especially since plants-as-medicine is one of the chief arguments of those who are trying to save the rain forest and other natural habitats.

The second—and contradictory—fact is that given all the impediments, it is amazing that so many plant-based drugs have been found. Among these impediments are the chemical complexity of plants; their toxicity; and the disparate, far-ranging, and often misleading uses made of them in traditional medicine.

However these facts are reconciled, the modern industrial world in the last half of the 20th century has been the only culture in recorded human history to move away from plants as the core of its medicines. This movement continues into the 21st century and occurs at the same time as tremendous growth in the number of pharmaceutical drugs. In 1998 more than 9,000 prescription drugs were available in the United States. As recently as the mid-1960s, there were only about 300.

The beginning of this book posed the question, "Why doesn't modern science reap more benefits from plants?" Tracing the story of medicinal plants over the past several thousand years has revealed the foundations of an answer.

Plant chemicals, like other chemicals, can be very toxic, which makes devising safe pharmaceutical drugs from them much more difficult than working with nontoxic substances. Researchers, furthermore, have had too many plants to study. Europeans, for example, have used more than a thousand plants to treat diabetes. The time and financial resources to identify—let alone explore—more than a small percentage of these possibilities have not been available. If traditional medical systems had used only a small number of plants, the pharmaceutical companies, government agencies, and others could have focused on them.

Even more important is that modern science has defined medicines—whether from plants or another source—as having only one compound that is bioactive. This approach solved a wide range of practical problems, such as the need to patent medicines and to standardize them. It has, however, limited plant-based pharmaceutical drugs to those derived from plants in which such a compound exists, and from which,

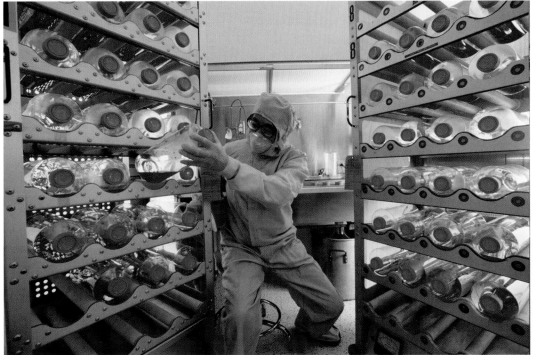

A researcher in a drug-production room maintains sterile conditions; technologically advanced facilities are an essential part of drug development. Bioactive chemicals in plants can be extracted, standardized, and processed to meet the highest standards set by modern pharmacology. Medicine's self-imposed need to work with one active compound at a time slows progress, and isolating plant compounds often changes or destroys their medicinal effect.

at a minimum, it has been discovered and can be economically mass produced.

The need for a single active compound is, even the strongest advocates of the status quo admit, extremely restrictive. Whether modern science could have picked another approach to plant-based medicines is for future historians to decide. Options other than the single active molecule certainly seem available. Whole plant and multiplant remedies, for example, could have been tested via epidemiological evidence (see Chapter 8).

Perhaps the most important impediment to more plant-based pharmaceutical drugs has been economic. More plants are not tested for their usefulness as drugs because they cannot be patented unless someone changes their chemical composition. Today, to bring a drug to market in the U.S. usually requires the expenditure of some 500 million dollars, in a process that can take up to two decades. Pharmaceutical companies are not willing to make such an investment if they cannot patent the resulting product. The science is there; the incentive is not.

Despite these realities, the romance of discovering medicines from plants persists. Drug development in a laboratory can seem unexciting compared to the search by explorers in remote tropical forests for plants that could save millions of lives. Add so-called savage, primitive peoples to the plot, and the story becomes irresistible. For the news media, such exploration has long been a saga that almost writes itself. In 1961 a newspaper headline in California read, "Researchers Use Jungle Drug in Fight Against

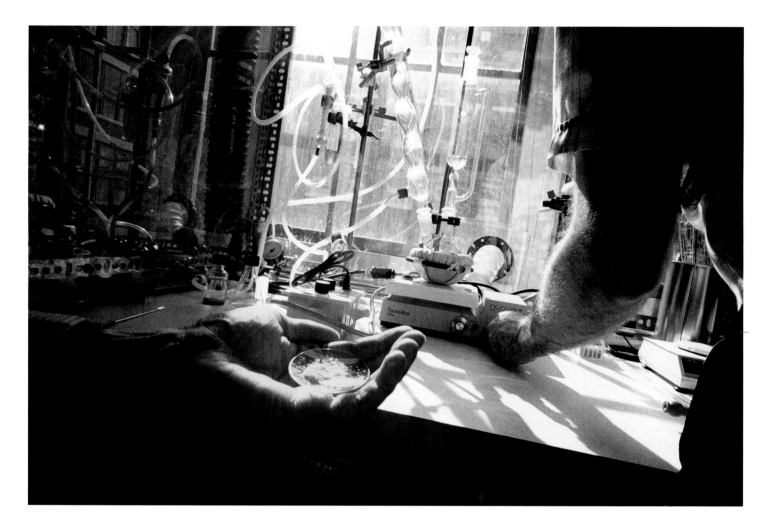

In a makeshift laboratory, researchers mix dry chemicals in an attempt to duplicate an experimental drug developed by a major pharmaceutical company. While traditional remedies and plant chemicals offer promising indications that they could be effective against the virus that causes AIDS, modern medicine has actually developed some effective treatments.

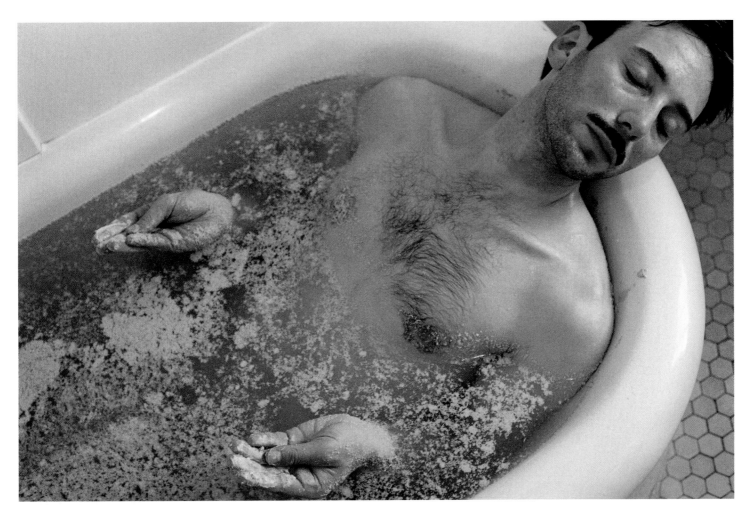

Many people, such as Thomas Avena, an HIV patient soaking in colloidal oatmeal and herbal oils, turn to herbal remedies in addition to the powerful drugs offered by mainstream medicine. Gathering data about the benefits of such approaches remains a major challenge to researchers. Whatever they contribute, herbal remedies cannot replace all that modern medicine offers.

Cancer," with the subhead, "Secret of Head Shrinkers." The story: A California doctor was "believed to be the only white man ever allowed to participate in the head-shrinking ritual" of a "fierce" tribe located in a remote, mountainous area of Ecuador. This doctor had cured a local medicine man's daughter of typhus. In gratitude, the medicine man had told him "the secret ingredients which shrink human cells."

Head shrinking, the doctor learned, can be accomplished using "eight basic ingredients," all plants. He grew them on a plantation the Ecuadorian government gave him for that purpose. Studies of these plants, the newspaper reported, demonstrated what scientists called "evidence of pronounced inhibitory effects in various types of cancers, including leukemia." Nothing came of the doctor's research.

The concept of magical medicines existing somewhere in the wilderness is comforting. People want to believe that the ultimate wonder drug is out there, like a holy, life-giving grail, waiting to be discovered. In the 1992 movie *Medicine Man*, Sean Connery played a botanist working in the Amazon. He had found and was studying what seemed to be an extraordinary plant remedy. "Six months ago, she [a Venezuelan] came to see me, a couple of lumps on her throat," he told a young scientist—of course, a beautiful woman—who had just arrived from the United States. "I sent her downriver…to the hospital there, and she made her own way back. It took her a month, and the nodes were almost double in size." Then, he continued, "two injections of that sample you just tested, and the lumps disappeared within a week." What made the lumps disappear, according to Connery's character, was "juju," a unique substance found in "sky flowers," which grew a hundred feet up in the forest canopy. Whether or not real-life juju waits in places like the Amazon, the search for such flowers does not play much of a role in the way pharmaceutical drugs are discovered today.

––––––––––

THE U.S. PHARMACEUTICAL industry spent about 24 billion dollars on drug discovery and development in 1999. Because of this investment, industry leaders see "on the horizon" new antibiotics and new drugs to prevent or treat malignant melanoma, breast cancer, diabetes, heart disease, Alzheimer's disease, depression, and osteoporosis. In the absence of a dramatic, unexpected breakthrough, none of these remedies will be based on plants.

The industry's vision of its future is high tech, built around technologies such as monoclonal antibodies and recombinant DNA therapy. Mapping the human genome could lead to entirely new categories of drugs. One possibility is the manufacture of drugs that use laboratory-made genetic material to interfere with the operation of

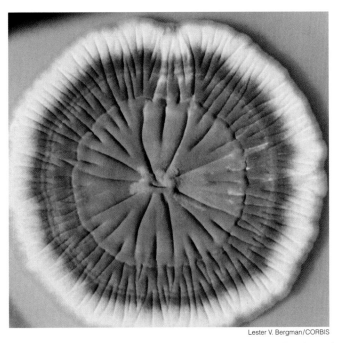

For centuries before modern scientists extracted the antibiotic penicillin from fungi such as this magnified colony of *Penicillium*, traditional healers used a wide range of molds to prevent and combat infections. None of these age-old practices has led to the development of a modern antibiotic drug.

genes—either human genes that are causing problems or the genes of disease-causing bacteria that have invaded the body. These substances are called antisense drugs because DNA has two strands—the sense and the antisense—and the drugs affect the antisense strand.

Some of these high-tech efforts could involve plants, not to obtain bioactive chemicals, but as factories that produce genetically manipulated material that has been added to them. One of the appeals of plants-as-factories is that they are inexpensive. Given sunlight, nutrition, and water, plants are essentially self-maintaining. Other possible production sources for genetically manipulated material—animals, bacteria, and viruses—can require more maintenance. Plants, furthermore, do not carry the virus that causes AIDS and other disease-causing agents, which can be found in animals.

Scientists have already genetically engineered tobacco plants, which they selected because tobacco's genetic structure is relatively easy to manipulate and because they have large leaves from which it is easy to extract material. Utilizing a bacterial or a viral carrier that spreads rapidly and without much difficulty through the plant, scientists have integrated bits of human genes into the genes of tobacco plants—which then manufacture a human protein or enzyme that can be extracted and used for medicinal purposes.

This procedure can produce complex human proteins, including a large number of human enzymes, hormones, growth factors, and even immune-system cells.

Another pharmaceutical possibility is to use plants to grow monoclonal antibodies, proteins produced by or composed of cells derived from a single cell that act against a specific antigen. Scientists inject a mouse with human cancer cells. The immune system of the mouse responds by creating an antibody that seeks and binds to the cancer cells. After isolating this antibody, scientists clone the gene that makes it, insert this gene into a type of bacteria, and inject these bacteria into plant cells. The plant then produces the antibody. This technique, which could be used to target specific human diseases such as lung cancer, could conceivably work well if the human immune system did not attack material produced by the plants. The alien antibodies could then reach—and combat—the cancer cells.

Plants and monoclonal antibodies could work together in another way: coupling a toxin—known to be effective against a particular type of cancer cell—to a monoclonal antibody that is designed to enter only that cancer cell. This approach could allow delivery of huge amounts of toxins to the cancer. One standard treatment for cancer now, chemotherapy, introduces toxins into the patient's system in hopes that enough toxins reach the cancer cells before the treatment proves intolerable to the patient.

Another sophisticated use of plants could be to add a human drug to the nectar of flowers by modifying a plant's genes to produce the drug. Bees would make honey from these flowers, and patients would eat the honey containing the drug. For certain medicines this method might allow patients to receive much higher dosages, at much lower costs, than would be possible using more traditional methods.

All of the above uses of plants raise important, and still unanswered, ethical questions because they blur the line between plants and humans. If plants that contain human genes get loose in the wild and reproduce, it could be an environmental disaster. Such plants, for example, could harbor pathogens that destroy existing species.

———

MOST PHARMACEUTICAL DRUGS TODAY still do not rely on such techniques. The drugs are discovered via "rational drug design," which emerged in the 1980s as researchers developed the capacity to identify biologic dysfunctions that can cause disease. With these dysfunctions—such as the low production of certain amino acids—in mind, researchers try to design the exact chemical grouping that will correct a specific problem. This is a lock-and-key approach. Researchers identify receptor sites on or within cells in various parts of the body and then try to find an agent that will go to and fill those sites—either to make something happen or to prevent something from happening by occupying the sites. Typical scientific articles reflecting the complexity of this method have titles like "Rational design of aromatic polyketide natural products by recombinant assembly of enzymatic subunits."

Rational drug design frees pharmaceutical companies from chemical prospecting—that is, finding bioactive substances in plants and other natural sources and then trying to see if they have any effect on human diseases. Instead, computers stimulate enzymes, and computer-based molecular models suggest the chemical structures of possible drugs. This rational approach is part of the overall trend away from research into plants and other natural products.

Many major pharmaceutical companies are now reducing or eliminating natural-products divisions, and of the 24 billion dollars spent in 1999 on drug discovery and development, only a tiny portion went to natural products. Only a small part of what was devoted to natural products, furthermore, involved plant research. Most money invested in natural products goes to investigate microbes, which yield antibiotics and are usually relatively easy to replicate and synthesize. Another major part of natural-product work is in researching venom from frogs, snakes, and other animals, all of which contain bioactive compounds. One example: When it faces danger, the Arabian saltwater catfish secretes a slime that promotes wound healing. Local people use it as a wound-healing agent. The slime, which scientists have found reduces healing time by a third, contains at least 60 proteins. Among other things, the proteins have demonstrated capacity to combat inflammation, cut pain, fight bacteria, clot blood, and stimulate the formation of new tissue. Although other catfish produce this slime, in the Arabian saltwater catfish it appears in the outer surface and is thus more accessible. But the chemically complex slime is difficult to synthesize. Modern medicine does nothing with it.

There are many reasons why pharmaceutical companies give plants a low priority. To collect plants and get them to the laboratory is expensive and labor intensive. Field work can be dangerous, and logistics can be cumbersome at best, relying on infrastructure such as old airstrips built by missionaries.

Processing and screening plants (see page 260) once they arrive in the laboratory requires an additional financial investment. And new problems appear once a plant tests well. Researchers worry about whether they can replicate an original sample to obtain an adequate supply. As has been seen in earlier chapters, the process of collecting is far more difficult than simply picking the plants. Variables such as time of year and day can be crucial. Plants are chemical factories, but their output may shift minute-by-minute as the temperature and the availability of water and nutrients change.

Some plants, furthermore, are exposed to cold, heat, darkness, chemicals, and other stresses during the journey from wild areas to the laboratory. These conditions can change their chemical makeup. That's why some experts now recommend extracting chemicals within hours of picking the plants. Such *(Continued on page 256)*

251

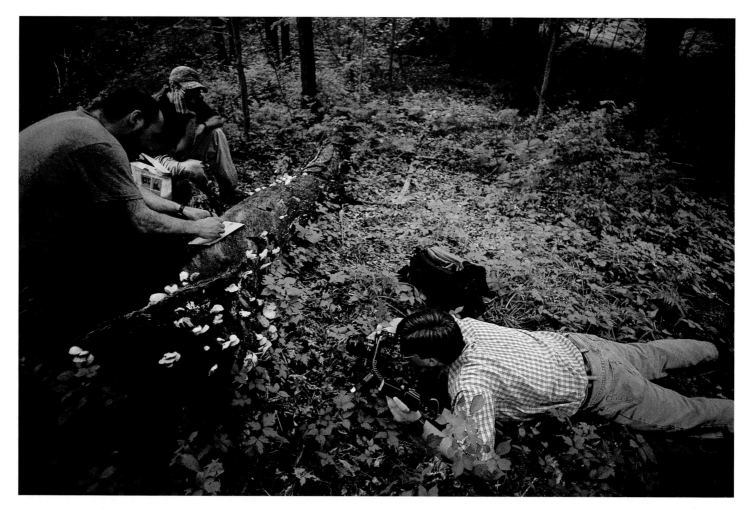

Experts from Cornell University collect specimens in the Lindsay-Parsons Biodiversity Preserve outside Ithaca, New York. They enter each specimen into a journal and photograph it in its natural environment. Such efforts help map biodiversity that still remains largely uncharted, even in terrain as familiar as New York State.

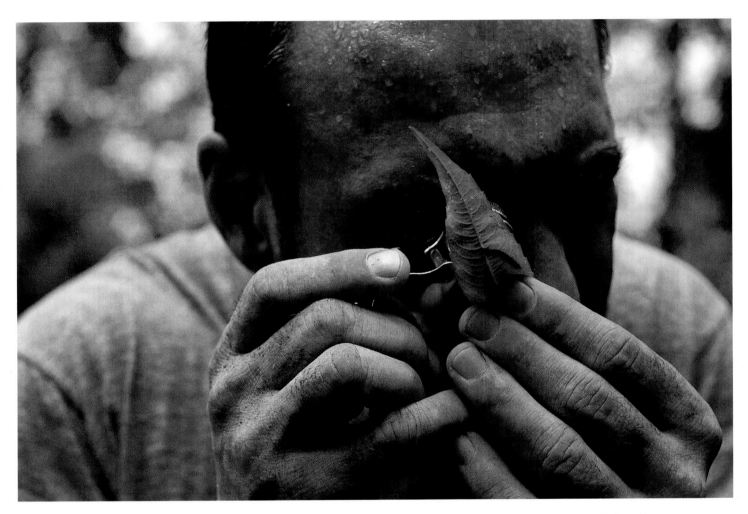

Fighting July heat, Cornell University specialist James Babcock scrutinizes a caterpillar on a leaf. As a boy Babcock spent many summers collecting plants with his grandmother, who knew all the medicinal herbs in their area. Now, he enters his findings on the project's website so that the information is available to everyone.

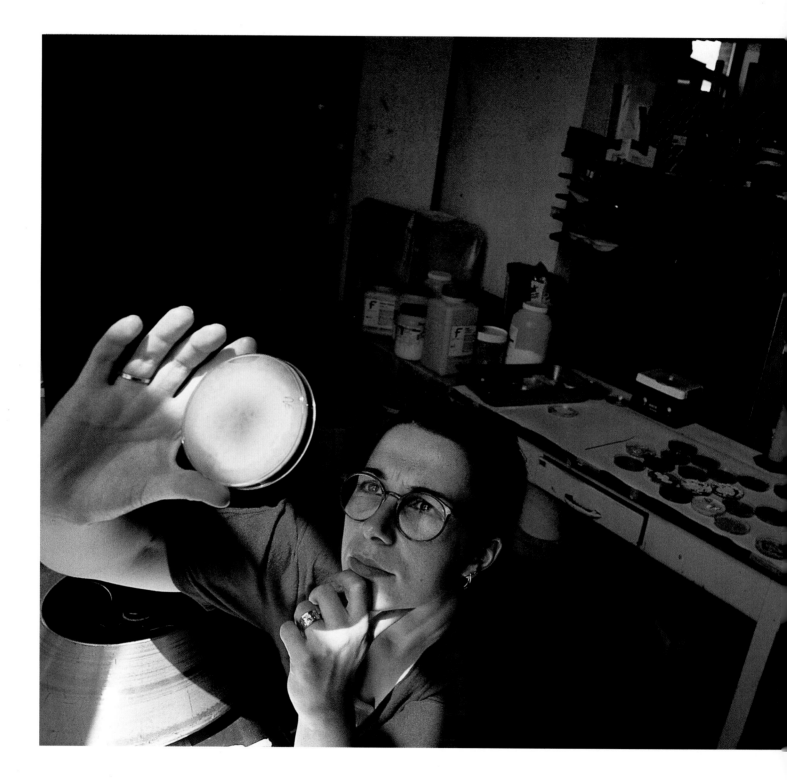

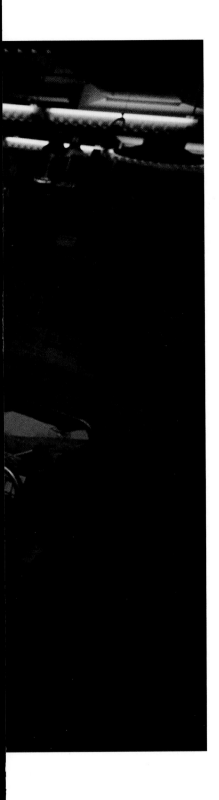

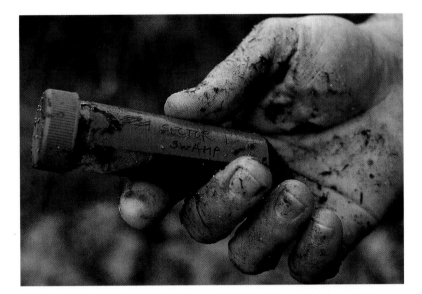

Her work in front of her, Sylvie Arnavielhe, a University of Alabama, Birmingham, microbiologist, studies a sample (left). Dr. Arnavielhe extracts DNA from specimens collected in the nearby forest. Work with genes of plants and other natural products offers extraordinary possibilities for advancing our understanding and for devising useful products such as pharmaceutical drugs from them. Recent work with plant genetics indicates that plants are much more complex than researchers had expected. A sample from an upstate New York swamp (above) may contain microbes new to science. Pharmaceutical companies often prefer working with such microbes rather than with plants. The cellular structure of microbes is simpler, thus easier to study, manipulate, and replicate.

quick extraction could be difficult to accomplish and could create even more expense.

––––––––––

Arguments about the ownership of information, knowledge, and ideas—and of life itself—add to the aforementioned biological, technical, and economic problems.

Traditional healers often hide information about remedies from fellow tribespeople as well as from outsiders. Albert Schweitzer, the 1952 Nobel Peace Prize winner who maintained a hospital in West Africa for four decades, noted in a memoir written soon after he arrived in Africa: "I hope in time to learn something more definite about these [traditional] 'medicines,' but it is always difficult to do so, because the knowledge about them is kept a strict secret. Any one who is suspected of betraying anything about them, and, above all, if it is to a white man, may count with certainty on being poisoned."

Such secrecy dates back to antiquity. In writing their medical papyri, Egyptian healers often used code names for plants.

Some people in the West have insisted that healing possibilities in nature are part of a global commons, a resource that belongs to humanity. When the first successful and safe polio vaccine was announced in 1955, CBS newsman Edward R. Murrow asked Jonas Salk, leader of the research team that developed it: "Who owns the patent to this vaccine?" Tens of millions of dollars had been spent on the vaccine, but Salk replied, "Well the people, I would say. There is no patent. Could you patent the sun?"

Salk's attitude is now out of fashion. U.S. law currently allows patents on any life-form that is changed by human action or ingenuity, and the World Trade Organization applies patent laws to all life-forms. Living matter that has been patented includes genetically engineered cotton and broccoli, cells from human umbilical cords, cells developed from genes found in a tribe living in a remote area of Papua New Guinea, and cells derived from material taken—without his knowledge—from a patient who demonstrated an unusual resistance to cancer.

Such patents, combined with the billions of dollars that can be made from pharmaceutical drugs, have bred concerns about biopiracy: Many developing countries worry that Western researchers and pharmaceutical companies will take local plants and knowledge, patent them, and keep the profits. These nations, which are rich in plants and knowledge but poor financially, are concerned about theft of their "green gold."

Partially in response to such concerns, more than 150 countries have signed the Convention on Biological Diversity of 1992, which says that a country owns the biological resources within its borders. The United States has not signed on the grounds that the convention does not contain adequate stipulations for preserving biodiversity and

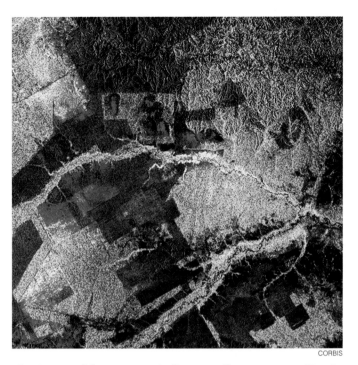

False colors in a radar image of Sumatran rain forests tell a true story: Purple and pink in the October 1984 photograph taken from the space shuttle *Endeavor* reflect clear-cut rain forest areas planted with palms and other commercial crops. In roughly the last century, about half of all the rain forests on Earth have disappeared.

that its poorly defined stipulations about national ownership would hamper biotechnological innovation. The Convention on Biological Diversity raises difficult questions. Some countries either do not have government offices responsible for negotiating profit-sharing agreements or have bureaucracies that make negotiating such agreements difficult. Remote areas where plants—and knowledge about them—are located are often part of traditional cultures that are in conflict with their country's central government. Who, then, gets money derived from pharmaceutical research? Everyone in the tribe? The village nearest where plants are obtained? The village healers?

Even when a traditional culture negotiates its own relationship with its central government, problems persist. Often these cultures are scattered in jungles and forests. The people have no bank accounts. When talk of money begins to spread, outsiders emerge from cities and other areas and claim that they, or others in the family, are members of the group and deserve part of the profits. International law related to ownership of the genetic contents of the plants, furthermore, remains vague. Are the knowledge of how to find and when to pick plants and the information on how to mix and administer them trade secrets that are protected by law?

Such issues have become emotionally charged in many countries, because those concerned know that they cannot stop what they call gene smuggling. Authorities have detained botanists leaving with plant samples, but all it takes to carry a plant's genetic code out of the country is a small piece of that plant.

Fueling the emotion is the fact that people from developing countries who have

Only ragged stumps remain of a wind-break in southern Peru, where pressure to use every square inch of land forces farmers to adopt practices that harm the environment and threaten many plant species. Loss of the sheltering line of trees, though it makes a handy perch for a schoolboy making friends with a dog, will encourage erosion and degradation of the land. Scientists may never know what medicinal benefits the forests lost to create such farmland may have offered.

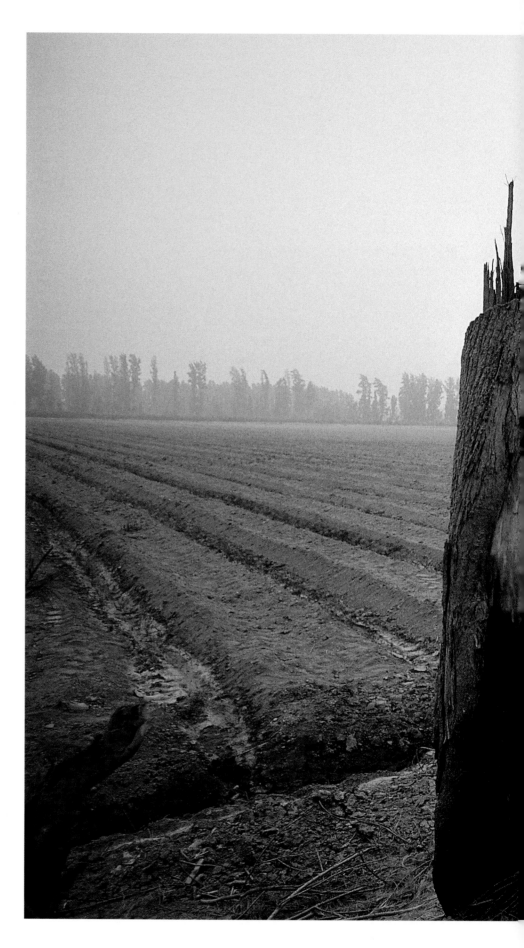

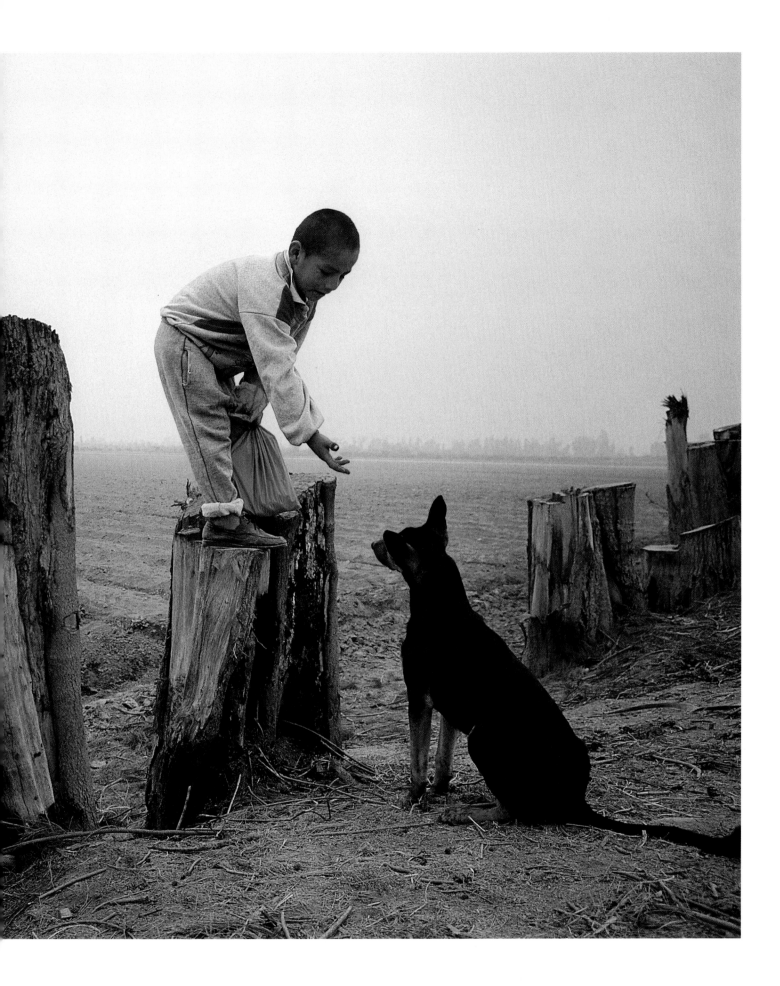

become citizens of countries such as the U.S. have taken out patents. One example of such opportunism is a patent for medicinal uses of the yellow-white powder from the turmeric plant. Conducting no new research, entrepreneurs essentially claimed to have discovered what people in India have known for centuries: that turmeric speeds up healing when put on wounds. The U.S. government eventually revoked a patent on turmeric when officials from India showed that the supposedly novel medical uses had been described in an academic paper many years earlier.

Another example of a plant from India on which a patent was granted is the neem tree, whose bark, seeds, and leaves have proven antiseptic and antifungal effects. People in India also use neem, which they call the village pharmacy, for dental hygiene and as a contraceptive. In Europe and the U.S. more than 35 patents have been granted on chemical constituents and compounds from the neem, whose name in Sanskrit, *sarva roga nivarine*, means "cure of all ailments." How many of these patents are for uses not documented in India remains a matter of contention.

In a July 1993 editorial, the *Hindu,* one of India's largest-circulation newspapers, calls the granting of such patents "theft" because medicinal use of the plants is "common knowledge and everyday practice in India." Noting that "biopiracy is an epidemic," the editorial argues that "if a patent system which is supposed to reward inventiveness and creativity systematically rewards piracy…it needs to be changed."

U.S. law allows an invention to be patented if it has not been published or patented in another country. It does not count use in another country as a reason to deny a U.S. patent. Nor does U.S. law recognize oral traditions. "…Even the folk knowledge orally held by local communities," the *Hindu* argues, "deserves to be recognised as collective, cumulative innovation."

———————

DESPITE ALL THE FAILURES AND IMPEDIMENTS to their use, plants retain an important place in modern drug development due to new screening technologies.

In the 1960s a pharmaceutical company could screen hundreds of plant compounds a year in search of biologically active molecules. Most testing consisted of injecting plant extracts into animals to see what happened. Leftover plant material was often destroyed after tests were run, even if it had come from remote places. In the late 1970s screening a hundred compounds a week was considered good. Now, thanks to improved screening techniques—known as high-through-put screening—it is not unusual for a company to screen hundreds of thousands of compounds a day and millions of compounds in a week.

These screens offer more than speed. New technology in creating cell lines—cells that can be grown endlessly in laboratory cultures—allows screening of a far higher number of compounds for their possible effect on a wider range of diseases. Whereas 1960s and 1970s screens looked at essentially one kind of human cancer, today's screens look at as many as a hundred types. A major problem for researchers has therefore become having enough compounds to screen. This has led to what is called combinatorial techniques, or combinatorial drug development, which allows researchers to make a new library of known compounds by changing and combining a diverse group of known chemicals. One experiment can create tens of thousands of compounds that had not previously existed. Researchers who make such new chemical combinations are looking for, among other things, new structures and interesting methods of bioactivity. They look at variables such as whether the compound binds to receptors and, if so, what kind of receptors.

Key to such efforts is having what scientists call a good lead compound or lead molecule—that is, one that can lead researchers to develop other compounds. Good lead compounds have a unique or interesting structure or have shown themselves to be strongly bioactive. Once scientists have such a compound, they can manipulate and modify it to get the new structures and methods of bioactivity that could eventually yield new pharmaceutical drugs. Compounds from nature often make excellent lead compounds because they offer a complexity beyond what humans, even armed with computer modeling and data banks, would think of doing. In compounds found in plants, nature may have put a nitrogen molecule off to an angle or added another hydrogen to the side as the result of tens or hundreds of millions of years of evolution.

But to serve as the sources for lead compounds, plants still have to be collected and processed to identify their active chemicals—the expensive, often frustrating, efforts that professionals call "find and grind."

One possible way to avoid these costs and uncertainties is biochemical farming: using chemicals that mimic stress to make plants produce desired compounds. Biochemical farming could be used for both the discovery of new chemicals and for the manufacture of chemicals that have already been discovered. Once identified, desired compounds of consistent quality and composition could be produced because the farmed plants would live in constant, controlled conditions. Plants used for such phytosecretion—the production of chemical compounds by a plant—could be grown in a water-based, or hydrogenic, medium rather than in soil. They could then be harvested more easily, because there would be no need to dig them up.

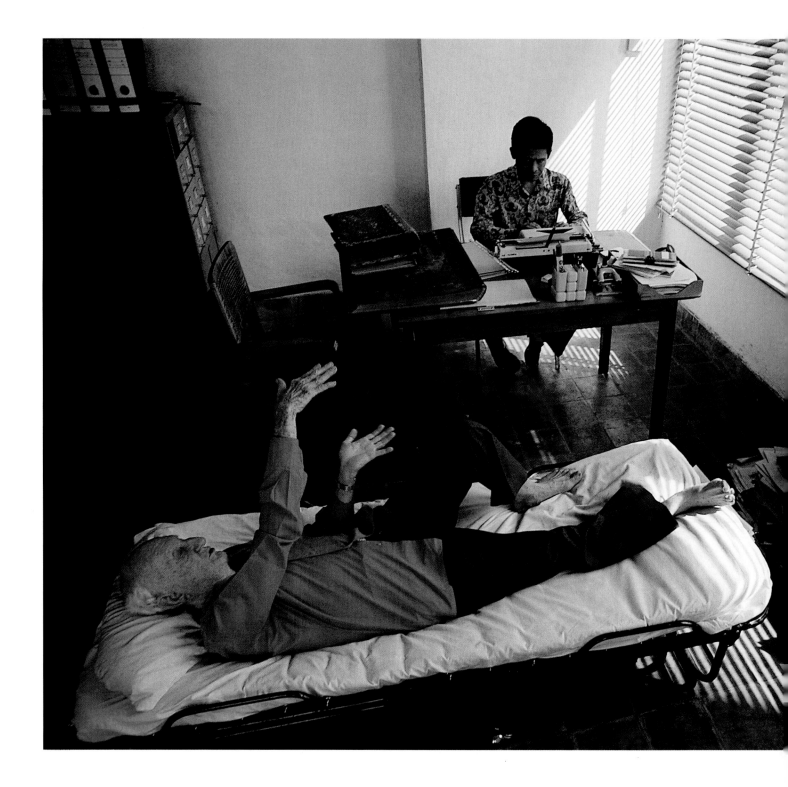

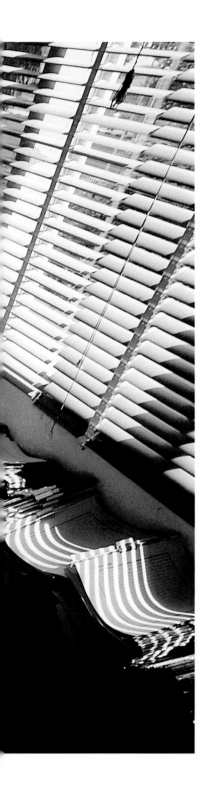

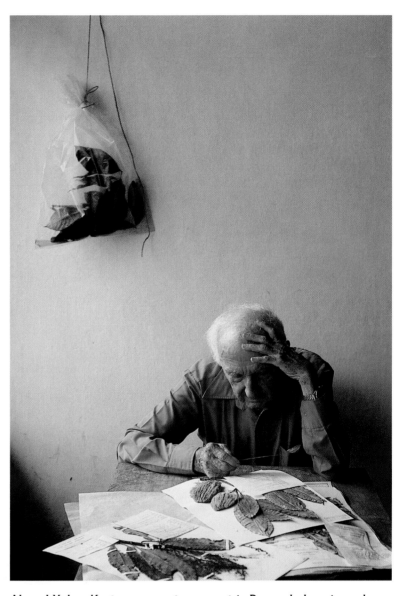

Ahmad Yahya Kostermans rests on a cot in Bogor, Indonesia, as he dictates to an assistant (left). Kostermans, now in his 80s, has studied the rain forest all his life. During World War II his knowledge of medicinal plants helped his fellow prisoners survive a Japanese prisoner-of-war camp. As part of his effort to make his life's work available to others, Kostermans organizes and labels his leaf collection. Full appreciation of what such knowledge offers may await future generations, whose technology—and conceptual approaches—can better handle the chemical complexity found in plants.

Despite advances in biochemical farming techniques, microbes can be much easier to work with than plants. There are many more varieties of microbes than there are plants, and these microbes are generally much easier to collect. No traditional societies claim ownership rights to the medicinal use of microbes—a sharp contrast to their increasing claims to own medicinal plants and knowledge of them.

Once a natural product such as a bacteria or a plant yields a promising bioactive compound, researchers may begin a race to synthesize it. The rewards for winning such a race include recognition, publication in respected scientific journals, and research money. And, if you learn how to build the molecule piece by piece, you may see ways to modify it and make it work better.

One such race occurred in the mid- to late 1990s with epothilone, a bacterial compound obtained from a sample of dirt, and commonly found, among other places, in decaying plant materials and the feces of some herbivorous mammals. Epothilone kills tumor cells in much the same way that paclitaxel does (from the Pacific yew tree; see Chapter 6). Examination of epothilone offered an opportunity to look at how it binds to the proteins of cancer cells' microtubules and to better understand how the microtubules function. Epothilone looked particularly promising because it can be produced less expensively in the laboratory and is much more active than the plant-based paclitaxel. Another advantage of epothilone is that it is a bit more water soluble, which means it may enter human cells much more easily. To enter human cells, paclitaxel must be administered along with emulsifying agents that can cause severe side effects.

Researchers have documented that for unknown reasons epothilone seems to generate much less resistance than does paclitaxel. Cancer cells can remove paclitaxel via a pump in their cells' membranes but seem unable to rid themselves of epothilone. The potential benefits to cancer patients are obvious, and the stakes for pharmaceutical companies are high: Worldwide sales for paclitaxel and related drugs in 1999 were about 1.8 billion dollars. If epothilone succeeds, it could decrease the role of one of the major plant-based drugs in the modern pharmacopoeia. Successful or not, the story of epothilone serves as a reminder that—despite the small percentage of pharmaceutical research money devoted to plants and other natural products—nature offers seemingly unlimited ways to kill cancer cells.

———

RESEARCHERS ONCE WANTED PLANTS for the natural chemicals they produce. Now they value plants for the information they provide. This fits well with the metaphor through which modern science increasingly perceives itself. During the industrial era, the prevailing wisdom tended to see humans as machines (see Chapter 6). It was not coincidence that plants were treated as chemical factories. As we enter a rapidly evolving information age, we define humans by the information encoded in our genes, and modern medicine increasingly moves toward reliance on those codes. It is thus not surprising that researchers, in turn, value plants as sources of information—and refer to nature preserves as "gene sanctuaries."

Nearly 400 years ago Shakespeare described plants as part of nature's "infinite book of secrecy." Now, as pharmaceutical researchers continue their search for new medicinal plants, they hope to learn to read—or at least copy from—this book before too much of it is destroyed.

A record number of plant species are disappearing or are endangered, including hundreds with known medicinal uses.

The principal killers of plants are destruction and fragmentation of wild areas due to population pressures, overexploitation, ineffective methods of farming, pollution, and demand for timber. A chunk of rain forest the size of New Mexico is destroyed each year. In the last century, as much as half of all the rain forests in the world have disappeared. And this is happening before Western scientists learn what lives there. Some 1.5 to 1.75 million species of organisms on Earth have been identified so far. That number keeps increasing, and could range as high as 100 million, because scientists keep finding more forms of life than expected in rain forests and in marine environments, which seem to have more biodiversity than exists anywhere on land.

If present trends continue, according to one estimate, more than half of all species on Earth could disappear by the year 2100. According to one analysis, 60,000 of the estimated 250,000 species of plants will be extinct by the year 2050. Another study postulates that 100,000 of 300,000 will be gone. Most of these species of plants still have not been named.

Fewer than 5,000 plant species have been studied in depth, less than one percent of all plants have been screened for possible medical effects, and only 10 to 15 percent of flowering plant species have been screened.

———

LOSS OF THESE PLANTS has a significance that far exceeds their disappearance before Western science tests them. As mentioned earlier, plants are the principal source of medicine for nearly two-thirds of the world's people. For many of these people, loss of biodiversity, although crucial, may be less important than loss of cultural diversity—which is disappearing at a faster rate. About one in every eighteen people on Earth,

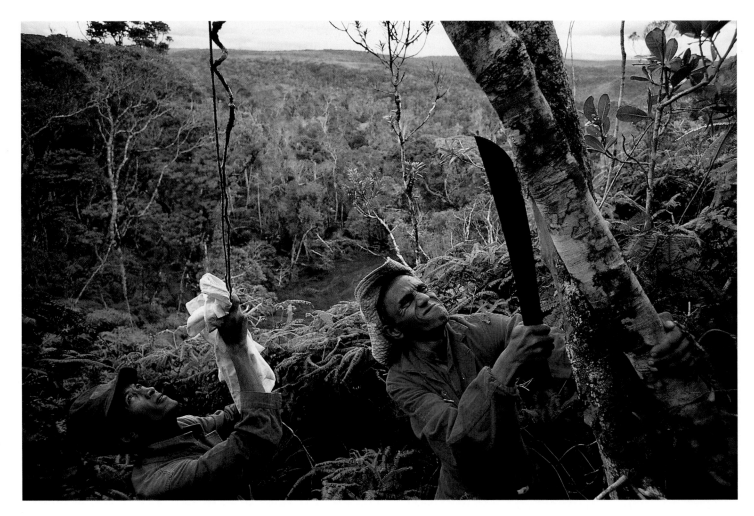

Two plant collectors in Madagascar gather samples in a rain forest soon to be mined. The samples will be sent to the National Cancer Institute, which screens more than 20,000 natural compounds each year. Many of these substances could offer lifesaving new drugs, but this promise may not become reality until medicine learns to take advantage of nature's offerings by using more than one bioactive compound at a time.

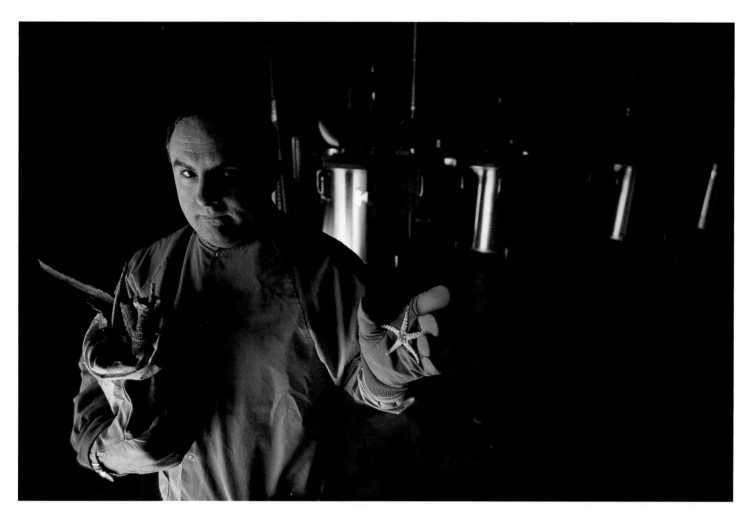

Subzero storage preserves samples at the repository for the natural-products laboratory of the National Cancer Institute in Frederick, Maryland. Dan Danner, technical manager of the lab, holds a bag of bark from Madagascar and a starfish. High collection costs—about 125 dollars a pound for plants and 350 dollars a pound for marine samples—discourage pharmaceutical companies from researching such life-forms, yet a sponge found in the Caribbean in 1954 led to the development of the AIDS drug AZT.

more than 300 million people, are members of what the United Nations calls indigenous cultures. This means they are rooted to identifiable portions of land, have lifestyles and economics to some degree cut off from the outside world, and speak languages that usually do not a have written form. Today, about 5,000 such cultures exist, but many are disappearing.

A good measure of this disappearance is the decline in the number of languages spoken. Of about 6,000 languages now used, 50 percent could be dead or near death by the year 2100. People living in the Amazon once had an uncounted number of languages, at least hundreds. Now they speak about 100 to 150, of which more than 80 percent are about to die. People in the region that is now the United States and Canada spoke about 300 languages when Columbus landed. Now the inhabitants speak 200, of which 135 have no speakers among the younger members of the groups.

Electronic communications, which some observers call "cultural nerve gas"; the economic lure of cities, now home to nearly half the world's people; and Western-style schools are killing these languages. Literacy defined as the ability to read and write is replacing other kinds of literacy, such as the ability to "read" the rain forest.

When a healer in such an indigenous culture dies, leaving behind no apprentice and no written documentation, it is as though part of a medical library has been burned. Such losses are occurring more and more often. In southern Africa a healer recently found an apprentice to train by dreaming which child it should be. The child's parents agreed, but how long can such practices continue? Will young people want to learn about forests that are disappearing? How many will accept the rigors of training in traditional medicine when schools and cities beckon?

Nongovernmental organizations now sponsor apprenticeship programs and have mounted other efforts to re-empower healers. These efforts have a direct impact on the search for pharmaceutical drugs from plants. If healers disappear before science develops the resources and sensitivity to learn from them, their knowledge may be lost forever.

———

LIMITED FINANCIAL RESOURCES MAKE it vital that researchers use the best possible methods in deciding what plants to collect for screening. The most well-known, but not necessarily the most pursued, approach is ethnobotany: the systematic study of how traditional societies use plants. Researchers apply an ethnobotanical—also called ethnomedical, ethnobiomedicinal, and ethnopharmacological—approach to Chinese and Ayurvedic approaches as well as to less systematized "primitive" medicine.

It is not unusual to see a news photo of an ethnobotanist smiling appreciatively as a

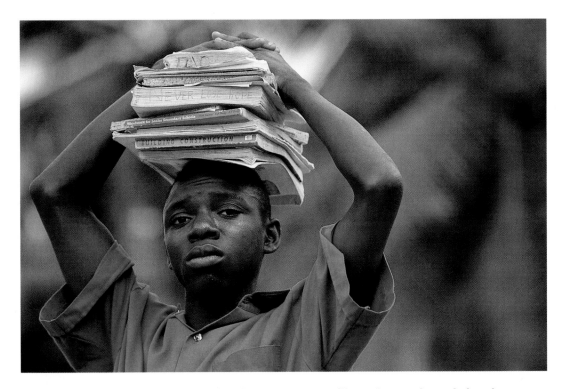

Textbooks contribute to the schooling of a young man in Ghana, but traditional plant lore learned from his mother and grandparents also constitutes a potentially important part of his education. Traditional healers, who rely on the oral transmission of knowledge, provide medical care for nearly two-thirds of the Earth's people. As traditional cultures give way to the modern world, such orally transmitted lore may be lost to future generations.

traditional healer administers a plant-based cure, but Western experts debate whether knowledge from traditional societies is important when seeking modern drugs. Some researchers dismiss traditional uses as folklore. They argue that the medicine practiced in such societies is usually misguided, ineffective, and based on ignorance of how the human body and medicines really work. As evidence they often cite the shorter life spans of members of these societies as compared to Western life expectancies.

Those who disagree say that prescriptions are based on thousands of years of experience and point to the modern pharmaceutical drugs discovered in the 19th and 20th centuries—nearly all of which were based on traditional uses of medicinal plants. Logic dictates, they say, that there must be many other effective plants that Western scientists have not yet identified.

Scientists are studying hundreds of possible cures based on the practices of traditional healers. Many produce false promises. In one typical example researchers collected 20 plants as instructed by a healer. Five of these plants showed activity against the virus that causes AIDS, about which the healer knew nothing. When researchers collected plants at random from the same area, only one was effective against the AIDS virus. Subsequent laboratory analysis showed that all of the positive results were due to laboratory errors.

In other studies the fruit of the West African bitter kola stopped growth of the

Ebola virus in laboratory tests. Ebola, which emerged from central Africa in the mid-1970s, causes high fever and massive bleeding, and it is usually fatal. Compounds in the bitter kola also proved to be effective against some types of the virus that causes the common flu. Traditional healers use the kola seeds primarily to combat poisons, and West Africans eat its fruit, often serving it to guests to welcome them.

In numerous similar studies of other plants recommended by traditional healers, extracts and active compounds from plants show activity against cancer, HIV, diabetes, eye disease, arthritis, and other major ailments. To date, however, these studies have not yielded one modern drug. Some studies may involve a miracle drug that is still working its way through laboratory and clinical trials, and future scientists, using more sophisticated technology and understanding, could eventually use other studies as the foundation for a major breakthrough. Or this research could remain what it essentially is today—a dead end.

In the meantime ethnobotanists and other scientists continue to report that traditional healers know much about plants that has escaped modern science. Physicians and medical researchers tend to dismiss such stories as anecdotal, unproved, and unverifiable despite of the ethnobotanists describing themselves being cured of fevers and vomiting.

Because symptoms in the jungle can have dozens of possible causes, the ethnobotanists' stories are most compelling when based on easily verifiable ailments such as insect bites or flesh wounds. In a typical example an ethnobotanist describes being bitten by numerous wasps. The healer accompanying him picks some plants and rubs them over the insect bites. All pain and swelling disappears.

When they do not come from trained scientists, such stories can sound apocryphal. One explorer, in a book published in the 1950s, described how a huge, poisonous snake bit him on the neck. The explorer said he expected to live four or five minutes. A native person, however, ran into the jungle, emerged with a mixture of plants, administered it, and the explorer quickly recovered.

Countless versions of similar stories can be told. Few are reported in the scientific literature. They represent a huge gap between the experiences of daily life in traditional societies and the workings of nature as understood by modern science.

————

OTHER METHODS OF DECIDING what plants to collect for screening include random collection of a wide variety of species. This option, often belittled in the professional literature, yielded paclitaxel, the last great medicine-from-plants success story.

A version of the random method is to select plants that seem to have mounted an effective defense against predators or competitors, which would indicate that the plants are producing powerful chemicals. If insects surround most plants in an area but leave one plant alone, that is a good indication of its defensive strength. A tree around which nothing grows but one kind of fern is also probably producing powerful chemicals.

Another possible method of selection is taxonomic: choosing plants from certain families, genera, species, or subspecies already known to possess interesting chemicals. Paclitaxel provides a good example of this approach. After it was found in the Pacific yew, and alternative sources were needed, researchers did not target other plants at random. They sought trees that are botanically related to the Pacific yew.

A fourth possible way to select plants for screening is geographic, collecting plants from areas with the greatest diversity. While temperate climates offer an array of interesting plants, most species grow in areas with tropical climates. A half acre of forest in the central U.S. has about 25 species of woody plants. The same amount of acreage in the western Amazon has nearly 300 species of woody plants. Because there is no winter, competition in the tropics is more complex and intense. Entities living in tropical areas must fight for light, space, and food all year long. Hot temperatures and the absence of a cold season that would curtail the growth of living things mean that there are more viruses, bacteria, and other microbes that cause plant diseases; more herbivores such as birds and insects; and therefore the greatest diversity in plant alkaloids and other defensive chemicals, as well as more plants that produce large quantities of these chemicals.

Perhaps the most important geographic environments still to be searched for medicinal plants are in the oceans and seas that cover 70 percent of the Earth's surface. Traditional cultures, even in island regions such as the Caribbean and the islands of southeastern Asia, rarely obtain medicines from underwater because so much is available, and easy to collect, on land. The only major exception is kelp, a plant that many traditional cultures use. It is an excellent source of iodine and helps prevent thyroid problems.

No underwater plant or animal yet furnishes a pharmaceutical drug, even though coral reefs are more biodiverse than tropical rain forests. One measure of their biological intensity is that a coral reef can have half a billion single-celled algae per cubic inch.

Because coral reefs are sites of constant chemical warfare as plants and animals fight for limited space, one of the principles of collection there is "if it's bright red, slow moving, and alive, we want it." The reasoning is that something red and stationary provides an inviting target for predators, and if the organism is alive it must be generating some effective chemicals. Other prime candidates for collection are creatures with soft shells. If an animal lacks a hard shell to protect itself, *(Continued on page 276)*

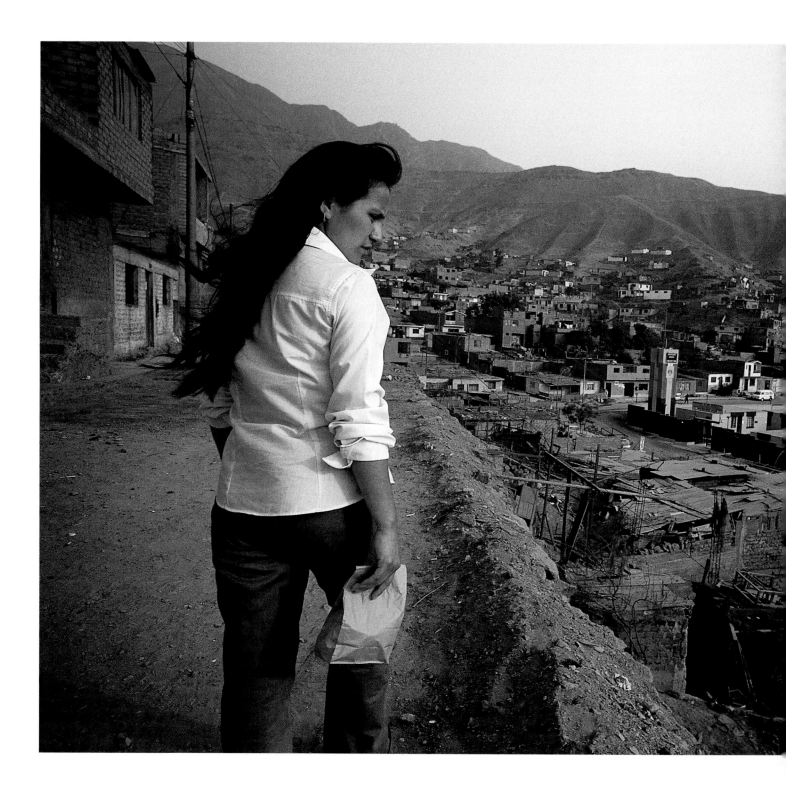

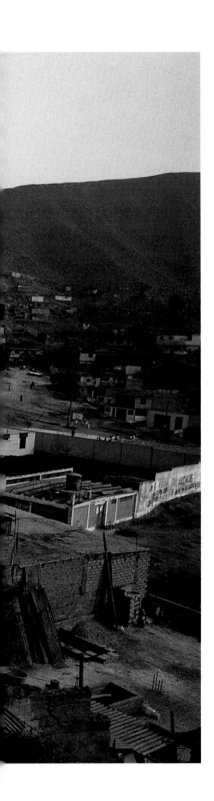

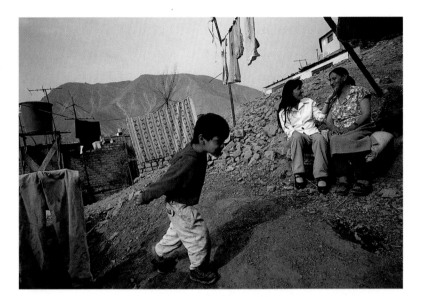

Poverty and poor sanitation foster the spread of drug-resistant tuberculosis in Comas, near Lima, Peru. Joelma Fuertes, who works for a government health program, delivers medicines to fight the disease (left). About half the world's people now live in cities, where many of them are too poor to afford modern medicines yet are cut off from traditional, rural-based healers. Curable diseases such as tuberculosis now are prevalent in areas like Comas. To cure the disease, patients must take a combination of drugs for 18 months after they are tuberculosis free, a grueling regime with painful side effects. Part of Fuertes's job is to develop relationships that encourage the patients to complete the full course of treatment (above). Many people in such neighborhoods have known only traditional healers and do not realize that they are likely to breed drug-resistant tuberculosis bacteria if they fail to take the full course of medications.

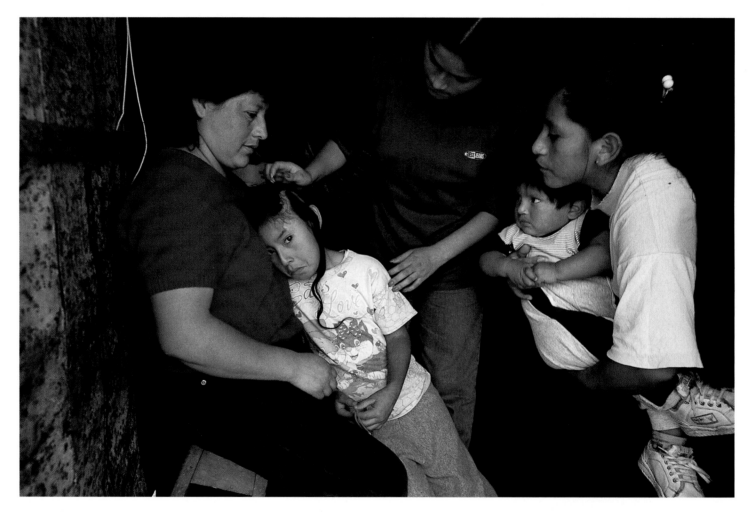

Scared and sorrowful, eight-year-old Janet Vasquez leans against her mother for comfort as health worker Naldo Angeles checks the girl for parasites. Such families usually move to urban areas looking for work. In the rural area they just left, these new residents of Lima, Peru, would rely on herbal remedies for problems like the parasites that now infest Janet.

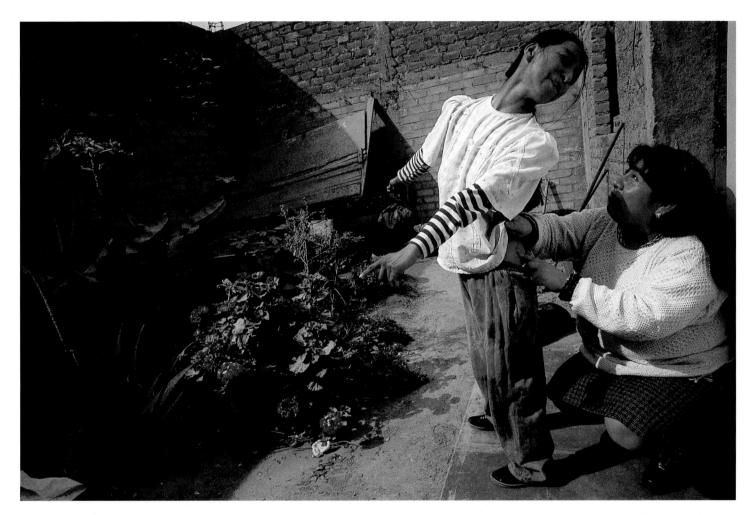

Janet Acuna, age 19, shows health worker Dalie Guerra in Lima, Peru, how the injection of antituberculosis drugs has caused painful bruising, a common side effect of the medicine. Traditional healers often provide herbal treatments that help ease the unpleasant side effects of modern medicines.

then there is a reasonable chance it relies on some kind of chemicals for defense.

The National Cancer Institute has more candidates for anticancer drugs from under the oceans than from tropical rain forests. None of these candidates is from a marine plant. The closest is halomon, a potential anticancer drug derived from a red alga found off the Philippines. According to current scientific thinking, red algae are not related to today's land plants, which all have the same basic metabolism as green algae and seem to have evolved from green algae.

Other possible pharmaceutical drugs have been derived from various marine life, including sea hares, sea squirts, sponges, mollusks, sea whips, tunicates, bryozoans, bugulas, and marine bacteria. The primary problem with researching such drugs, particularly those derived from organisms found in the ocean depths, is obtaining an adequate supply.

———————

A FINAL METHOD of selecting plants for screening is to choose plants used as medicine by various animal species, all of which have survived far longer than humans have existed.

Chinese myths describe how deer and dogs eat certain plants when they get sick, how birds peck at certain roots when they have accidentally touched poisonous berries, and how monkeys stop bleeding by making a ball of leaves and placing it on wounds. In one Chinese story a farmer encounters a snake that has been wounded and watches as another snake brings it a piece of a particular kind of grass. The farmer finds that the grass works to seal human wounds. This, according to the legend, is the source of a particularly effective wound-healing mixture of herbs.

Behavior with an apparent medicinal purpose can be found throughout the animal world. Rats, for example, eat clay after ingesting very toxic plants. The clay absorbs the poison. Much of this behavior, of course, does not involve plants. More than 200 species of birds sometimes hold an ant in their bill and rub the ant through their feathers. The ant may possess chemicals that help the bird fight parasites.

Researchers have noted most animal self-medication in primates such as gorillas, baboons, monkeys, and chimpanzees. Chimpanzees sometimes seem to eat particular plants in unusual ways. They suck juice out of the pith and spit out the rest. Do they do this because the plant has chemicals that acids in the stomach would neutralize, but which can be absorbed through mucous membranes of the mouth? Chimps also swallow the leaves of a particular plant whole, and hairs on the leaves scrape parasites from the animals' digestive systems. Other primates seem to eat a certain plant one way for food and another way when self-medicating. The apparently self-medicating behavior usually occurs only in the rainy season, when pest and bacterial infections are at their worst. The primates also sometimes seem to force themselves to eat leaves that taste bad or are extremely bitter, and they eat some plants that have no obvious nutritional value.

Most of the plants involved in the animal behavior cited above are high in bioactive chemicals. Their primary impact on animals seems to be to kill bacteria, cause the expulsion of parasites, combat lethargy or lack of appetite, correct bowel irregularity, and regulate the production of reproductive chemicals. Local people use most of the same plants for a wide range of purposes, many of which are similar to the plants' evident effects on animals. A female elephant eats leaves from a tree in the Boraginaceae family and shortly afterward goes into labor. Local women use the same leaves for the same purpose.

Studies indicate that some animal self-medication may be learned rather than innate. Chimpanzees in some areas of Africa, for example, dab leaves onto wounds, a behavior not seen among the same kind of chimpanzees living elsewhere. Likewise, bears chew roots of a lovage plant, spit it onto their paws, and rub it on their fur. Do they do this to kill bacteria and viral infections? No one knows. Navajo, who have lived near these bears for countless centuries, use this same plant in their medicine. According to their myth, the Navajo learned about the plant from bears.

Whether self-medicating behavior is learned or instinctive, however, is not as important as whether it actually exists. Some scientists remain skeptical about what they see as an unnatural intentionality ascribed to animals. They say that observers see what they want to believe.

One scientist proposed the following scenario: "A chimpanzee, for its science-fair project, analyzes the remains of a potato chip bag discarded by a person in Topeka. Among the chemical constituents in the potato chips, the ape finds one compound that, when analyzed in a test tube, displays anticholera activity. Does that mean Topekans can prevent or cure cholera by eating potato chips?"

Chances are, however, that animals have significant lessons to teach. Attine ants maintain gardens of fungi that they eat. The ants carry a particular kind of bacteria on their bodies. These bacteria produce an antibiotic that kills parasites that infest the ants' fungal crops. This fact in itself might not be worthy of much attention, except that the bacteria belong to a genus—the *Streptomyces*—that provides more than half of all antibiotics humans have ever developed.

While growing antibiotic resistance threatens to reach crisis proportions for

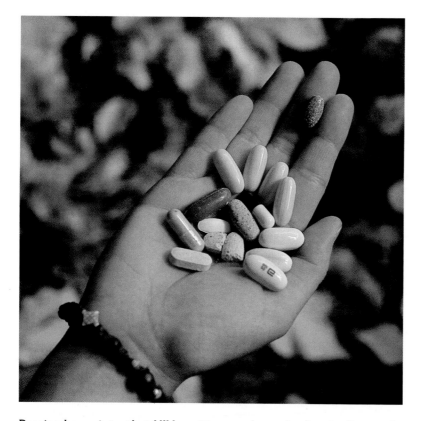

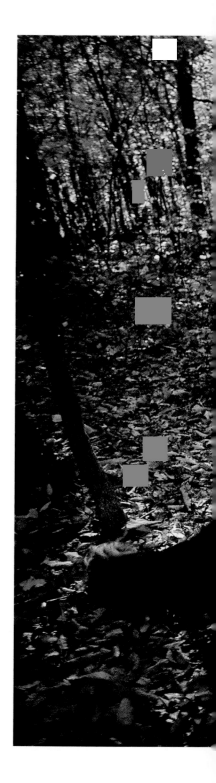

Proving her point—that HIV-positive people can lead active lives and contribute to society—Dawn Averitt, accompanied by her dog, Guinness (right), hikes the 2,160-mile-long Appalachian Trail from Maine to Georgia (left). Her exercise and attitude probably help combat the disease, and she diligently takes all the anti-HIV drugs (above) her physicians prescribe. Drug combinations, growing more common in medicine, essentially replicate the basic approach taken by nature: Numerous bioactive substances interact with each other while having an impact on the human body.

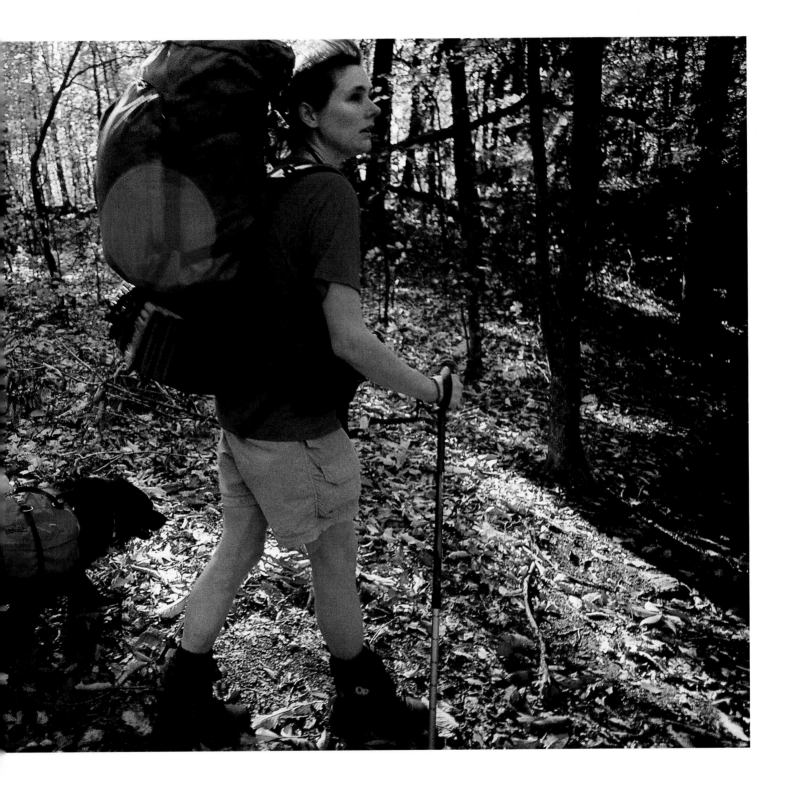

humans, ants seem to have been using antibiotics for perhaps millions of years without triggering resistance. How have they done it?

————

A FEW PLANTS BEING STUDIED today may become superstars like the rosy periwinkle and the Pacific yew. Given that advanced screening capability began to emerge in the mid-1980s, and the fact that it usually takes more than a decade for a new drug to receive approval for clinical use, some in-the-pipeline drugs might be available soon.

Among contenders is Calanolide A, derived from one *Calophyllum lanigerum* tree. This tall evergreen grows in Sarawak, the Malaysian portion of the island of Borneo, and its wood has numerous colors, ranging from yellow brown to deep red, which makes it particularly attractive as lumber. Calanolide A, which has been synthesized, has been extremely effective at killing the virus associated with AIDS.

Other possible drugs that fight cancer and the virus that causes AIDS include 9AC, or a-amino-camptothecin, a derivative of camptothecin, an alkaloid found in a Chinese ornamental tree; harringtonine and homoharringtonine from a small Chinese evergreen tree; phyllanthoside, from a tree native to Central America; (1)-calanolide B (costatolide) also from *Calophyllum lanigerum*; conocurvone, from a shrub that grows in Western Australia; and ellipticine, from a bush native to Fiji. Other drugs—such as michellamine B, from the leaves of a vine that grows in Cameroon, and ipomeanol, obtained from a fungus that grows on sweet potato plants—have shown promise but seem to be too toxic for human use. Clinical studies using some of these drugs have been dropped, at least for now, because of their extreme toxicity. Some of these substances are being given to patients in countries where drug regulations are less strict than in the United States. At a minimum, these chemicals may stimulate scientists to create synthetic variations that prove effective.

————

WHILE ALL THIS SCIENTIFIC work grinds on, the news media continue to whet appetites with variations of the lost-miracle-cure story.

A typical lost-miracle-cure tale goes something like this: Ethnobotanists explore a remote rain forest. They are the first, or among the first, outsiders to enter the region. They take leaf, bark, and berry samples from a particular tree. Perhaps they identify this tree after building a relationship with a local healer, or maybe humans have never used the tree before. It makes no particular impression on them, and it is among hundreds of plants they sample.

Upon returning home, ethnobotanists submit these samples for testing and go on

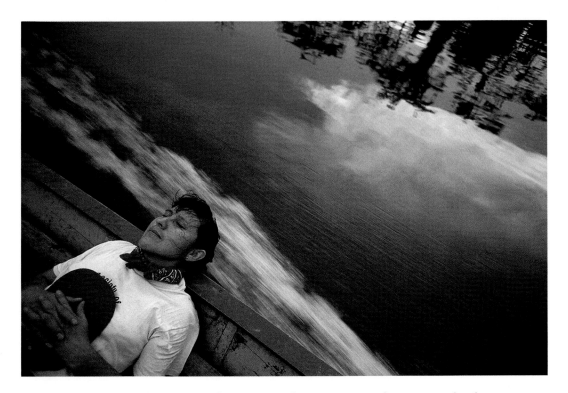

Elsa Meza, who works for a major pharmaceutical company, snatches a nap as her boat moves farther into the Amazonian rain forest of Peru. She gathers plant specimens, often with the advice of local healers, to be sent to the United States for laboratory testing of their potential as drugs. Plant collectors must work with the host country's permission; without it they commit what has come to be called "biopiracy."

to their next assignment. Then a call comes from the pharmaceutical laboratory. Bells are going off. "Where did this tree come from?" people at the laboratory ask. "It has a novel molecular structure with new ways of acting against cancer." Or, maybe it seems to provide human cells with 100 percent protection against the virus that causes AIDS. Laboratory scientists need more samples in order to continue their work.

Another ethnobotanical team returns to the same rain forest to get more samples from the tree. But something is wrong. The area is no longer wild. It looks barren. A logging company has cut down most of the trees, including the one they are looking for. All that remains where it stood is a stump. Trees almost like it are still standing, however, and the ethnobotanists take samples. They test well but are not nearly as potent as the now forever-gone tree.

This story has elements of a classic fairy tale—the quest for a lifesaving potion, a journey into unknown dark areas, destruction by unseen forces, and universal lessons. It also involves a forest, which is often the site of magical events in dreams.

Such stories make good news copy because they are so appealing. Who doesn't want to believe that "juju" is out there, waiting to be found? Anyone who has suffered from a major disease, or who has loved someone who suffered from a disease such as cancer, knows what just one new magic bullet could mean.

Many of the facts in these lost-miracle-cure *(Continued on page 286)*

A villager in Milagro, Peru, holds the heart-shaped leaves of a *sangre de drago*—dragon blood—tree, which is named after the blood-red color of its sap. Traditional healers use this sap to treat a range of ailments including cuts, ulcers, bronchitis, diarrhea, and dental problems. Dragon blood also contains compounds with strong antiviral capability.

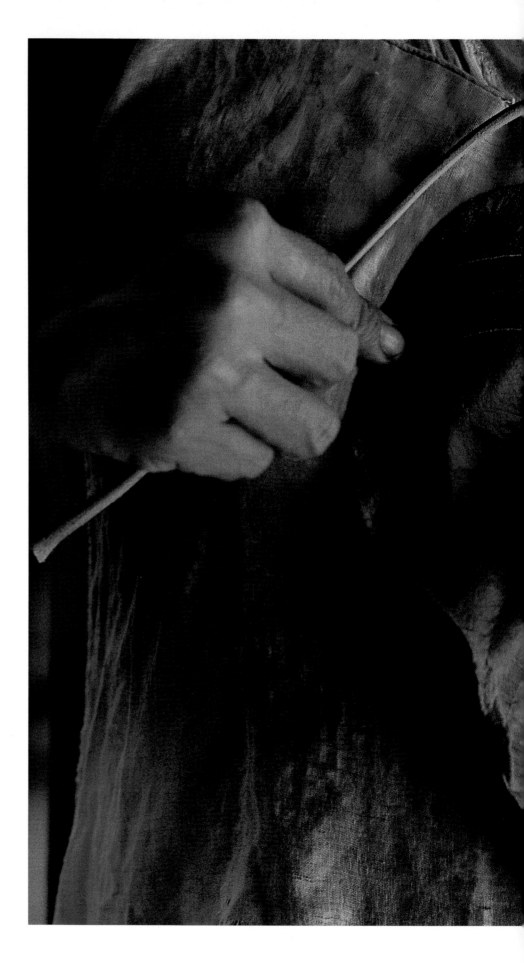

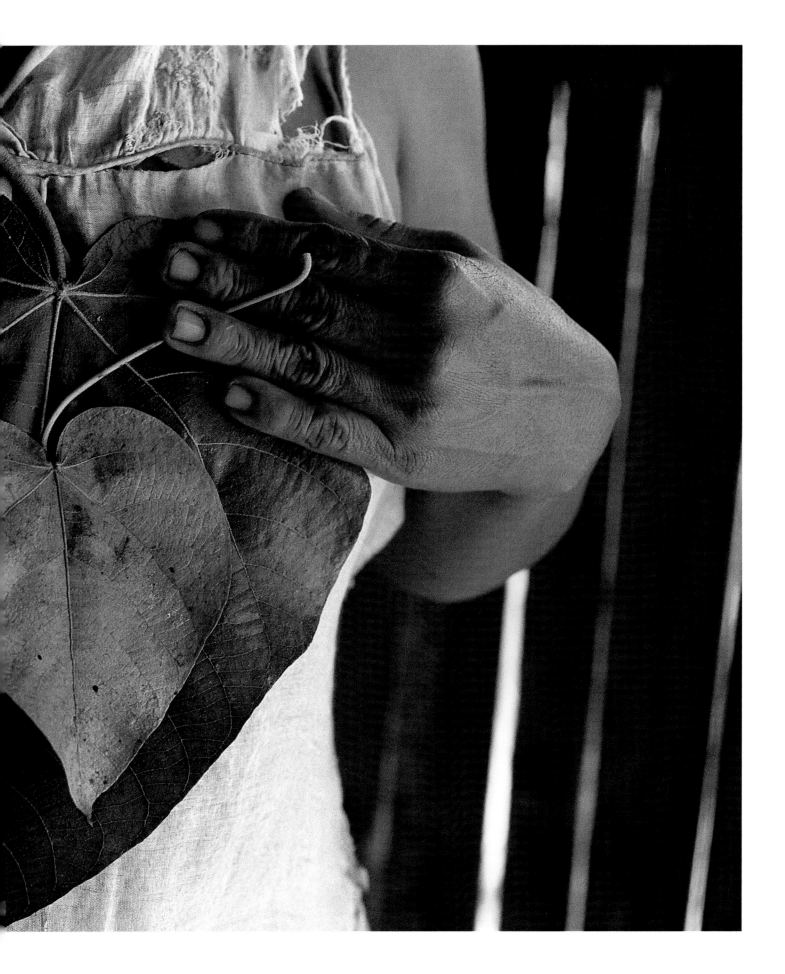

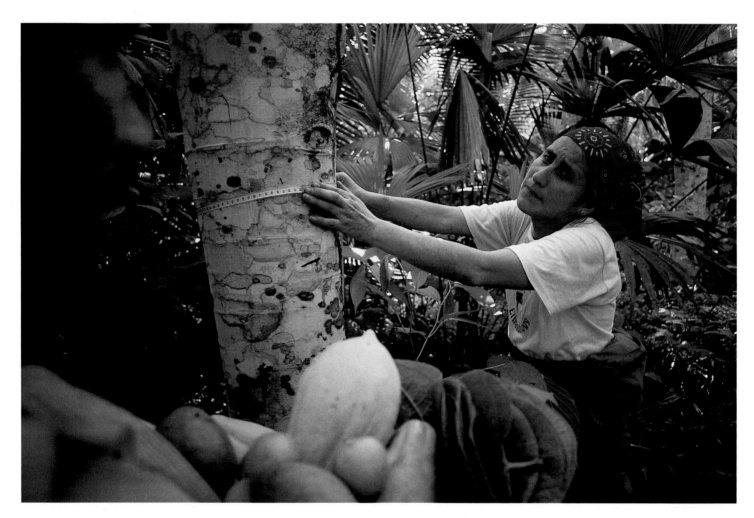

Measuring a dragon blood tree, Elsa Meza urges villagers in Milagro to wait for it to mature before extracting the sap. Pharmaceutical research has shown that the sap can be an effective treatment for diarrhea. It acts on the secretory mechanisms of the intestinal tract.

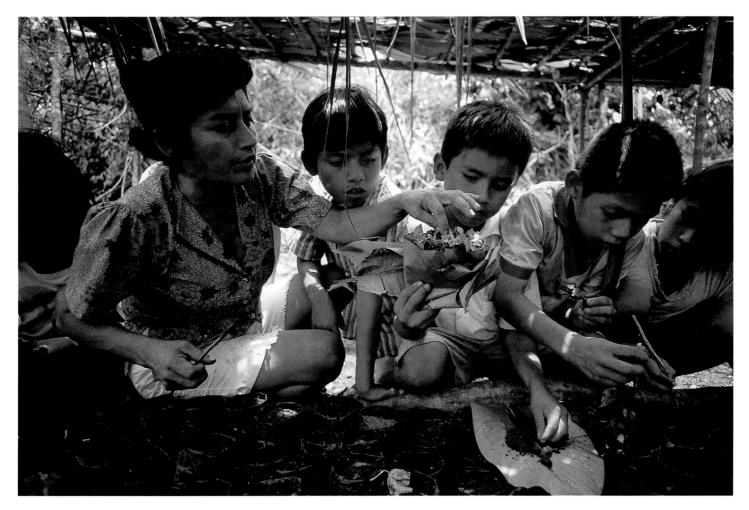

Local teacher Celia Pishagua guides her students as they plant dragon blood seedlings in Milagro. When the trees mature, the villagers will profit from their hard work. Preserving biodiversity and stimulating young people to care about it are essential if local cultures—with their knowledge of medicinal plants—are to survive.

stories are true. But the tales have more to do with psychology, our need for hope, and the dynamics of the news profession—the need for exciting copy—than they do with drug discovery. They ignore the real-life ending. Even if the tree cited above had been rediscovered in good shape, and even if the laboratory scientists had received all the samples they needed, given the record of modern science's relationship with plants, chances are overwhelming that no drug would ever be developed.

———

To find exciting plants achieves little if the plants are then judged solely on whether scientists can isolate and replicate one of their active components.

Ernest Hemingway's warning, never to confuse movement with action, seems applicable here. Screening provides considerable movement. Plants are gathered and checked, money is spent, jobs are created, numbers are added, scientific papers are published, and numerous plant chemicals demonstrate activity against disease. But how much action, in the form of actual treatments for disease, is there?

Never before has a society collected so much information about medicinal plants that it is unable to use.

Perhaps one solution is to improve screens, the gateway through which all plant chemicals must pass. It may become possible, for example, to detect plant chemicals that boost the human immune system. So far, this has proved to be too difficult because of the immune system's inherent complexity. To test for chemicals that affect a specific cancer is, by comparison, much simpler. These tests can expose the cancer cells to a compound and measure with relative ease whether the cancer has been adversely affected. Screens for plant chemicals effective against chronic conditions like arthritis, or useful in treating a wide range of genetic disorders, have likewise eluded researchers. But that does not mean they always will. Improved screens may someday identify plant chemicals that inhibit the growth of cancer cells, as opposed to killing them, thus opening up a range of less toxic cancer treatments.

Despite such possibilities, modern medicine may never utilize the full medicinal power of plants unless it devises a way to move beyond reliance on the single active compound.

The latest advances in modern medicine help keep a premature baby in Seattle, Washington, alive. Also essential to her well-being is contact with her father. Heart-to-heart, skin-to-skin contact reduces the baby's stress and heart rate. The role of herbal medicine in this emerging balance between high technology and the natural basics remains to be seen.

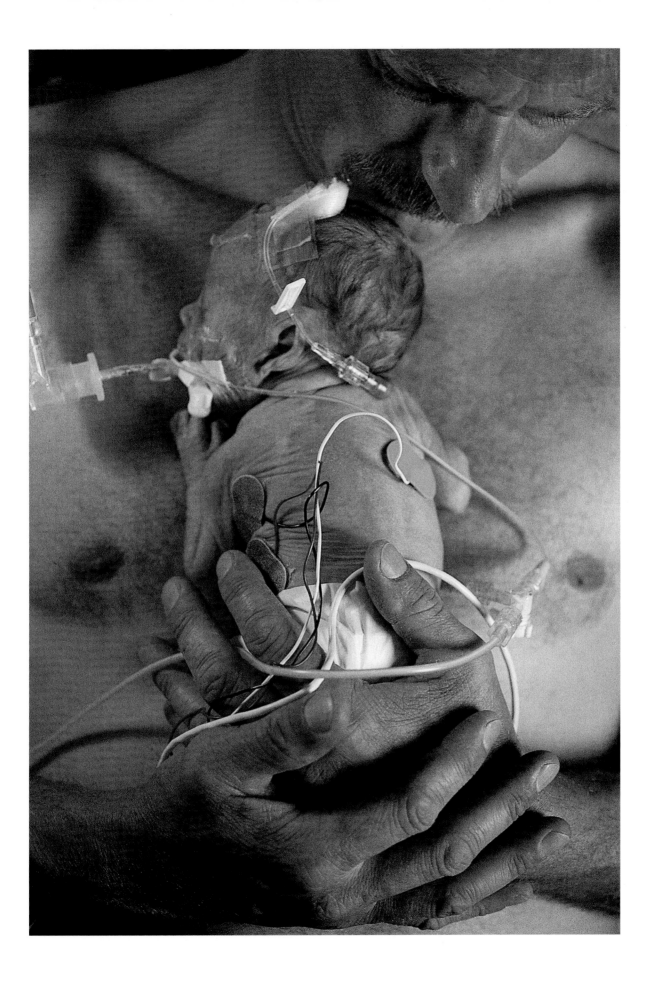

CHAPTER EIGHT

Can Herbs Heal You?

Studies in laboratory animals show that green tea can reduce or eliminate malignant tumors. It contains epigallocatechin gallate (EGCG), a compound that inhibits an enzyme called urokinase—which cancer cells need in order to grow and spread. Black tea, which is most commonly consumed in the West, comes from the same plant as does green tea but has no documented anticancer effects. Black tea leaves are allowed to oxidize and ferment before drying, which eliminates much of the EGCG. Green tea leaves are steamed immediately after picking. This process removes the enzyme that promotes oxidation, thus preserving the EGCG.

Epidemiological evidence shows that cancer rates, particularly gastrointestinal cancers, are very low throughout parts of China, Japan, and other Asian countries in which green tea is popular. Whether consumption of green tea contributes to these low cancer rates remains unknown.

Bioactive chemicals in flowering plants—some of the most complex chemicals in all of nature—helped them survive whatever killed the dinosaurs. Processing will soon transform this freshly cut batch of calendula, mint, orange peel, chamomile, and other blossoms into an herbal remedy. Such medicines can fight disease and stimulate the body's own healing powers in ways that modern science is just beginning to understand.

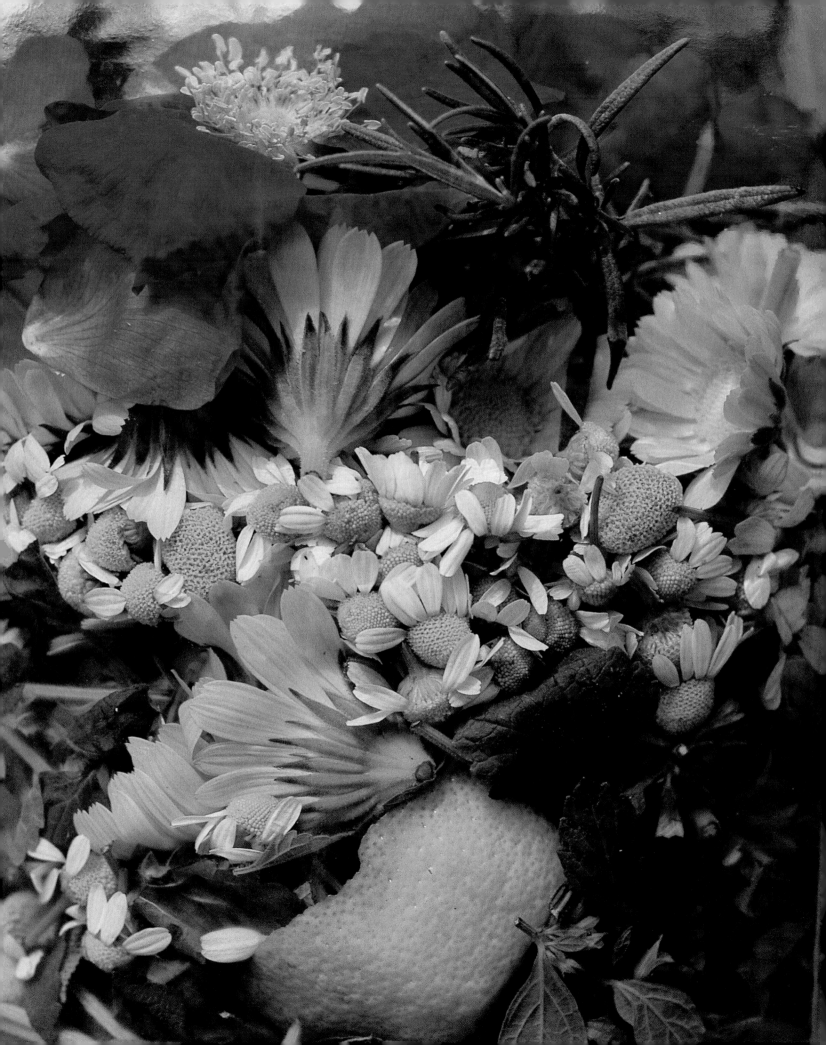

MODERN SCIENCE MAY be making a fundamental mistake by looking for the single active compound. Such efforts could be doomed to failure, like opening a radio and trying to find the one component piece that produces the sound. Scientists could focus more on the whole plant and combinations of plants, with their uncounted and unidentified bioactive compounds that act upon each other as they interact with the human body. The study of whole plants and combinations is rare—largely because single active compounds, particularly those that have been modified, are easiest to patent and because FDA regulations encourage this approach.

Furthermore, pharmaceutical companies and other research institutions have invested tens of billions of dollars in laboratories, equipment, and other facilities devoted to finding single active compounds. To them, successful research consists primarily of the synthesis and manipulation of individual molecules.

Some scientists, however, have conducted studies that take a broader view of plants. These studies meet and maintain high standards of accuracy—including what pharmacological researchers consider their most exacting procedure: the randomized, double-blind, placebo-controlled trial.

In this type of trial, which came into use in the 1950s and has dominated Western medicine since the 1970s, patients are randomly divided into two groups. Neither the subjects nor the doctors know who is receiving medicine or a placebo, essentially a sugar pill with no pharmacological effect. Placebos can be especially important when testing botanical medicines because skeptics often say that any positive effects of these medicines are derived from the power of suggestion. Some botanicals work, these skeptics say, not because they have any physiological effect, but because people believe they will work, thus prompting their own bodies to generate compounds that promote healing.

In the last decade of the 20th century, a series of double-blind, placebo-controlled studies focused on a plant used to treat one of mankind's most common viral infections, hepatitis B, which can remain dormant for years but may lead to chronic liver disease and liver cancer. A vaccine against hepatitis B, available since the early 1990s, does nothing to help about 300 million carriers, most of them in developing countries.

In the late 1980s an international team of scientists headed by Baruch Blumberg, who won the 1976 Nobel Prize in medicine for his work on infectious viral diseases, used written and oral sources about traditional healing to identify nearly 2,000 plants used to treat jaundice, a symptom of hepatitis. The researchers sorted these plants by species and use-patterns, then selected some 150 species whose use seemed to be

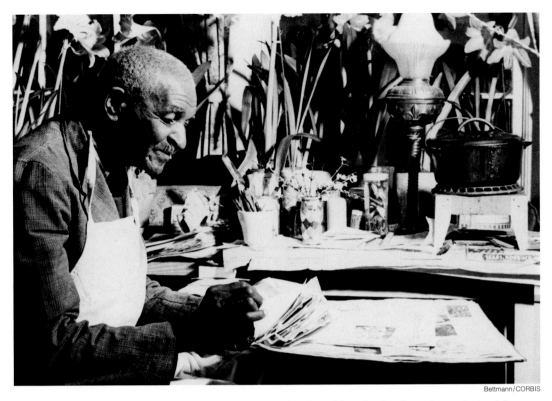

Bettmann/CORBIS

Botanist George Washington Carver (1864-1943) developed hundreds of products derived from peanuts, soybeans, and other plants. Carver believed that peanut oil improved a traditional treatment for respiratory problems. He developed a peanut product for treating coughs, sore throat, and bronchitis as well as other illnesses.

supported by the most convincing evidence. The plants came from Europe, North America, the Caribbean, and Asia.

Of these 150 plants the scientists decided that the most promising was *Phyllanthus amarus*, a plant from India that Ayurvedic healers have used for more than 2,000 years to treat jaundice and other illnesses. The researchers did not identify the active principles in *Phyllanthus amarus*. Instead, they extracted a combination of chemicals that in laboratory tests bound themselves to, and presumably disrupted, the replication or development of the hepatitis B virus.

As the scientists prepared for human trials, they knew that using the extract of the plant and measuring its presumed effect on the virus could fail to capture the full impact of *Phyllanthus amarus*. Their approach certainly was a far narrower view of the plant than is designated in ancient Sanskrit and Tamil literature, which always specifies using whole parts of the plant, such as its flower. But the study design gave scientists variables they could define, standardize, observe, and measure.

The extract, taken in a capsule three times a day by human carriers of the hepatitis B virus, produced dramatic results. As reported in the prestigious journal *Lancet*, surface antigens for the virus, essentially the biological effect of the virus's existence, disappeared from the blood of two-thirds of the people treated with the plant extract. Only one of 23 people in the control group, who took placebo capsules, experienced similar results.

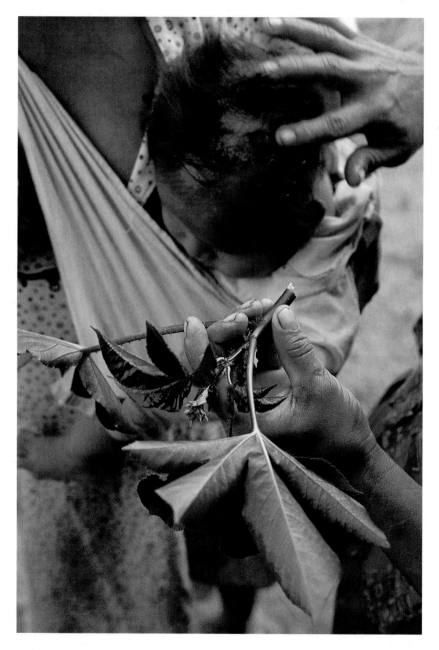

In Milagro, Peru, plant sap eases skin problems such as the infected mosquito bite on a baby's scalp (above). Science has not tested most herbal remedies like this one, but no other type of medical treatment is available for this baby and many other sufferers. A woman in Madagascar coats her face with paste from the root of the *tomotamo* plant, a member of the ginger family (opposite). The paste makes skin smooth, tender, and younger looking—and also provides protection against sunburn.

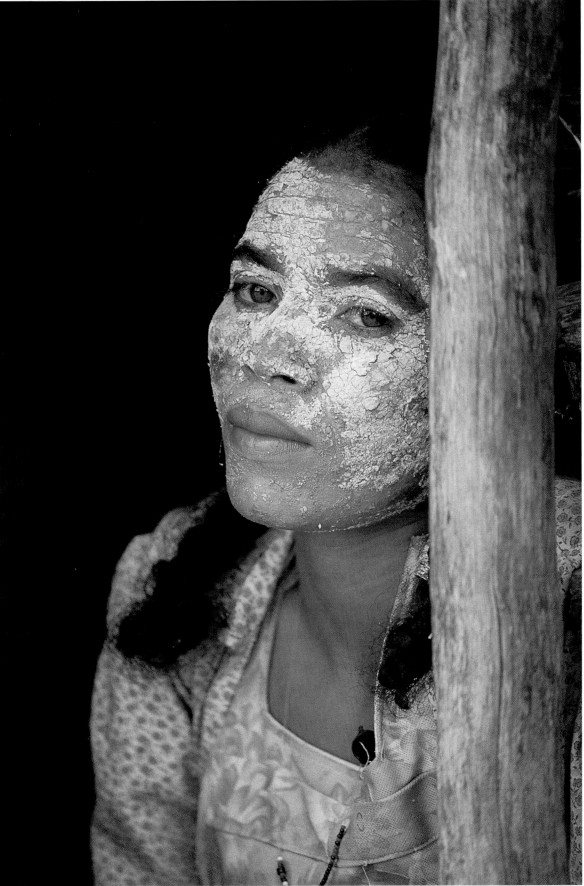

293

Encouraged by the results, other researchers tried to replicate them. In some studies the *Phyllanthus amarus* seemed to act against the virus; in others it did not. Numerous explanations were offered. Because the plants used in these studies were grown in different places and collected at various times, they may not have contained the same levels of bioactive molecules. Some studies used plants grown in India; others used plants grown in China. Drying and shipping the plants could have affected their chemical potency.

Whatever the reason for the ambiguous results, they ended major clinical trials of *Phyllanthus amarus*. It was, in addition, difficult to raise money for research into a remedy that would have had a limited market in developed countries, whose citizens have been immunized against hepatitis B. Researchers in Hong Kong and mainland China, however, have created a new pill consisting of *Phyllanthus* and Chinese herbs. They claim this pill can inhibit reproduction of the virus associated with hepatitis B, prevent the liver from becoming too fibrous, and improve liver function. While never stating that this pill cures hepatitis B, they promise it can keep the rate of hepatitis recurrence low. The cost per patient is up to 2,000 dollars a month. Such pills may offer patients access to healing plants that could save their lives, but the potential for abuse is clear. People who carry a deadly virus and worry about developing a fatal illness are asked to pay as much as 24,000 dollars a year for a remedy whose effectiveness has not been proved.

––––––––

STUDIES OF BOTANICAL REMEDIES that treat skin diseases offer less ambiguous results. One study conducted in England in the early 1990s used a combination of Chinese herbs to treat atopic dermatitis, a disease of unknown origin that is characterized by red, thickening, and scaling patches of skin, usually on the face, feet, and hands. All the herbs—including burra gookeroo, dictamnus, peony, rehmannia, licorice, potentilla, nepeta, and clematis—were processed into a drink according to the dictates of ancient Chinese pharmacopoeias.

In an article published in *Lancet*, the researchers explained that this herbal treatment dates back thousands of years, but that they did not adopt the basic principles of traditional Chinese medicine. "Rather," they said, "we applied Western methods of clinical diagnosis" and used the herbs as a "conventional drug prescription." The Western doctors, for example, used the exact same herbs on every patient. A traditional Chinese doctor would have prescribed an individualized combination of the herbs, as well as different changes in diet, for each patient.

All patients participating in the study had severe cases of atopic dermatitis that modern medicine had been unable to help. Patients in the control group drank the same amount of a placebo combination of herbs with "no known benefit to atopic dermatitis," but which had "a similar smell and taste to the active treatment."

One of the advantages of studying skin diseases is that results are relatively easy to see and measure. As reported in *Lancet*, every patient taking the Chinese herbal experienced "a rapid and continued improvement in both erythema [redness of the skin] and surface damage scores…." This study demonstrated, the authors concluded, "that TCHT [traditional Chinese herbal therapy] affords substantial clinical benefit in patients whose atopic dermatitis had been unresponsive to conventional therapy."

The authors reported that "an understanding of the pharmacological basis for the beneficial effect" of these plants is "limited," but emphasized that the plants are known to have anti-inflammatory, sedative, and immunosuppressive effects. The plants also could have stimulated the patients' genes to produce particular enzymes.

A similar study examined the effect of Chinese herbs on children with severe atopic dermatitis. Ten herbs were ground, boiled, and given orally. A placebo group took carefully selected herbs just as the patients in the adult experiment did. The results were promising: improvement in condition for 91.4 percent treated with the Chinese remedy and 10.6 percent in the placebo group.

In a follow-through to both studies, researchers found that patients who continued to take the Chinese herbs over a protracted period "maintained the benefits of the therapy with minimal side effects," and that those who discontinued the treatment "experienced a decline in their condition."

Other studies, also published in major Western medical journals in the 1990s, document how Chinese herbs, combined and prepared according to traditional Chinese specifications, have proved successful in treating eczema. As with the treatment of atopic dermatitis, how and why these herbs worked remains unknown. One of the principal components of the eczema treatment was the tree peony flower, whose alkaloids constrict capillaries connected to the kidneys—which would have no identifiable effect on eczema.

———

PUBLICATION OF SUCH STUDIES is still unusual in a Western scientific community devoted to the single active compound. Remedies with numerous active compounds, however, are far from new to modern science, which increasingly relies on multimodal treatments, the use of more than one drug at the same time. One prominent example is the "AIDS cocktail," a combination of several types of drugs. Other combinations include chemotherapy cocktails to treat cancer; treatment with four or more antibiotics to cure tuberculosis; and simultaneous use of two or more drugs to treat heart attacks, malaria,

An increasing number of studies report that fruits and vegetables—like those sold by a street vendor in Luxor, Egypt—combat disease. Epidemiological studies in the United States document that people who eat certain levels of fruits and vegetables have significantly lower rates of cancer, heart attacks, and strokes. Researchers have identified a range of plant chemicals that may be responsible.

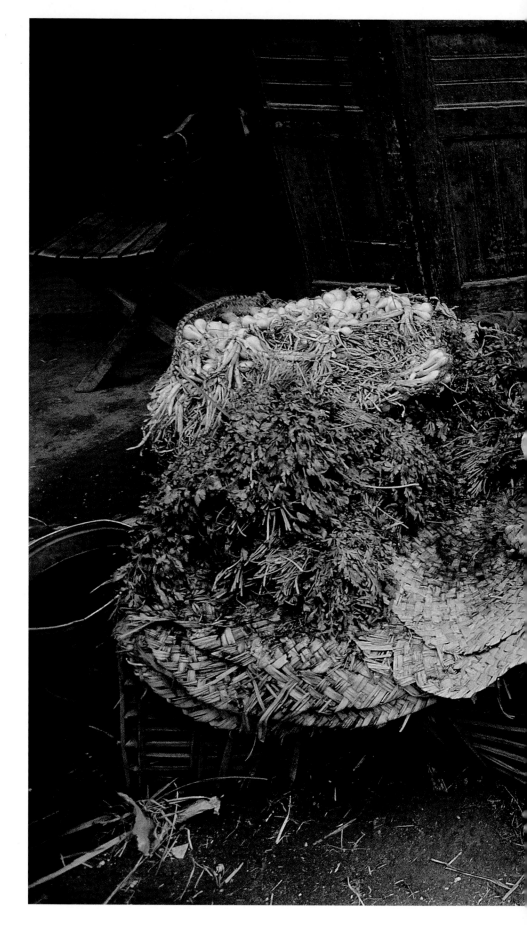

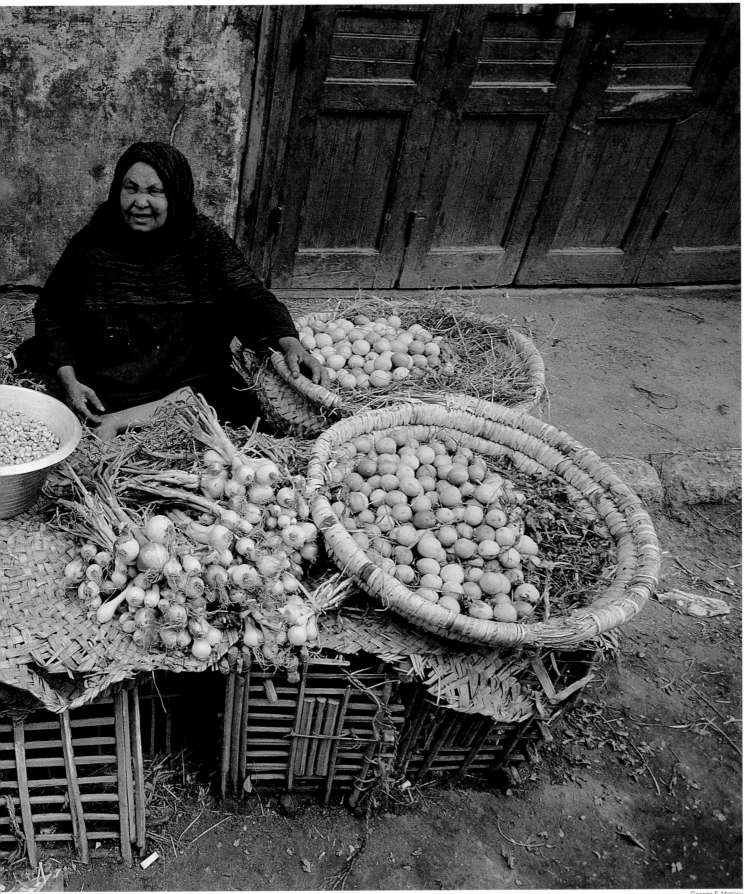

297

rheumatoid arthritis, chronic hepatitis C infections, and diabetes. Such multimodal treatments usually combine unrelated drugs that act in different ways on different parts of the body. Treatment for difficult cases of diabetes, for example, may combine two standard drugs, one that reduces the liver's production of blood sugar and another that makes muscles more sensitive to insulin.

In every case of multimodal treatment, doctors do not know how the drugs interact with each other or act in unison upon the human body. Many of the multidrug treatments, furthermore, have never been tested in double-blind studies. Doctors have simply found that their patients do better when taking the drugs in combination. Success with such combinations is fostering further experimentation. "I like their synergy," says one doctor who has started to use two antibiotics together to treat certain infections. He, like all doctors using multimodalities, follows a model set by botanical medicine: Use a complex prescription and judge it by results, not by knowing exactly what it is or how it works.

It is impossible to know whether malpractice lawsuits may arise from multimodal treatments whose effects have not been documented or whether modern medicine's use of such multimodalities indicates a willingness to move beyond a reliance on the single active molecule. Change in attitude and expectation comes hard to all professions, and the process by which accepted wisdom changes can be slow and painful. Full exploration of multimodalities—and botanical medicine—may have to await the passing of the generation that grew up with the belief that good medicines are magic bullets. Jacques Monod, who won the 1965 Nobel Prize in medicine for describing the genetic regulation of enzyme and virus synthesis, says that the scientific community often reacts in two stages to a new idea. First, people say that the new idea is absurd, and then they call it obvious.

———

IN THE MEANTIME, evidence of the extraordinary power of another type of multimodality continues to mount. Hundreds of studies document with unexpected consistency the powerful effects of chemicals in fruits and vegetables, and all support the same conclusion: The more fruits and vegetables people eat, the less likely they are to suffer heart attacks, strokes, or cancer—the three biggest killers in the United States. Some of the results offer surprises. For example, chocolate, its fat and sugar content notwithstanding, has chemicals that may act as a cardiac stimulant and lower the risk of heart disease.

Much evidence about the impact of fruits and vegetables comes from studies that gather information on behavior, such as diet, as well as on disease, over long periods of time. "The Nurses Study" conducted by the Brigham and Women's Hospital in Boston has followed the medical histories of 121,701 nurses since 1976. Such epidemiological

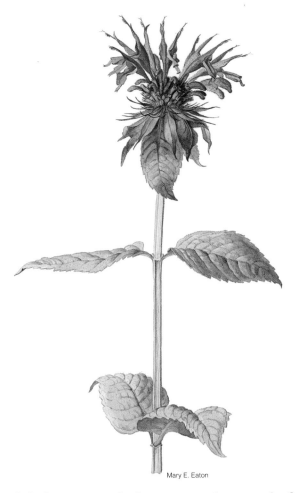

Mary E. Eaton

The fragrant aroma of the bergamot—also known as scarlet monarda, Oswego tea, and bee balm—resembles that of orange blossoms. Native Americans use bergamot to treat a wide range of ailments including coughs, cuts, headaches, and chills. Many people today use a related species to combat digestive problems.

studies have a proven record, but care must be taken to interview people in a timely manner and to avoid jumping to conclusions even when relationships seem obvious. A Scottish scientist in the late 18th century observed that slaves locked in cargo holds of ships often developed scurvy—and concluded that one cause of the disease was the lack of fresh air. Scurvy is actually caused by Vitamin C deficiency.

Epidemiological insights also come from patterns within entire societies. The cow-herding Masai people of east Africa, for example, eat 2,000 milligrams of cholesterol a day, double to quadruple the average American intake, yet Masai have low cholesterol levels and little heart disease. The plants they eat along with meat may lessen the negative effects of, or break down, cholesterol.

Logically, it makes sense that fruits and vegetables fight disease. If substances from plants such as the Madagascar rosy periwinkle and the Pacific yew kill cancer, why shouldn't plants that people eat as food do the same thing? Not much is known, however, about precisely how and why this disease-fighting effect occurs. The reasons are difficult to pinpoint because plant foods, like medicinal plants, consist of hundreds, and perhaps thousands, of chemicals.

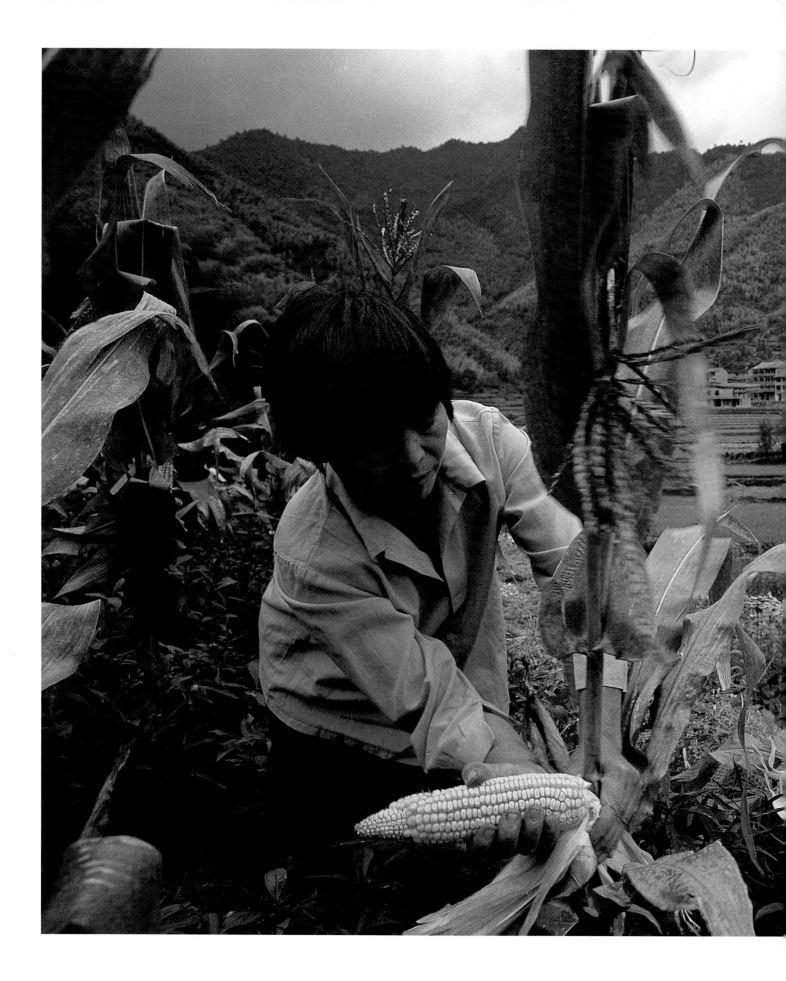

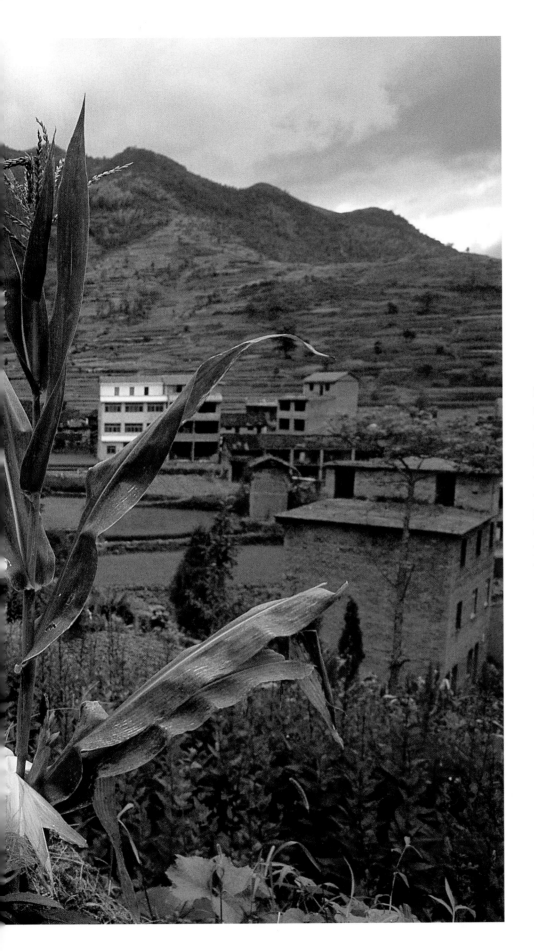

Farmers in northeast China, like their counterparts throughout most of the developing world, often cultivate food and medicinal crops side-by-side. Numerous medicinal herbs grow behind this woman picking corn. The herbs will be sold to local healers and in the markets of nearby cities. As the developing world becomes more urban, most people continue to depend on traditional herbal medicine.

It is possible that what seem to be active agents in food only indicate other chemicals that have not been identified, but studies suggest that a variety of known compounds are responsible. These compounds are called nutriceuticals, a word coined in the early 1990s to describe components in dietary fruits and vegetables that may have little or no food value, but that help prevent and treat disease.

The concept of fruits and vegetables as medicine has an important precedent in vitamins, which were called "accessory food factors" when first identified in the early 20th century. Lack of sufficient vitamins can result in debilitating and often-fatal diseases such as scurvy and beriberi, just as lack of sufficient nutriceuticals can lead to disease.

Well-known nutriceuticals include alpha-carotene, beta-carotene, beta-catechins, canthaxanthin, deguelin, ellagic acid, indoles, isoflavones, lutein, lycopene, phenethyl isothiocyanate, rypotoxanthin, and sulforaphane; and potential stars include conjugated linoleic acid, fucoxanthin, inositol hexaphosphate, klevitone, and protocatechuic acid. Many of these compounds are gaining repute as new findings generate attention from the news media. Which will prove to be the best disease-fighters must await the results of ongoing research, but in the meantime the ways in which they work are becoming better understood. Many nutriceuticals are antioxidants, which neutralize free radicals—molecules that have an unpaired electron and are highly reactive—produced when cells burn oxygen to create energy. Experts estimate that free radicals attack the average human cell ten thousand times each day, causing great damage. They can change free-flowing cholesterol into another version of cholesterol that sticks to the walls of arteries and contributes to the diseases of aging such as osteoporosis, cataracts, macular degeneration, and mental decline.

Other disease-preventing compounds in fruits and vegetables include detoxifiers, which prompt human cells to produce enzymes that neutralize carcinogens, agents that cause cancer. Detoxifiers can attach themselves to carcinogens and remove them from cells, promote repair of damaged DNA, block formation of premalignant cells, and stimulate the liver to produce enzymes that eliminate cancer-causing molecules from the body.

Fruits and vegetables also contain disease-fighting vitamins, such as A, C, and E, as well as important minerals such as calcium and zinc. Further health benefits of the plants come from compounds that regulate cell actions and from hormone regulators such as phytoestrogens that mimic the activity of human hormones.

Phytoestrogens—estrogens produced by soy and a range of other plants including flax, alfalfa, yams, broccoli, cauliflower, and brussels sprouts—provide one possible

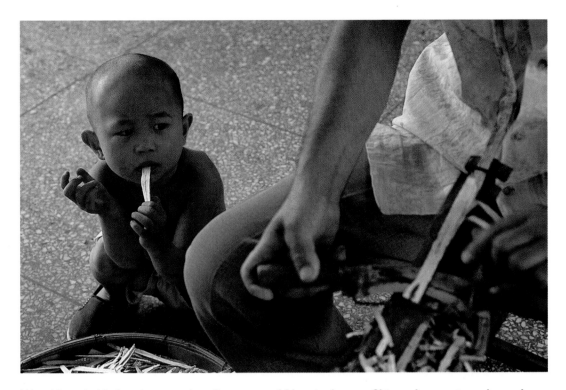

Watching nimble hands at work, a four-year-old boy in Anguo, China, chews astragalus as he studies a worker slicing the root into paper-thin strips. The dried slivers will be sold in Anguo's bustling marketplace. Chinese traditional medicine uses astragalus as a diuretic and to stimulate the immune system. Research shows that it does cause bone marrow to produce more microbe- and virus-fighting cells.

example of why plants produce bioactive compounds. By mimicking mammal estrogen, phytoestrogens, which seem to have only one-thousandth the chemical power of mammal estrogen, help protect plants by reducing the fertility of grazing animals. Plant production of phytoestrogens, in fact, is often highest during animal mating season.

In human females phytoestrogens may reduce the chances of breast cancer and other estrogen-related diseases by attaching themselves to estrogen receptor sites. This decreases the intensity of chemicals accumulating at these sites and thus decreases the likelihood of disease developing. Such actions may be particularly important to women in Western societies. They now menstruate at an earlier age and for a longer time than they did in earlier eras, thus increasing their risk of developing estrogen-related diseases by extending the number of years their breast, and other, cells are exposed to estrogen. Phytoestrogens also seem to provide anticancer protection to males, whose testosterone produces estrogen, which in turn can contribute to prostate cancer.

These processes can become complicated because estrogen consists of a steroid compound that produces various hormones, some of which can be powerful carcinogens. Some phytoestrogens seem to act against these more dangerous hormones.

———————

THE EFFECTS OF CHEMICALS such as phytoestrogens on cancer provide a prime example of how nutriceuticals can act to prevent, as opposed to treat, disease.

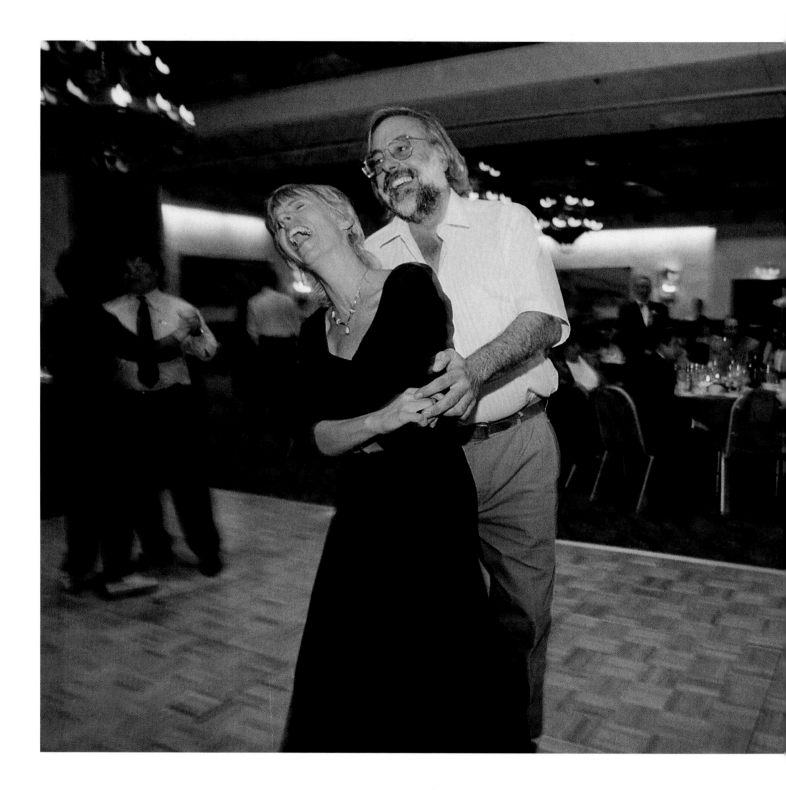

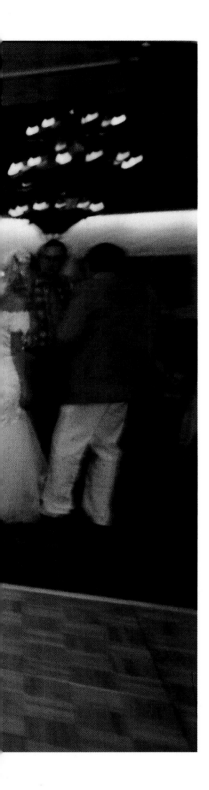

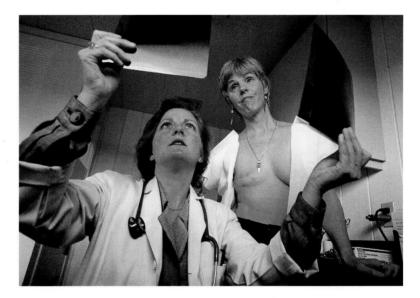

Reading the results of scans evokes a grimace from mastectomy patient Jessica Allen of Santa Fe, New Mexico (above). She battled breast cancer courageously, using surgery and other offerings of modern medicine in combination with more traditional healing techniques such as herbs. She also embraced Native American healing ceremonies based on meditation and intensive prayer. Although the medical treatments and alternative therapies did not ultimately save her life, they probably allowed Jessica more time to experience joy, as she did dancing at her brother's wedding (left).

Archaeological evidence indicates that humans have always combated cancer. Hippocrates called the disease *karcinos*, the Greek for crab, an apparent likening of the pain of the disease to that of being pinched by a crab. Galen, in accordance with his belief in humors, saw the cause of cancer as too many, or improperly flowing, fluids in the body.

Traditional Chinese healers view cancer as a disease that develops because weak or toxic blood cannot nourish body tissues. Deficient blood, in their view, allows pollutants to accumulate in tissues until they become toxic and form malignant tumors. The Chinese advocate using botanical medicines, acupuncture, and other means to detoxify and purify the blood, and then rebuilding it with good nutrition.

Cancer treatments in Europe during the Renaissance included arsenic, mercury, silver, copper, and zinc. None, according to available evidence, did much good. The modern use of chemicals to treat cancer, commonly called chemotherapy, began after World War II, when researchers discovered that mustard gas, which had proved deadly during trench warfare in World War I, is particularly lethal to cells that divide frequently. Some chemotherapeutic drugs most widely used today are close relatives of mustard gas.

Few of these older treatments contributed to the modern scientific understanding of cancer, a condition in which cells endlessly divide and grow. Carcinogens enter cells and disrupt metabolism, causing them to reproduce past their normal life span. Healthy cells die after dividing about 50 to 100 times.

Countless steps must occur before cancer appears, and chemicals from fruits and vegetables can interrupt every one of them. For some cancers, diet during childhood may be especially important. For others, diet could become important as age and cancer risk increase. Many plant chemicals seem to attack cancer when it is most vulnerable, at the earliest stages, which can be 20 or 25 years before anyone first notices it. People who eat soy, for example, have high levels of genistein, a compound that blocks the growth of connective blood vessels for tumors, thereby killing them. Plant chemicals may also stimulate the body's own mechanisms, including detoxification enzymes and tumor-suppressor genes, at least a dozen of which have been identified.

Through such actions, fruits and vegetables are effective not only in preventing cancer but also in helping to fight cancer that has already developed. Cabbage, for example, has a compound called indole-3-carbinol, which slows the growth of certain cancer cells, and citrus fruits have limonene, which seems to inhibit and kill some types of cancer. Many studies suggest exciting possibilities that require further investigation. Breast cancer patients with low levels of alpha-linolenic acid, for example, seem more likely to have the cancer spread. Flaxseed oil provides this acid and may help contain the cancer. Other studies suggest that some nutriceuticals may enhance the effect of cancer chemotherapy and other mainstream cancer treatments.

––––––––

WHILE EATING FRUITS and vegetables is good for a person's health, getting the most out of them is not always simple. How a food is prepared can affect the levels and bioavailability of nutriceuticals. Cooking may destroy them, or it might release a particular chemical, making it more available to the body. To cook garlic seems to eliminate many of its disease-fighting chemicals, but cooking tomatoes significantly increases the availability of lycopenes, chemicals that are effective against some cancers. Studies, furthermore, document that fruits and vegetables ripened on the vine can have higher levels of nutriceuticals, and that eating fruits and vegetables grown organically can mean ingesting fewer harmful toxins and hormones.

The existence of nutriceuticals raises questions about the difference between a food and a medicine. If a food is ingested primarily for medicinal purposes—such as cranberry juice, which curtails the ability of infection-causing bacteria to cling to the walls of the urinary tract—does it become a medicine?

This question is not academic because obtaining therapeutic amounts of food may require extracting chemicals and transforming them into medicines. Most people are probably unwilling to eat several cloves of fresh garlic every day, even though chemicals in garlic lower cholesterol, combat hypertension, and may help fight stomach cancer. Hence, a leading brand of garlic pills contains "aged garlic extract" that claims to deliver chemicals without causing upset stomach or "garlic breath."

Extracts of garlic and other foods deliver far more of the disease-fighting compounds than people can get from eating those foods. The limonene in oranges, for example, seems to slow the formation of tumors and shrink existing tumors. But to get effective levels of limonene someone might have to eat 400 oranges every day. The same is true for nuts, many of which are high in compounds such as ellagic acid, a health-promoting antioxidant.

The very chemical that fights disease may make a food difficult to eat. Sulforaphane in broccoli stimulates enzymes that detoxify chemical carcinogens, but it gives it a bitter taste, perhaps to discourage animals from eating the plant. The broccoli available in stores has been bred to have a milder taste, which makes it less effective against cancer. Research possibilities include new methods of cultivating broccoli sprouts, which can be high in chemicals similar to sulforaphane without the bitter taste; and the creation of a broccoli pill containing concentrated sulforaphane or a synthetic version that has similar effects.

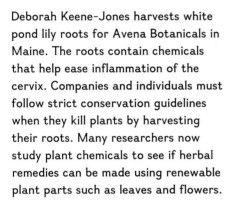

Deborah Keene-Jones harvests white pond lily roots for Avena Botanicals in Maine. The roots contain chemicals that help ease inflammation of the cervix. Companies and individuals must follow strict conservation guidelines when they kill plants by harvesting their roots. Many researchers now study plant chemicals to see if herbal remedies can be made using renewable plant parts such as leaves and flowers.

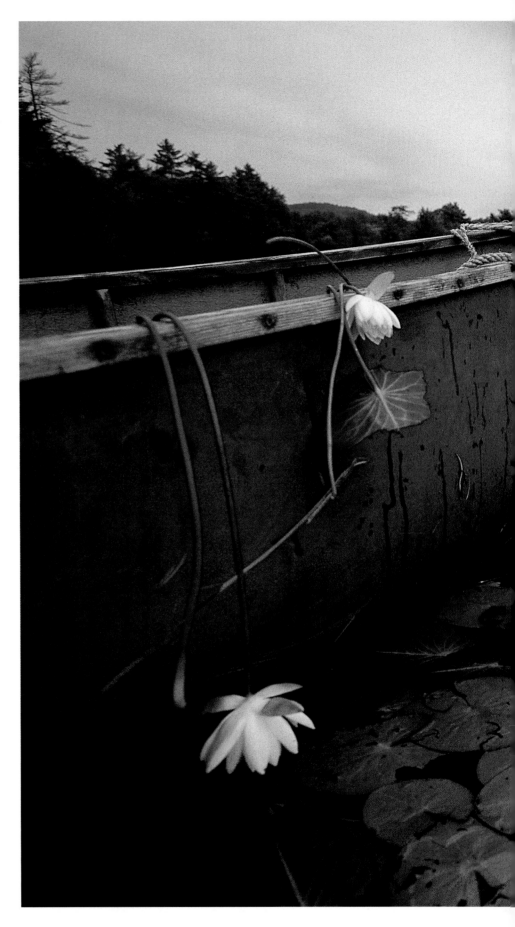

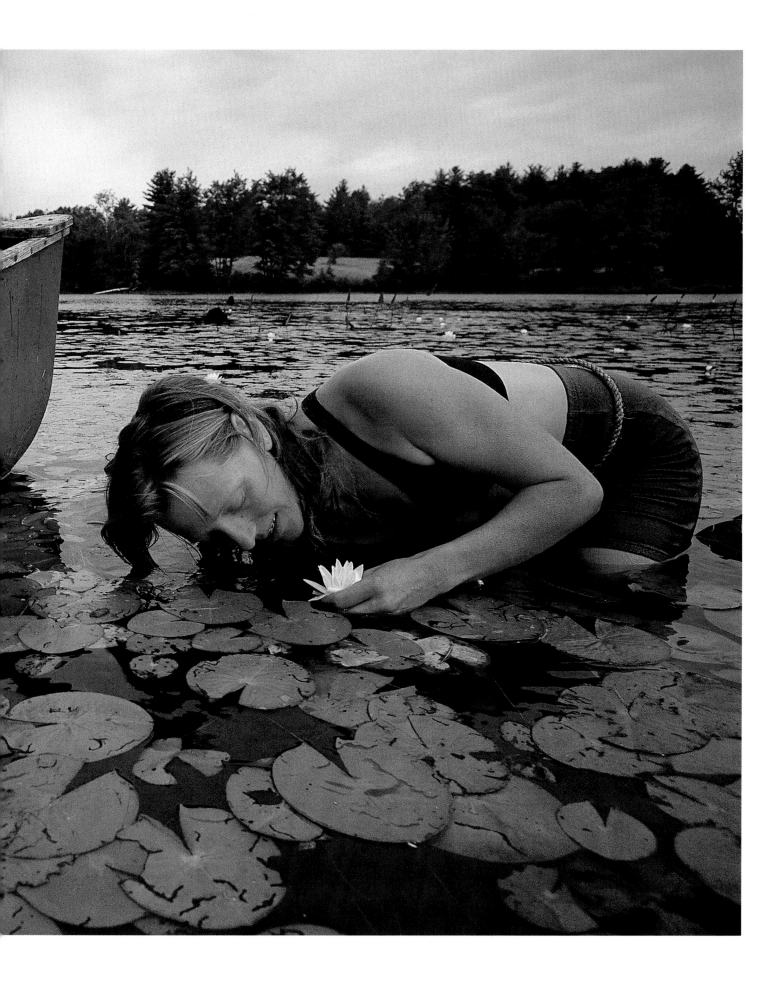

Such pills would transform broccoli into a concentration of cancer-fighting chemicals—perhaps even into a magic bullet. This might work well, but it could sacrifice the benefits, many perhaps not yet identified by modern science, found in the natural package known as broccoli. There may, in fact, be no way to obtain all the benefits of bitter-tasting broccoli without eating it.

————

THE WHOLE PLANT versus single-active-compound argument has become perhaps most emotional in debates about medicinal uses of cannabis, more commonly known as marijuana. Written references to medicinal uses of marijuana date from at least 15th-century B.C. China. These sources mention its use in the treatment of malaria, constipation, rheumatic pains, absentmindedness, and female disorders. Western scientific articles published in the 19th century include claims that marijuana can help treat depression, glaucoma, insomnia, asthma, nausea, and anorexia. More recent studies indicate that marijuana helps lower pressure within the eye, which can help people with glaucoma keep their vision; control muscle spasms, which is crucial for people with multiple sclerosis, spinal cord injury, epilepsy, paraplegia, and quadriplegia; and combat nausea and pain for people enduring chemotherapy.

Much of the debate centers around whether a pill consisting of tetrahydrocannabinol (THC), a compound extracted from marijuana, achieves these results just as effectively as smoking marijuana, without the risks of addiction, health problems, and law-enforcement complications. Advocates of using the whole plant point out that marijuana has about 400 known compounds, any number of which might be necessary to maximize its medicinal benefit. One possible solution to the problem is the use of prescription-only marijuana patches that could deliver the same chemicals as the smoke, but without the toxins. Medical marijuana has attracted considerable attention—e.g., in the late 1990s, voters in California, Arizona, and the District of Columbia overwhelmingly authorized its use—in part because botanical medicines are gaining in popularity.

Despite the frequent absence of reliable guarantees about safety, quality, and honesty of claims, more and more people are expressing faith in a "green bullet." Americans spent 13 to 15 billion dollars in 1998 for herbals, vitamins, and minerals—an increase of about 30 percent in just one year. Such sales may make these products the fastest growing items in America's mass-market retail trade, and they have triggered a movement of botanical medicines from health food stores to drugstore and supermarket chains.

The growing popularity of botanical remedies—which some experts now call the invisible mainstream—can also be seen in the large number of magazines, newsletters,

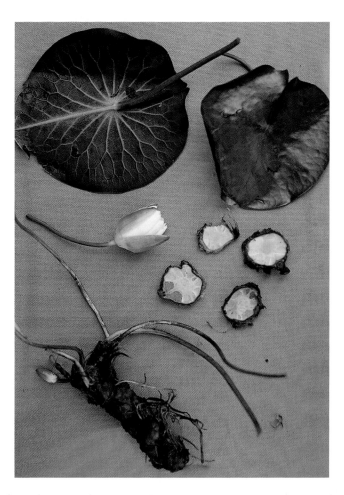

Dissecting a pond lily tuber reveals that its shape resembles a woman's reproductive organs. Herbalists, guided by what they called the doctrine of signatures, believed that the shape of a medicinal plant indicated what ailments it might treat and how it should be prescribed.

websites, radio programs, and books devoted to them. The goal in *Resident Evil 2*, a 1998 video game, is to stop the spread of an evil virus. In the game's action, green herbs increase health, blue herbs act as antidotes to poison, and red herbs are most cherished. Combining red with green herbs increases the green herbs' ability to improve health.

Developing countries, particularly those with emerging Western-oriented middle and upper classes, are experiencing the same growth in the popularity of botanical medicines. Wild ginseng is being depleted in the U.S. because of demand for it in Asia, where many people regard it as a cure-all. A black market in wild ginseng, now called "green gold," has spawned ginseng poachers in Virginia and North Carolina.

Overharvesting of medicinal plants is a serious problem. The Convention on International Trade in Endangered Species of Wild Fauna and Flora (CITES), a 146-nation consortium formed in 1975, lists goldenseal, which has annual sales of more than 250,000 pounds in the U.S. alone, as threatened. Harvesting of black cohosh and other root crops is also a cause for concern. In Africa harvesting of bark from the *Pugeum africanam* tree, which has become popular in Europe and the United States as a treatment for prostate problems, threatens the tree's long-term presence.

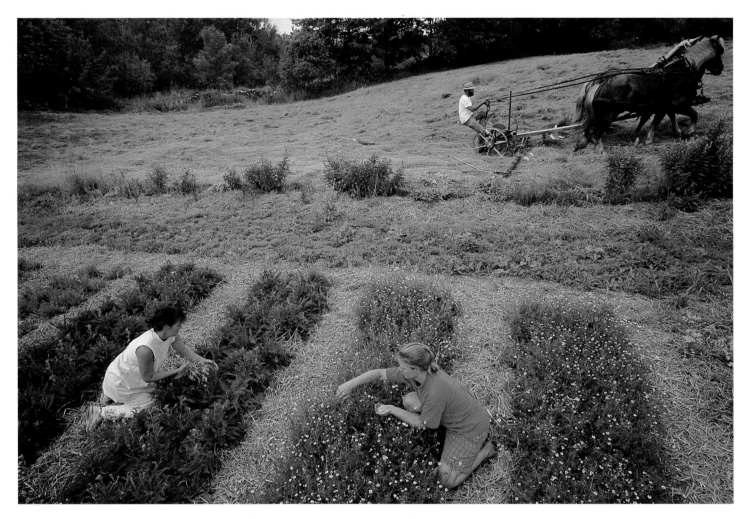

Traditional methods hold sway at Avena Botanicals, where workers harvest chamomile flowers by hand and horses pull a gardener's mower. The cut hay will act as an organic fertilizer. Chamomile helps promote a healthy scalp, relieves stress and nervous stomach, and helps teething babies.

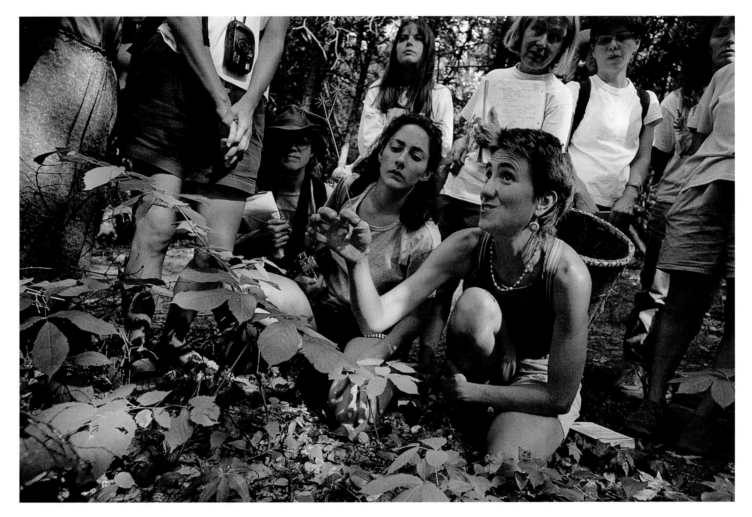

Deb Soule, founder and owner of Avena Botanicals in Rockport, Maine, teaches regular classes about medicinal plants. Most of her students are women who want to use herbs for themselves and their families. Annual sales of herbal remedies in the United States and Europe now total billions of dollars, and experts expect the figure to increase significantly each year.

USE OF BOTANICAL MEDICINES is increasing in part because major pharmaceutical companies and manufacturers of home products have started to invest hundreds of millions of dollars each year in advertising and marketing. But underlying the popularity of botanical remedies are fundamental societal shifts: Prosperity and improving lifestyles mean that people expect to live longer and better; former members of the baby boomer counterculture have an instinctive connection with medicine they regard as more natural; and new technologies such as the Internet make it much easier to generate and disseminate information about medicinal plants. Physicians have lost much of their function as information gatekeepers.

Another relevant societal shift is a self-help psychology that has expanded to the health field, part of a larger challenge to authority figures such as doctors. Adding to their alienation from the medical establishment is people's disappointment with prescription medicines. Despite huge and continuing increases in spending on prescription medicines—in industrial societies spending on prescription drugs has tripled in the last ten years to 110 to 120 billion dollars a year—many drugs have been largely ineffective against acute illnesses such as cancer and chronic conditions such as arthritis. This failure has prompted people to seek alternative sources of medicine.

FUNDAMENTAL TO THE growing popularity of herbs seems to be nostalgia for a time when humans lived closer to the earth, without the complexities and contradictions of contemporary life. A book written by Dr. Seuss, *You're Only Old Once!*, published in 1986, opens with a poem that captures this nostalgia well:

> *One day you will read*
> *in the National Geographic*
> *of a faraway land*
> *with no smelly traffic.*
> *In those green-pastured mountains*
> *of Fotta-fa-Zee*
> *everybody feels fine*
> *at a hundred and three*
> *'cause the air that they breathe*
> *is potassium-free*
> *and because they chew nuts*
> *from the Tutt-a-Tutt Tree.*

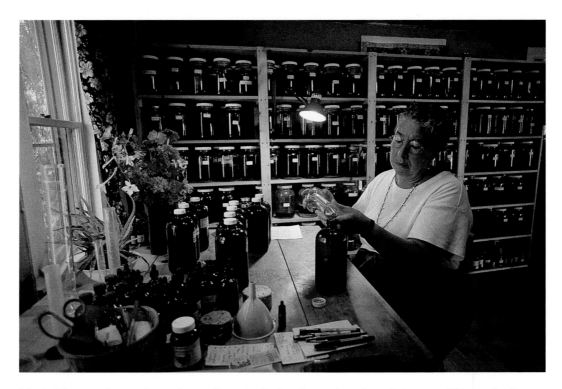

Maria Marta, who works at Avena Botanicals, bottles a plant-based tincture. This method of preparing herbal medicines probably has not changed for hundreds of years. To identify all the chemicals in such remedies and to document their exact effect on the human body remains beyond the technological capability of modern science.

This gives strength to their teeth,
it gives length to their hair,
and they live without doctors
with nary a care.

With desire for a renewed closeness to the Earth have come changing attitudes toward what has been regarded as superstition. In Bram Stoker's 1897 novel, *Dracula*, Lucy, a well-to-do young woman, is about to go to bed in her London apartment. Dr. Van Helsing, an expert on "obscure diseases," wants to protect Lucy from vampires, so he offers her huge bouquets of white flowers, which he describes as "medicines." Van Helsing hangs them around her bedroom window and wraps them around her neck.

Lucy laughs and throws them to the floor. "Why these flowers are only common garlic," she says.

"There is a grim purpose in all I do, and I warn you not to thwart me...," Van Helsing responds. "There is much virtue to you in so common a flower." Is the virtue Dr. Van Helsing describes the product of superstition, or does it symbolize ancient wisdom

FOLLOWING PAGES: Hands filled with healing herbs contain, clockwise from upper right, small yellow blooms of St. John's wort, used to help relieve some types of depression; echinacea to boost the immune system; feverfew to ease migraine headaches; plantain to relieve stings and burns; and calendula to help heal skin wounds.

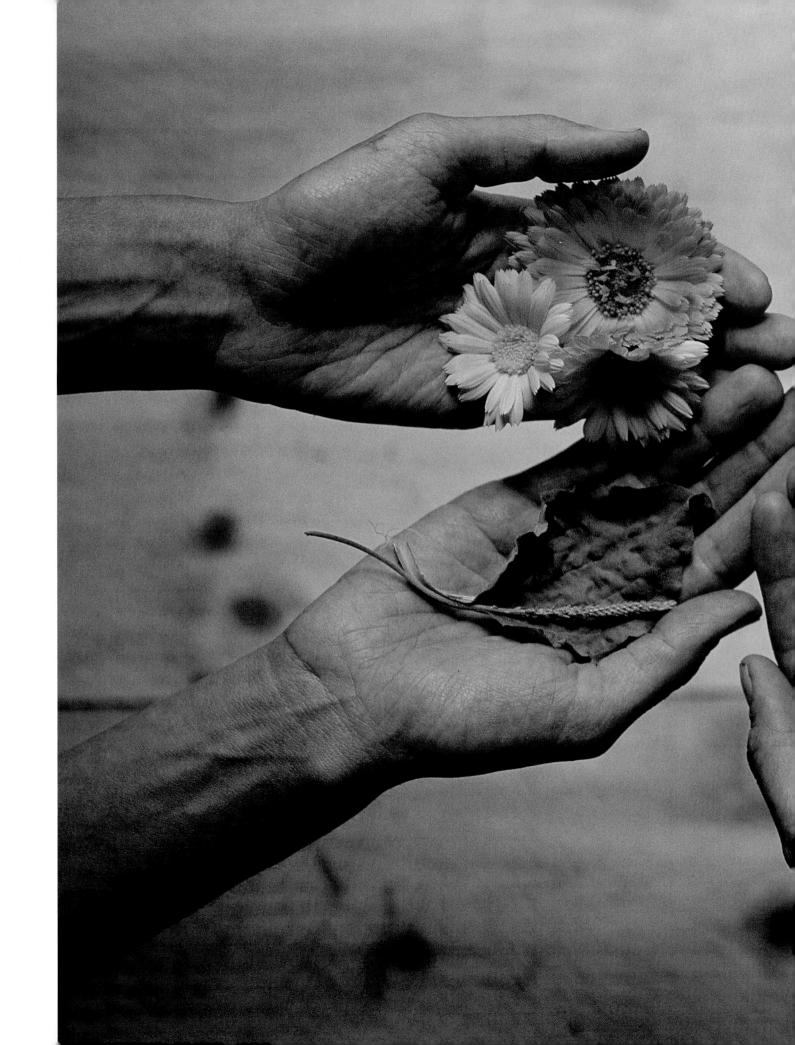

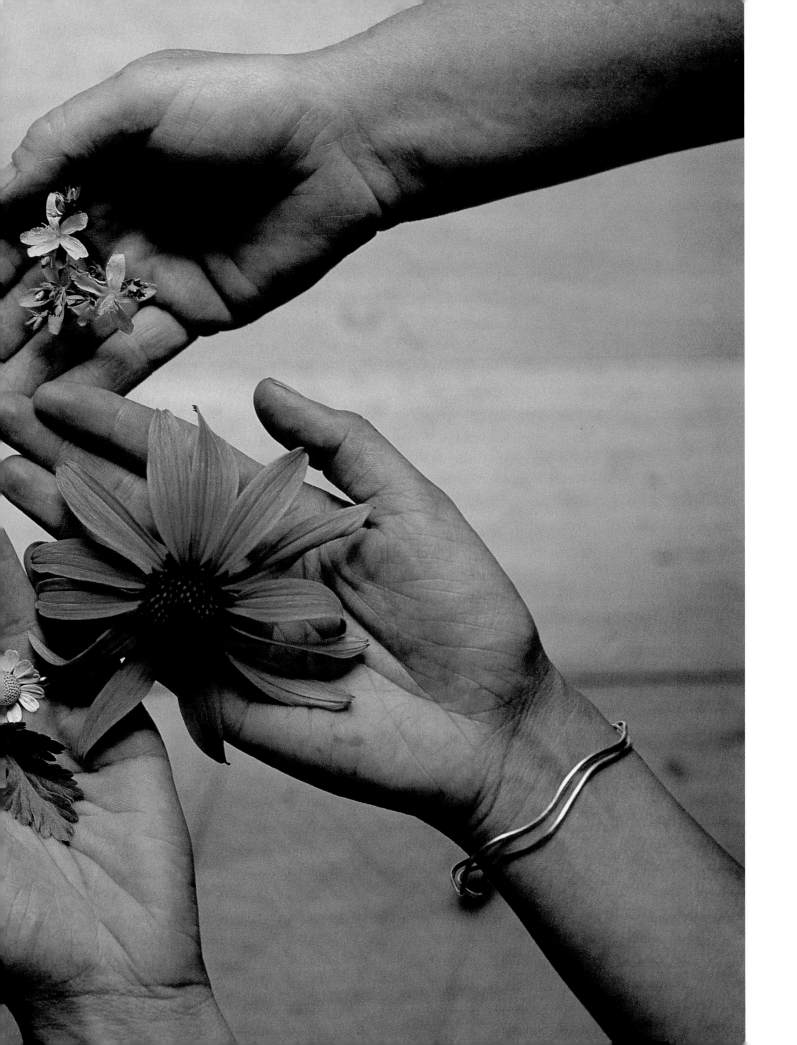

about garlic's healing powers? Are Lucy's laughter and her rejection of the garlic the acts of a rational, educated person, or those of someone closed to new ideas? In the novel removing the "common flowers" exposes Lucy to great danger, but modern readers have usually sympathized with Lucy's attitude—until recently, when scientific analysis confirmed Dr. Van Helsing's assertion that garlic possesses a special power.

Attitudes toward "primitive" healers are also changing. Until recently, most references made in Western writing to traditional healers have been derogatory. One study conducted in the 1960s examines Zulu healers in southern Africa. The author records their use of several hundred plants and concludes that they are "groping in the darkness of profound ignorance…." Seeing their medical practices, he says, is like stepping back in time because, he asserts, they live in "a state of life so primitive" that anything lower could not be considered human.

Westerners often call such healers witch doctors, linking them to witchcraft and other magic arts. As recently as the 1970s, experts often regarded traditional healers as mentally ill for claiming to turn into wild animals, communicate with plants, experience visions about what treatment to give, and receive instructions from dead ancestors during dreams. After spending long periods of time with traditional healers, one scholar compared them to acute schizophrenics. Both, he said, demonstrate "grossly non-reality-oriented ideation, abnormal perceptual experiences, profound emotional upheavals, and bizarre mannerisms."

Now, as part of the general movement toward botanical remedies, the view of traditional healers is changing. Western scholars and members of the general public are more willing to overlook what seems like irrationality. They find that these healers have a knowledge about how to identify and use medicinal plants that modern scientists cannot match.

Resurgence of respect for traditional healers is also occurring in developing countries due to groups such as the Oxford University-based Global Initiative For Traditional Systems of Health (GIFTS). GIFTS works with governments and local groups to conduct research, institute training and education programs, and formulate policy initiatives that help people appreciate the value of traditional medicinal systems. Such efforts are, from one perspective, part of a larger push to overcome the legacy of colonialism, which taught people to discard their own culture in favor of Western science. GIFTS's mission is partly born of necessity. One example: Most of the 22.4 million HIV-positive people in Africa, which has 75 percent of the world's AIDS cases, rely on locally originated botanical treatments.

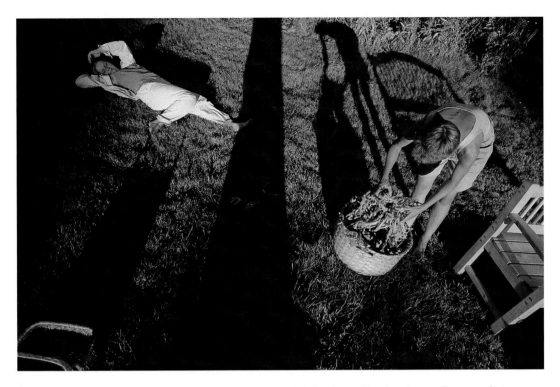

Summer shadows lengthen as Deb Soule works with a basket of herbs. Avena Botanicals is one of the few companies that harvest and process herbs totally by hand. This method adds to the costs but helps maximize quality and reliability. Ensuring that herbal remedies are what they claim to be remains a major problem.

Even though exaggerated claims about botanical cures for AIDS have been made, many of these treatments relieve opportunistic infections associated with AIDS and help people regain weight and strength. Such results confirm the need for further research and suggest that botanical remedies have much to offer.

―――――――

DESPITE, OR PERHAPS BECAUSE OF, its growing popularity, botanical medicine generates skepticism. It is not necessarily true, as many people assume, that medicines from plants are always safer and have fewer adverse side effects because they are natural. Processing can move a botanical away from what nature created. "Our extracts are so pure, they're five times more potent than the original plant," boasts one manufacturer.

Botanical remedies, furthermore, can contain powerful chemicals. Their mild side effects can include headaches and stomach distress, and they can be highly toxic, causing permanent damage and even death. Plant chemicals can change heart rate, blood pressure, and glucose levels. They can interfere with anesthesia during surgery, magnify or decrease the effect of prescription drugs and treatments such as cancer chemotherapy, affect male and female fertility, and produce birth defects.

The most common concerns about botanical remedies involve the need for accurate, complete, and understandable labeling, and for uncontaminated products. Americans, for example, now spend about 300 million dollars a year on echinacea, and Europeans also spend a huge amount—annual sales in Germany alone are well over 30 million dollars. Emphasizing that no one even knows "for sure what the 'best' dosage is," *Consumer Reports* magazine in 1999 analyzed popular brands of echinacea. Their findings: Up to a 500 percent variation exists in the amount of compounds—such as caffeoyl-tartaric acid, chlorogenic acid, cichoric acid, and echinacoside—that can serve as markers for echinacea's bioactivity. Even pills in the same bottle sometimes showed significant differences.

––––––––

SOME OF THESE COMPOUNDS vary depending on the species of echinacea used and whether chemicals were extracted from the leaf or root. Herbal advocates say that such variations are not always "bad," while other people reject herbal remedies because they lack scientific precision. "When herbal medicine devotees become aware that any useful ingredient in their unregulated leaves, stem, and root mixtures can be isolated and made available as regulated drugs, labeled with full information about content and proper dosage, they will begin making fewer trips to the health-food store," one expert on bogus science writes. Nonetheless, the unquestioned power of many botanical remedies means that they are not part of ongoing arguments about conventional versus alternative medicine.

In a recent public debate Arnold Relman, editor-in-chief emeritus of the *New England Journal of Medicine*, described much of alternative medicine as based on "irrational or fanciful thinking" and theories that "violate basic scientific principles…." Relman, however, did not attack what he terms "herbal therapy." Such therapy, he said, should not be in "fundamental conflict" with mainstream medicine because "many plant-derived materials have been proved to have important biological effects." But, because herbal products are not regulated by the FDA, the preparations, Relman says, "are highly variable in content purity and potency." Relman called for "many more control studies comparing standardized herbal preparations with conventional pharmaceuticals…."

Few professionals involved with botanical products would disagree about the need for more studies. At issue is whether botanical products need to meet the same placebo, double-blind standards imposed on pharmaceutical drugs, usually at a cost of hundreds of millions of dollars per drug, or whether different kinds of tests can produce useful information. That a plant has been used safely for hundreds or thousands of years, for example, could be accepted—as it is in much of Europe—as evidence that it is not toxic.

Studies of botanical remedies can be conducted only if someone pays for them. One solution comes from James Duke, a botanist who retired in 1995 after 30 years as a U.S. Department of Agriculture specialist in medicinal plants. Before a pharmaceutical drug can be approved, Dr. Duke suggests, its manufacturers, who test it for toxicity and effectiveness, should be required to test it against any botanical remedies that might provide the same benefit.

Such studies are especially important because some manufacturers of herbal products sometimes make emotional and unprovable claims. Patients with diseases such as cancer or AIDS and their families are often barraged with "new drugs" and "plant cures" promising, "You Do Not Have to Die!"

Magazines that are oriented toward botanical medicines and mailings that come after subscribing to such magazines yield a stream of advertisements with proclamations like these:

"A synergistic combination of nutritional supplements that work together to begin to purge your circulatory system of crusty plaque and debris."

"Regulate Blood Pressure Naturally."

"Free Yourself From Joint Pain Naturally."

"Midlife as nature intended."

"I feel like a kid again."

"We have to get older. But does that mean we have to age?"

"Guaranteed Better Health…Only $5!!"

"Experience the difference in how you feel in just 15 minutes."

"Utilize the power of Mother Nature to combat the effects of Father Time."

"Very Rare Ancient Chinese Super-Healer Now Available!"

"I really expected to be dead by now."

"Know this information or be prepared to die."

Some of these advertisements tell people they need a particular botanical remedy to protect the investment they have already made in other botanicals: "People take herbs and stay sick, because they do not know how to cure with cayenne pepper," one warns.

Some new products are based on the pharmaceutical industry's development of the anticancer drug paclitaxel from the Pacific yew tree. "New! VitaYEW," says one mailing, which contains a "Special Limited Time Introductory Offer!" for remedies from "An Ancient Tree That Became a Modern Miracle." Telling potential customers that paclitaxel "is only one constituent out of hundreds of health-promoting natural compounds that the Pacific yew tree contains," the mailing describes how Native Americans use the yew as a "tea for treating kidney problems, tuberculosis, liver deterioration, ulcers and digestion."

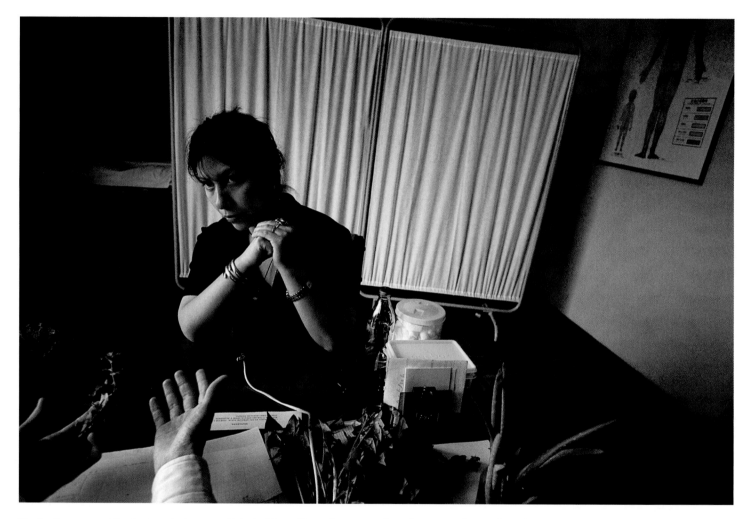

Rocio Cuya, a patient at a state-run clinic in Lima, Peru, listens as her doctor explains that she can treat her headache and insomnia either with pharmaceutical drugs or with herbal remedies. Basically, the modern drugs promise more dramatic results but often have negative side effects.

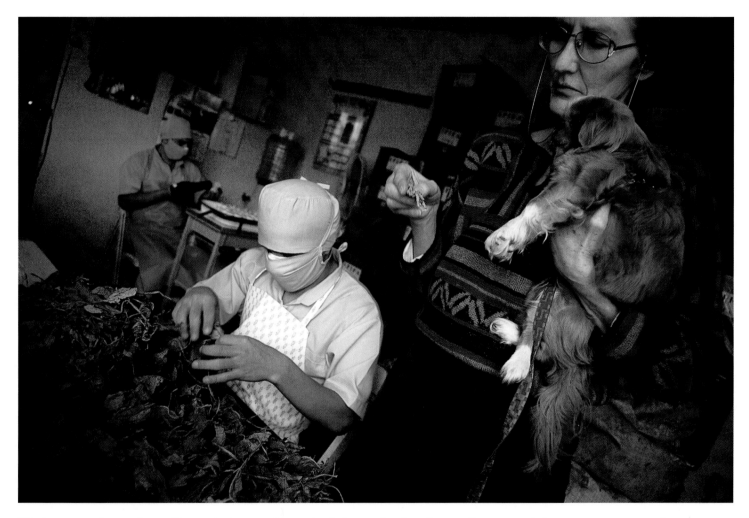

Workers at a clinic in Lima, Peru, which specializes in herbal remedies for chronic illnesses, including cancer, wear masks to protect themselves from inhaling too much plant dust as they sort specimens. The dog visited briefly while Constanca Barera, his mistress and owner of the clinic, checked the quality of a shipment of comfrey.

WHILE HERBAL LABELS in Europe usually offer explicit information, product labels in the United States must include disclaimers such as, "This statement has not been evaluated by the Food and Drug Administration. This product is not intended to diagnose, cure, or prevent any disease." These warnings have essentially evolved in response to the Dietary Supplements Health and Education Act of 1994. More the product of political compromise than of science, this law addresses labeling and claims, not the safety or efficacy of botanical remedies. According to the act, "herbal dietary supplements" cannot make health claims about a specific disease or health-related condition. They can say, for example, that a particular botanical remedy "helps maintain cardiovascular function and a healthy circulatory system," but cannot state that it "helps prevent heart disease."

Over-the-counter (OTC) medicines, which the FDA defines as drugs safe enough not to require a doctor's prescription, are another area of confusion. Of the hundreds of thousands of OTC medicines in the United States, fewer than a dozen rely on plants as a principal ingredient. Among these are aloe, cascara sagrada, and psyllium as laxatives; peppermint oil for coughs; red pepper for skin pain and inflammation; slippery elm to soothe mucous membranes; and witch hazel as an astringent.

Other regulatory options exist, among them those currently used by many European countries. Germany is the only industrial country to have a government agency, called Commission E, that examines botanical medicines for safety and efficacy. Commission E has rated 600 to 700 medicines that consist of plants or combinations of plants, using a standard of "reasonable certainty"—in contrast to the full certainty imposed on drugs by the FDA. Sources of information that Commission E considers valid include traditional use, chemical analysis, laboratory studies, clinical and epidemiological studies, patient case records, and unpublished data. Approval from Commission E means that government health programs will reimburse the costs of a botanical remedy if it is prescribed. Disapproval and lack of approval can come from determination of excessive risks or from lack of evidence of efficacy.

BECAUSE U.S. FEDERAL LAW does not allow therapeutic claims on labels and most insurance companies still do not provide reimbursement for visits to healers trained in botanical medicines, many people are forced to rely on word-of-mouth anecdotes, advertisements, salespeople, the news media, and information generated on-line. Too much information can become a problem. A search for 1998 and 1999 stories about dandelion, an important but far-from-popular botanical medicine, yielded 40 articles on

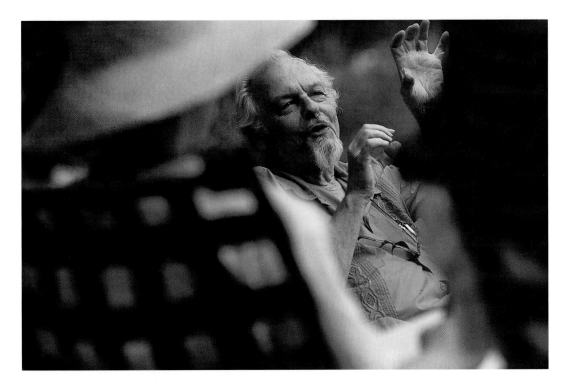

For three decades botanist Jim Duke was one of the U.S. Department of Agriculture's most respected experts on herbal medicines. Duke wants pharmaceutical companies to test new drugs, when appropriate, against herbal remedies to see which are really most effective.

MEDLINE, the National Institutes of Health database, and 80 articles on the Dow Jones Interactive news clipping service.

To determine which sources are reliable and to transform data, claims, and stories into useful and reliable knowledge require hard work. It is rarely wise to simply gather flowers or pick something off a store shelf and use it. People must make sure that botanical remedies are safe for their health circumstances and must not use plants as an excuse for self-diagnosis. Certain plants, for example, may temporarily relieve symptoms such as increased frequency of urination that may indicate prostate cancer, which is curable if detected early enough.

Unfortunately, many people do not want to invest the time and energy needed to learn about botanical medicines. They either rush into using them, often not discussing this with their doctors, or they do nothing in hopes that a doctor will eventually tell them what to do.

Botanical remedies require that doctors, too, work hard. Most doctors have not been taught about plants in medical school and do not feel qualified to give their patients expert advice. Physicians who search their professional journals find warnings, such as the potential effects of botanicals on prescription drugs. But, as indicated above, medical literature increasingly presents evidence that plant-based medicine must become part of standard care. One recent article on heart disease in the *Archives of Internal Medicine* documents how botanical medicines can be useful in the treatment of congestive heart failure, hypertension, angina pectoris, atherosclerosis, cerebral and peripheral vascular disease, venous insufficiency, and arrhythmia.

TENS OF THOUSANDS of studies examine the bioactive compounds in plants. Many have titles such as "Effects of Different Processed Products of Radix *Angelica sinensis* on Clearing Out Oxygen Free Radicals and Anti-Lipid Peroxidation" and "Specificity of the Tonoplast Transport of the Oleanolic Acid Monoglycosides in the Vacuoles from *Calendula officinalis* Leaves."

A large percentage of these studies have few practical implications because they involve the effect of plant chemicals in laboratory cultures and on animals. Nonetheless, the broad effects of botanical remedies are clear. They can kill microbes and fungi, and they have a proven impact on each of the human body's basic systems: digestive, circulatory, respiratory, reproductive, urinary, nervous, endocrine, muscular-skeletal, integumentary (skin), and immune. Some plants, such as astragalus and echinacea, suggest new mechanisms for medicinal action: They boost the human immune system's ability to fight disease-causing agents such as bacteria. Modern pharmaceutical drugs, in contrast, directly attack bacteria.

In general, botanical remedies differ from pharmaceutical drugs in at least four important ways. To a larger degree than is true for pharmaceutical drugs, botanical remedies are not as effective for all people. This may be in part because botanical remedies are less standardized and because much less is known about how they work. Most botanical remedies are usually also slower-acting than pharmaceutical drugs, more mild in immediate impact, and much more useful for chronic—as opposed to acute—conditions. This does not mean, however, that they cannot help ameliorate health problems also treated with pharmaceutical drugs.

The following brief summaries provide an idea of what research to date indicates botanical remedies can do. None of the summaries is complete, and all should be used only as a stimulus to learn more. (See also Plant Profiles, which begins on page 337.)

ALOE juice acts as a laxative, and aloe gel, cream, and lotion help heal first- and second-degree burns.

Active compounds include aloin, barbaloin, and aloe-emodin, which are cathartics. Aloe has antiprostaglandins that reduce inflammation. Its chemicals also increase the movement of lymph fluids and blood to areas of skin that have been burned.

ANGELICA root stimulates the appetite, relieves mild stomach discomforts, and is used with certain kinds of angina, chest pains caused by atherosclerosis. It is taken as a fluid extract or as a tincture, an extract in an alcohol medium.

Angelica contains at least 15 compounds that act as calcium-channel blockers, which cause smooth muscles in the uterus, intestines, arteries, and elsewhere to relax. Angelica can curtail the activity of intestinal worms, kill fungi, trigger the secretion of gastric juices, and combat stomach spasms. Studies also indicate that it can lower blood pressure.

———

ECHINACEA fights viruses, stimulates the immune system, and is especially effective against flu, yeast infections, herpes, and inflammatory diseases. Echinacea is usually taken as a capsule, extract, or tincture.

Echinacea helps prevent bacteria from entering uninfected cells. Polysaccharides in echinacea stimulate the immune system by activating phagocytes, such as spleen cells and white blood cells, which ingest microbes such as bacteria and viruses. Echinacea may also act like interferon, the body's own antiviral compound.

———

FEVERFEW prevents and treats headaches, including migraine, cluster, and premenstrual headaches. It may also combat inflammation and pain associated with arthritis and other problems for which aspirin might be used. Unlike aspirin, feverfew has little negative effect on the stomach although some people report gastric upset. It is usually taken as capsules or as a tea.

One of feverfew's active constituents, parthenolide, appears to inhibit production of certain chemicals, including the hormone serotonin, normally released during a migraine attack. Feverfew helps relieve arthritis symptoms by inhibiting the release of prostagladin and other enzymes from the white cells that are found in inflamed joints.

———

GARLIC kills bacteria, fungi, and parasites; boosts the immune system; and helps prevent cancer, heart attacks, and strokes. It is most commonly taken as a capsule.

Garlic contains sulfur-containing compounds, such as diallyl-trisulfide and the allylsulfides, which seem to facilitate excretion of carcinogens from the body and to slow the growth of some cancer cells. Garlic also contains at least a hundred other compounds that are reported to inhibit platelet aggregation in the arteries and lower cholesterol and other risk factors for heart attack.

———

SAW PALMETTO helps combat urinary problems associated with benign prostate

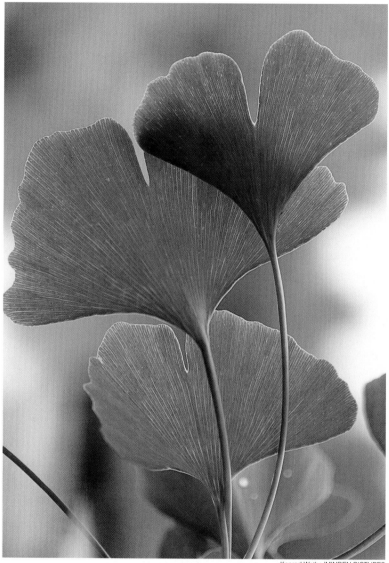

Konrad Wothe/MINDEN PICTURES

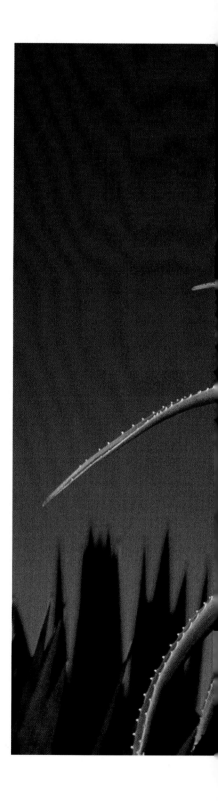

Aloe leaves surround blooming stalks in Madagascar's Spiny Desert (right). Since ancient times healers the world over have used aloe—primarily its juice and leaves—to treat a wide range of ailments. Taken internally, chemicals in aloe have a laxative effect. Aloe juice on burns, frostbite, and other skin wounds helps them heal. Extracts from gingko leaves (above) can treat circulatory problems such as arteriosclerosis and high blood pressure. Scientists have demonstrated that gingko increases memory performance and learning capability.

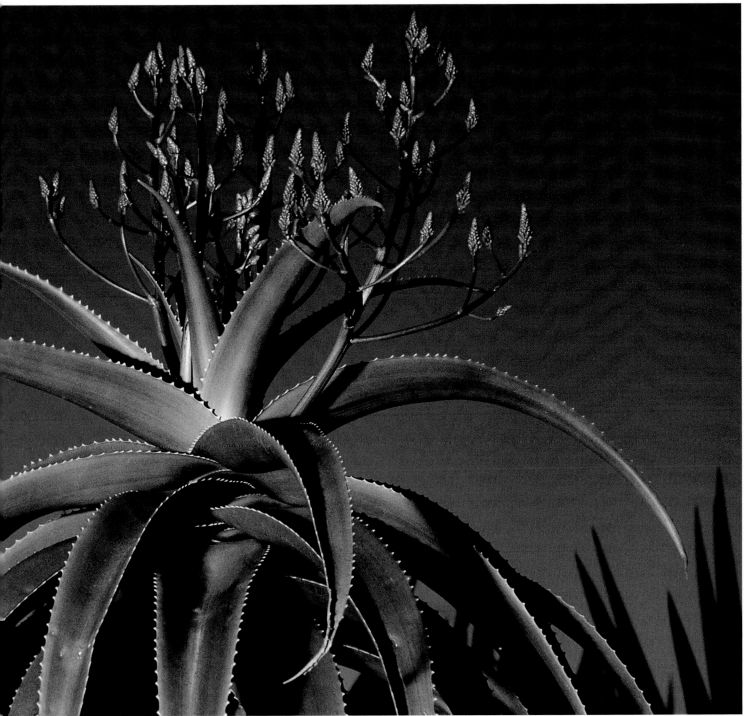

enlargement. An extract from the berries is usually taken as a capsule.

Chemicals in saw palmetto berries inhibit the conversion of testosterone to dihydrotestosterone (DHT), a hormone that helps sperm reach maturation and promotes a healthy prostate. DHT levels are often elevated in men with benign prostate enlargement. Studies also show that saw palmetto extract has antiallergenic and anti-inflammatory activity.

———————

CHANGE IS UNAVOIDABLE. Neither advocates nor opponents, nor those who are oblivious and indifferent, can ignore the new role of botanical medicines. With billions of dollars now spent each year, powerful institutions have begun to shift toward their use.

In the U.S., supermarket and drugstore chains are now advertising that their pharmacists are experts on vitamins and herbals. The United States Pharmacopoeia, which issues official standards for pharmaceutical drugs, publishes monographs describing, among other things, the identified active ingredients in dozens of widely used herbal remedies. More health insurance companies—catching up with Europe, where reimbursement for herbal remedies is common—are providing coverage for botanical medicines and for healers familiar with them. Pharmaceutical companies and other large corporations are acquiring companies that produce botanical products. The legal profession is talking about ways to patent botanical medicines based on variables such as unique formulas and manufacturing techniques. The FDA is discussing new options such as judging botanical remedies through clinical trials that are shorter and cheaper and that do not require the extensive chemical data currently demanded for substances to be recognized as pharmaceutical drugs. More and more scientific papers on herbal remedies published in Europe and Asia are becoming available in English.

In the meantime, an understanding of what 17th-century poet John Milton called the "strange and vigorous faculties" of plants continues to grow.

A plant's chemical-based defense system, recent research has documented, can be as complex as the human immune system. Plant defenses even have chemical memory. After combating a particular disease-causing virus, a plant can retain a resistance to that virus and related microbes. Among other components of plant defenses is the capacity to order cells near an invader to die, exuding poisonous, acidic chemicals. Some cells stiffen to exclude and wall off invaders, while still others produce the equivalent of antibiotics.

Sophisticated plant defense mechanisms include those that time the greening of

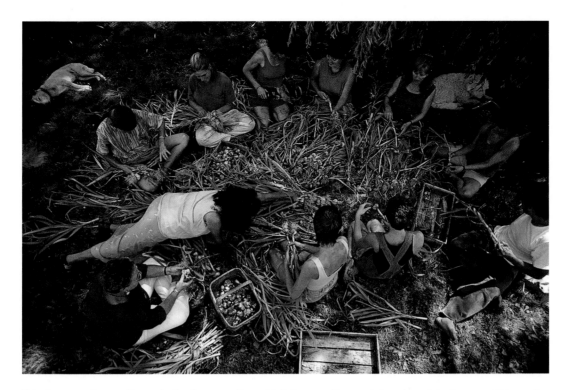

Workers at Avena Botanicals clean garlic, which has antibacterial and antiviral properties and helps prevent cardiovascular disease. Most plants are best harvested at times of the year and day when their chemicals are most potent. This garlic was pulled from the ground in the morning after the first three layers of the stalk had turned brown.

leaves to the absence of herbivores and the production of chemicals that protect plants during constant exposure to sunlight. The chemicals responsible for such defensive actions may have beneficial effects on humans, as could plant capabilities that go far beyond defensive functions. Many plants generate an amino acid called glutamate that they use for internal communications. Humans also produce glutamate, which serves as a chemical messenger in the brain. Other instances of commonality are evident in the apparently countless ways that plant-generated chemicals bind to human receptors. Licorice, to cite one example, produces glycyrrhizic acid, a compound that binds to human kidney cells—which respond as if it is aldosterone, a chemical that the adrenal glands release to combat low blood pressure. These links between plants and animals may be coincidences, but growing genetic evidence indicates that they are vestiges of the time billions of years ago before plants and animals evolved in different directions.

There is much to learn. "The best part of our knowledge," Oliver Wendell Holmes, Sr., told Harvard University medical students in 1861, "is that which teaches us where knowledge leaves off and ignorance begins."

It is at what Holmes called the "points of contact between our ignorance and our knowledge"—more specifically, our knowledge that plants offer far more than is available from their single active molecules and our ignorance about how to understand and utilize their amazing complexity—that we can most usefully begin.

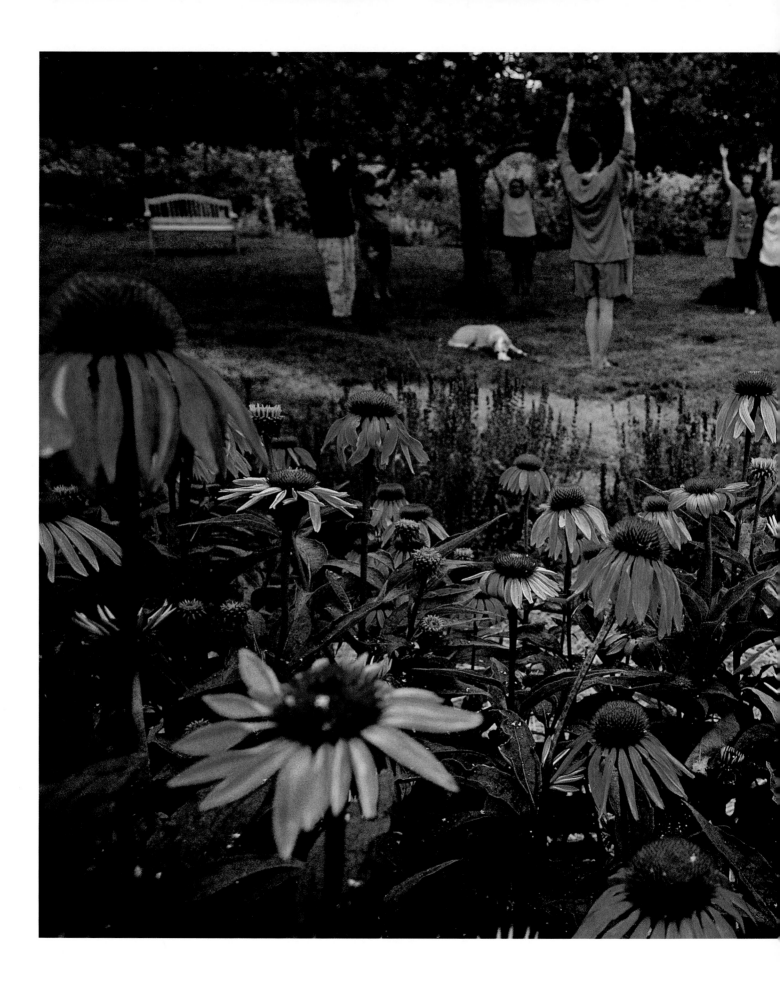

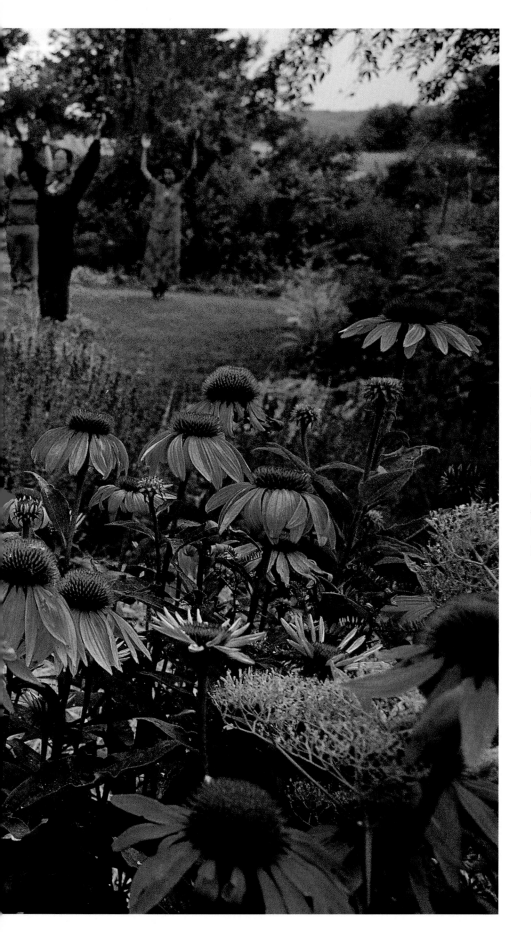

Beyond vivid blossoms of echinacea, whose chemicals boost the human immune system, students at Avena Botanicals learn *chi gong,* an ancient Chinese philosophy that combines movement, meditation, and healing. Chinese and other Asian approaches to health, which often include the use of herbal remedies, continue to gain popularity in the West.

Flying Serpents and a Nobel Prize

On the counter next to me, as I enjoy a late-night snack in the kitchen, is a bouquet of dried milk thistles that I picked near our house. Their prickly green leaves grew brown as they dried out, and their heads burst open to reveal puffy white down attached to tiny seeds.

Although people had been using milk thistle as a medicine for at least 2,000 years before I began working on *Nature's Medicine*, to me it was only a weed that invaded our backyard. Now I see beauty, grace, mystery, and power—a capacity to protect and cure.

Milk thistles caught my attention because their ripe seeds contain numerous compounds—such as silydianin and silybin—that protect and cleanse the liver. Among other things, they stimulate the production of new liver cells and keep toxins from entering.

In *Remembrance of Things Past* novelist Marcel Proust says that changes in perception like mine are the only true voyage of discovery. True voyages, he says, consist not of going to new places but of seeing with new eyes.

My voyage of discovery has lasted several years, and my vision has changed tremendously. When I began this book, I focused on why we do not derive more pharmaceutical drugs from plants. My frustrated awareness that places like Madagascar offer extraordinary cures that we somehow manage to neglect remains valid. But a much broader perspective, one that goes beyond pharmaceutical drugs to demand full utilization of all that botanical medicine offers, is necessary. Much is within what poet Robert Browning calls "man's reach."

The best way to begin is to end the attitudes and practices that separate medicinal plants and modern science. This separation is a historic anomaly. Throughout the countless years that humans have existed, we have enjoyed a growing closeness with medicinal plants. The only exception is the last half of the 20th century in industrialized societies, particularly in the United States. Here, ironically, modern science has dramatically increased our understanding of plants while pulling our medicine away from them.

———

My hope is that the growing popularity of herbal medicines and the medical profession's increasing awareness of how much plants offer will soon end this separation. Science—which continues to increase our understanding of plants, the human body, and the amazing chemical bonds that link us—can lead the way. One goal should be achievements that attract a Nobel Prize in medicine for work related to the medicinal use of plants, something that has never happened.

Specific steps should include the following:
Adding the study of plant chemicals to medical and pharmacy school curricula; developing a view of the human body that includes non-Western concepts such as the flow of energy along meridians; improving techniques for extracting chemicals from plants and refining the technology that allows standardization; and growing beyond dependence on the single active molecule through conceptual breakthroughs that draw together botany, molecular biology, genetics, chemistry, pharmacology, and medicine.

To narrow the gap between medicinal plants and modern medicine requires that we overcome economic constraints and generate new expectations. We must...
• Preserve cultural and biodiversity to ensure that our children and grandchildren inherit what they may possess the wisdom to appreciate.
• Rethink definitions of progress to embrace research and insights that bring us closer to natural processes rather than presuming mastery over nature.
• Change government regulations, patent laws, and insurance policies to encourage the development of medicines not defined by the single active compound.

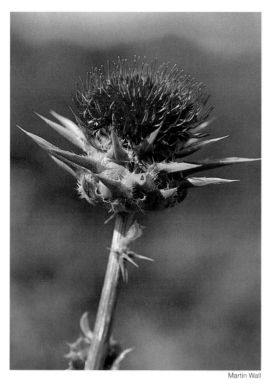
Martin Wall

Milk thistle blooms on a sturdy stalk. Its seeds contain chemicals that keep toxins from entering the human liver.

• Conduct public health campaigns and launch other educational efforts that emphasize prevention, with plants providing one of the primary tools.

———

CIRCUMSTANCES TODAY IN many ways resemble those surrounding the legendary city of Ubar. Located in the Arabian desert, Ubar enjoyed enormous wealth because it provided the Roman Empire with frankincense, which the Romans relied upon for medicine, cooking, and religious ceremonies. The price for this frankincense, according to legend, was kept artificially high because Ubar maintained a monopoly. Although traders from Ubar brought frankincense out of the desert along a road sometimes as wide as a ten-lane freeway, outsiders never traveled to the city. They believed, as Herodotus wrote in his *Histories*, that the "frankincense trees" were "guarded by winged serpents."

The Romans did not have to worry about flying snakes. The Arabian desert is home to numerous poisonous snakes, some of which leap up but none that can fly. More importantly, the Romans could have grown their own frankincense. They did not because they were convinced that frankincense emerging from the desert was the best and only frankincense possible.

As we enter the 21st century, our flying serpents are economic structures and imperatives—worries about patents and profits, and the 500-million-dollar investment that must be made before a drug reaches the market. These modern-day serpents keep us from conducting the research and clinical trials that must be completed before we better utilize plants—for both prevention and treatment.

We have somehow made the manufacturers of pharmaceutical drugs our Ubar, distant places upon which we must rely for medicines. But plants are telling us that so much more is available. Like the Romans who eventually realized that they could grow their own frankincense, we can look, figuratively at least, to our own backyards.

When I pull out pieces of the milk thistle, tannish seeds with a black dot and a white tip fall out. The seeds are thin, about as long as a pencil eraser. Even after all this time and study, they still amaze me. They look insignificant, yet I have a cousin and friends with hepatitis whose livers they help protect. These simple seeds transform how the world looks to me. Maybe what I am feeling is an affinity to plants that lies deep within all of us. In his *Alchemical Studies,* Swiss psychologist C. G. Jung discusses the image of "the wonder-working plant" that appears in the "unconscious."

How did wonder plants get imbedded into our unconscious? Bonds tying us to plants and our commonality with them, both of which scientists are now documenting, must come from more than coincidence or a quirk of fate. God, or nature, or whatever words we use to denote the originating and driving force responsible for life, has placed an extraordinary gift on this planet with us.

To believe this, we need not regress to the much-disproved and easily mocked doctrine of signatures, which held that God had placed clues in plants that would help us see how to use them. Plant parts that looked like human hair, according to this doctrine, would combat baldness. A much broader view is possible. Benjamin Rush, a physician who signed the Declaration of Independence and was friends with Thomas Jefferson, argued that "the Creator" had put on Earth natural remedies for all disease. After working on this book, it is hard to disagree with him.

Joel L. Swerdlow
Washington, D.C.
February 9, 2000

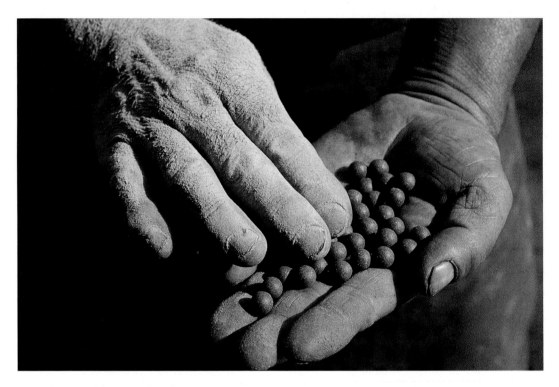

A worker in the Tibetan Medical and Astrology Institute in Dharmala, India, holds pills made from a dried herbal mixture. If present trends continue, modern science may never understand the healing effects of such remedies—especially those made from more than one plant.

An Introduction

Presented in this section of *Nature's Medicine* are 102 plants arranged alphabetically by Latin name. This selection of plants—many of which are featured in the text of this book—serves two purposes: It provides a framework for appreciating these particular medicinal plants, and it is representative of the many hundreds of other plants that help preserve human health and treat disease. On page 338 is a list of these plants by their common names and the page numbers on which they appear.

We selected the plants profiled here for a wide range of reasons. They are a mixture of the familiar and the surprising. Various plants affect each of the major systems that make up human physiology, and many serve as treatments for ailments that range from minor indigestion to cancer.

Included here are plants that have led to pharmaceutical drugs now at the core of modern medicine; others are candidates for new drugs. Other plants, which come from many cultures and geographical areas, have been crucial to the still evolving relationship between modern science and medicinal herbs.

Some of the profiled plants are prominent in homeopathic medicine, some of the plants demonstrate how common foods and spices can be medicines, and some are plants used by animals for self-medication. Although mushrooms are no longer classified as plants, two well-known mushrooms used historically for healing and currently the focus of intensive research are included.

Each plant description includes a section called "Folklore and Traditional Uses." In it you will find both fables and facts, including some of the rich history of mankind's experience with medicinal plants. From dandelion to deadly nightshade, this section of each profile provides insights into the myths and realities of healing herbs.

The "Medicinal Uses" section documents, among other things, the rapidly growing body of science that confirms the incredible healing and health-promoting power in plant chemicals. In reference to a plant's active constituent elements, we use the term "principle" in an unfamiliar way: to denote, according to the dictionary, "an ingredient (e.g., a chemical) that exhibits or imparts a characteristic quality."

This group of Plant Profiles is not meant to be a compilation of the 102 most popular medicinal plants. Neither is this section of the book intended to be used as a guide for self-medication. Care must be taken because many of these plants are poisonous or otherwise harmful if taken internally or if not prepared correctly. Some are illegal unless obtained as part of a prescription medicine. Just because chemicals from plants are "natural" does not mean that they are always safe. Please let your doctor and other health practitioners know which herbal remedies you are taking.

See the "Additional Resources" section for suggestions on how to learn more about these and other medicinal plants.

Two artists created the paintings of the plants featured in this section. Jane Watkins painted all except those on pages 339-L (left), 342-L, 348-R (right), 353-L, 354-R, 355-L, 358-L, 360-R, 361-L, 366-L,369-L, 370-L&R, 371-L&R, 372-L&R, 373-R, 375-L, 377-R, 386-R, 387-R, 388-R, which were done by Mary E. Eaton. Brief biographical notes on the two artists appear on page 394.

Achillea millefolium

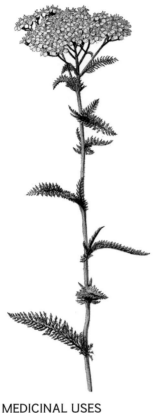

COMMON NAMES
Yarrow, Milfoil, Nosebleed,
Woundwort, Stanchweed

LATIN NAME
Achillea millefolium

FAMILY Asteraceae

PARTS USED
Leaf, stem, flower

DESCRIPTION
Yarrow is a creeping perennial
that reaches about three feet in
height, with small flowers of
various colors and thin, fernlike leaves.

HABITAT
Yarrow is indigenous to
Europe and parts of Asia, but
it is now cultivated in temperate regions all over the world.

**FOLKLORE
AND TRADITIONAL USES**
Yarrow was found in a Neandertal grave that dates back
60,000 years, along with other
herbs still used medicinally. It
is impossible to know whether
the yarrow was there because
the deceased was a healer or
because it was used as part of a
ritual. It is known, however,
that the Chinese used yarrow
stalks in consulting the I
Ching, also called the Yarrow
Stalk Oracle. The Celts used
the plant in divining the
weather and the thoughts
of others. This belief in the
fortune-telling powers of
yarrow has persisted in Britain
to modern times. Young people, it is said, sometimes put it
in their bed to induce dreams
of their true love.

MEDICINAL USES
Yarrow's Latin name comes
from the legend that Achilles
cured wounds with yarrow
during the Trojan War. The
plant has been used since
antiquity to stanch the wounds
of war, a fact that gained it the
name *herba militaris*. Such use
is supported by scientific evidence: Achilleine, the yarrow
component, has been shown to
arrest internal and external
bleeding. Yarrow has other
medicinal uses, such as relieving gastrointestinal ailments,
reducing fevers, stimulating the
appetite, and treating throm-
boses. Chamazulene, found in
yarrow's essential volatile oil,
acts as an anti-inflammatory,
an antiallergen, and an antispasmodic.

Aconitum napellus

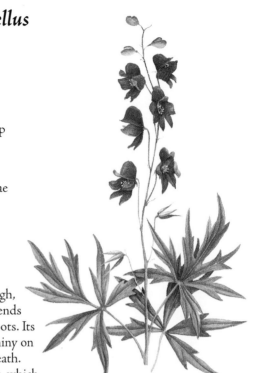

COMMON NAMES
Aconite, Monkshood,
Wolfsbane, Soldier's cap

LATIN NAME
Aconitum napellus

FAMILY Ranunculaceae

PARTS USED
Root, rhizome, stem,
leaf, flower

DESCRIPTION
A perennial shrub that
grows two to six feet high,
aconite's erect stem extends
from thick, tuberous roots. Its
dark green leaves are shiny on
top and lighter underneath.
Helmet-shaped flowers, which
bloom in summer or fall, are
usually purplish blue.

HABITAT
Aconite species can be found
in Europe, North America,
Asia, and Africa.

**FOLKLORE
AND TRADITIONAL USES**
The name *Aconitum* may be
derived from *akone*, meaning
"cliffy" or "rocky," because it
tends to grow in such areas.
According to Greek mythology, aconite became poisonous
from the foam that dropped
from the mouth of Cerberus,
the gatekeeper of hell, when
Hercules dragged him up from
the nether regions. Medea,
priestess of the goddess
Hecate, attempted to poison
her stepson Theseus using
aconite so that her birth son
could inherit her husband's
throne. Aconite is believed to
be among the ingredients of
"flying ointments," potions
used by witches to create the
sensation of flight.

MEDICINAL USES
Aconite was formerly used to
treat pain, arthritis, inflammation, fever, skin diseases, and
neuralgias. Aconite works very
quickly, becoming active just a
few minutes after being taken
orally. Alkaloids found in the
plant have analgesic or anti-
inflammatory properties.
Aconite is widely and safely
used as a homeopathic remedy
for physical or psychological
stress. Aconite root, however, is
extremely poisonous. As little
as a teaspoonful of it or its
preparations can cause paralysis of the cardiac muscle or respiratory center. For this reason,
despite its having been used
throughout history, it is not
currently recommended by
Germany's Commission E, a
group of German experts on
herbal remedies who evaluate
plant medicines for efficacy
and safety.

Allium sativum

COMMON NAME
Garlic

LATIN NAME
Allium sativum

FAMILY Alliaceae

PART USED
Bulb

DESCRIPTION
A perennial, garlic grows as tall as two to three feet, with a straight stem. Leaves are long and flat, and the flowers are mainly white. The bulb consists of several cloves, grouped together in a membrane that is papery white.

HABITAT
Although garlic now grows worldwide, it originated in Central Asia. It does best in a rich, sandy, moist soil in sunny areas.

**FOLKLORE
AND TRADITIONAL USES**
Garlic has a place in folklore all over the world. A Muslim legend describes garlic springing up in the left footsteps of the devil as he stepped out from the Garden of Eden after the fall of man. Yet in eastern and southern Europe, garlic is regarded as protection against evil spirits. A superstition in ancient Greece dictated that runners in a race should chew garlic to prevent competitors from getting ahead.

MEDICINAL USES
Garlic has been used medicinally since the time of the ancient Egyptians. During the

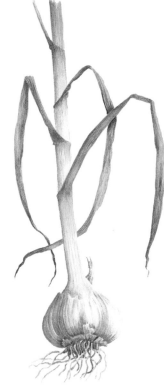

1920s in Switzerland, researchers isolated the inert chemical alliin from garlic. When crushed or chewed, alliin is transformed into the antibiotic allicin, the substance responsible for garlic's characteristic odor and pharmacological qualities. Worldwide studies have shown garlic's effectiveness against myriad diseases. Studies in Britain indicate that garlic reduces cholesterol, blood pressure, and the likelihood of internal blood clots. Other scientific studies show that dietary garlic, as well as onion and other allium vegetables, may prevent stomach cancer. Garlic has also been shown to strengthen the immune system in people with AIDS.

Aloe barbadensis

COMMON NAME
Aloe vera

LATIN NAMES
Aloe barbadensis, A. vera

FAMILY Liliaceae

PART USED
Leaf

DESCRIPTION
An evergreen perennial, true aloe has fleshy gray-green leaves with spiny edges that grow directly from the root with no stem. The leaves taper toward the end and have spiny edges. The colorful flowers are tubular.

HABITAT
Aloe species are indigenous to Africa and also grow on islands in the southern Mediterranean and in the West Indies. Aloes need only a moderate amount of water.

**FOLKLORE
AND TRADITIONAL USES**
The name "aloe," meaning "bitter and shiny substance," derives from the Arabic *alloeh*. Called the "plant of immortality," aloe has been found in the wall carvings of ancient Egyptian temples. After Alexander the Great learned of aloe when he conquered Egypt in 332 B.C., he had an army secure the island of Socotra, where it grew, to ensure that only his soldiers would benefit from its healing power. In Mecca many graves have aloes planted nearby, symbolizing the patience needed during the

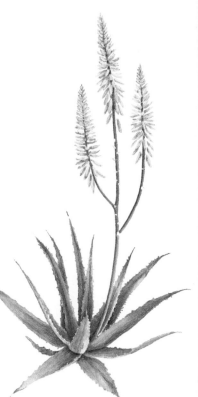

time between burial and resurrection. Aloe gel is the product used most frequently in the cosmetic and health-food industries.

MEDICINAL USES
Aloe's most important ingredients—aloin, barbaloin, and aloe-emodin—are responsible for its cathartic action. The Chinese and ancient Greeks prescribed aloe for constipation, and today aloe is still prescribed by physicians as a laxative. Aloe is considered a powerful healer for external burns, scrapes, and sunburn. In laboratory tests, aloe-emodin has shown signs of being able to combat leukemia. A European study also suggested that aloe gel can reduce the blood sugar levels in people with diabetes.

Ananas comosus

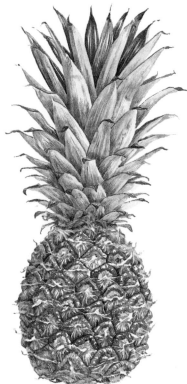

COMMON NAME
Pineapple

LATIN NAME
Ananas comosus

FAMILY Bromeliaceae

PARTS USED
Fruit, leaf

DESCRIPTION
A perennial, the pineapple plant grows about two to four feet tall. The reddish yellow fruit has a scalelike surface surmounted by a crown of stiff, spiky leaves. Pineapple is the only cultivated fruit whose stem runs completely through it.

HABITAT
The pineapple is native to South America but is now grown in North America, Cuba, South Africa, Australia, and the Philippines.

**FOLKLORE
AND TRADITIONAL USES**
In Brazil tribal peoples have always regarded pineapple highly and have used it as a staple food and as an ingredient in some wines. When early explorers brought the pineapple back to Europe, its sweetness and unusual appearance made the fruit a symbol of royal privilege. In the American colonies, the pineapple symbolized friendship and hospitality. And hosts who could provide such a rare and exotic fruit made a statement about their high social standing. Pineapples were so popular in colonial America that confectioners rented them to households by the day.

An enzyme found in pineapple is now used as a meat tenderizer. It is said that the fingerprints of pineapple cutters can be obliterated by excessive exposure to this enzyme. The leaf of some varieties is a source of piña fiber for embroidery thread.

MEDICINAL USES
Pineapples have been used in traditional tropical medicine for ailments ranging from constipation to jaundice. Without fresh fruit on board, sailors who came across pineapple in the early days of European exploration escaped scurvy by eating it, a rich source of Vitamin C. Pineapple contains bromelain, a protein-splitting enzyme that has been shown to increase bleeding time and reduce the aggregation of platelets. Bromelain also has proved effective in killing parasites such as worms.

Angelica sinensis

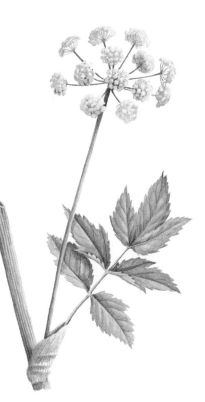

COMMON NAMES
Dong quai, Chinese angelica

LATIN NAME
Angelica sinensis

FAMILY Umbelliferae

PARTS USED
Root, rhizome

DESCRIPTION
A perennial or biennial, dong quai grows to more than six feet tall and produces greenish white flowers. The root is brown, large, and white on the inside, with ten or more tentacle-like branches extending from it.

HABITAT
Indigenous to Asia, dong quai grows in damp mountain ravines, meadows, banks, and coastal areas. It requires a deep, moist, fertile soil in shade or full sun.

**FOLKLORE
AND TRADITIONAL USES**
Angelica got its name by its association with divine protection against sorcery. This use dates back at least to the 1500s, when John Gerard said it was "available against witchcraft and enchantments," a belief that still persists in parts of rural America. Early American settlers considered the plant so valuable that they imported its seeds from England. In China, dong quai is known as the "empress of herbs" and also called *dang gui*, which means "proper order," in reference to its medicinal qualities. It is one of the most widely consumed herbs in China. During that country's Cultural Revolution of the 1960s and 1970s, wild supplies of dong quai were exhausted, and people began to cultivate it. Dong quai is often used to make soups and teas. It is also a flavoring agent in liqueurs, such as Chartreuse, and in gin.

MEDICINAL USES
According to traditional Chinese medicine, dong quai has a balancing effect on the female hormonal system. Also called "female ginseng," it is used to treat many gynecological problems, namely irregular or delayed menstruation, premenstrual pains and cramps, menopausal hot flashes, and uterine bleeding. Dong quai's chemical constituents stimulate uterine contractions and, therefore, should not be used during pregnancy. Its coumarin derivatives affect blood coagulation, act as antispasmodics, and dilate blood vessels. It is used as a blood purifier and in the treatment of rheumatism, ulcers, and hypertension.

Aralia racemosa

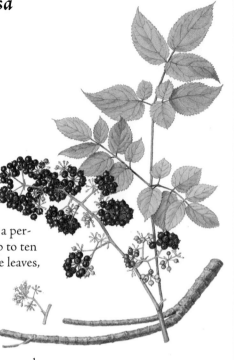

COMMON NAME
American spikenard

LATIN NAME
Aralia racemosa

FAMILY Araliaceae

PARTS USED
Root, rhizome

DESCRIPTION
American spikenard is a perennial bush growing up to ten feet in height with large leaves, small greenish white flowers, and red or purple berries.

HABITAT
The species *Aralia racemosa* is found from central Canada to Virginia, but other types of spikenard grow elsewhere in North America.

FOLKLORE AND TRADITIONAL USES
Native Americans ate the aromatic spikenard roots and young leaves in soups and other dishes. Related to ginseng, wild sarsaparilla and other species of spikenard were used as flavorings in teas and root beer. Another plant called spikenard and related to valerian was found in perfumes in ancient times. According to the New Testament, Mary Magdalene applied it to Jesus' feet.

MEDICINAL USES
This herb's current use for coughs and skin conditions is based on traditional applications. Native Americans of various groups used American spikenard and related species for a variety of ailments, including as a tea for backaches. Decoctions of the roots and bark helped women with menstrual problems or prolapsed uteruses. People of both sexes used spikenard for conditions that in colonial times were called humors in the blood. They also treated pulmonary and respiratory infections such as coughs and tuberculosis with spikenard. Poultices of American spikenard were put on wounds, swellings, and burns. This plant contains a volatile oil, tannins, and diterpene acids. It was included in the *National Formulary of the United States* from 1916 to 1965.

Arnica montana

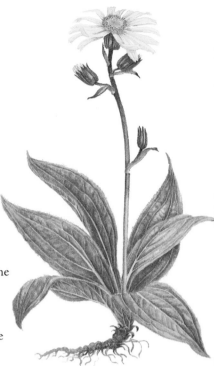

COMMON NAMES
Arnica, Mountain daisy, Mountain tobacco, Leopard's bane

LATIN NAME
Arnica montana

FAMILY Asteraceae

PARTS USED
Flower, rhizome

DESCRIPTION
A perennial, arnica grows one to two feet tall and bears orange-yellow, daisylike flowers. Oval leaves form a flat rosette near the surface of the soil.

HABITAT
Arnica is indigenous to Europe, western North America, southern Russia, and Central Asia.

FOLKLORE AND TRADITIONAL USES
Arnica is known as the mountain daisy, a flower associated with foretelling future loves. People pluck its petals and say, "she loves me, she loves me not," with the last petal's message delivering the final word. In Victorian times daisies symbolized innocence, a symbol that remains today with the expression "fresh as a daisy." Native Americans mixed a species of arnica with ocher and parts of a robin to make a love potion. After this mixture was made into a powder, a person would go into a river and, mentioning the name of the desired sweetheart, would smear it on his face. Arnica is currently an ingredient in hair tonics, perfumes, cosmetics, and antidandruff preparations.

MEDICINAL USES
Arnica's medicinal properties were discovered independently by Native Americans at an unknown date and by Europeans by the end of the 16th century. To treat his angina, German philosopher Johann Wolfgang von Goethe drank arnica tea. Russian folk medicine uses arnica to treat uterine hemorrhages. More than a hundred different preparations with arnica extract are marketed in Germany. It is commonly used externally for acne, rashes, cuts, bruises, and sprains; as a gargling solution, it may help relieve flu symptoms. The plant has been shown to be an analgesic and an anti-inflammatory, most likely due to sesquiterpene lactones. Arnica should never be taken internally except in the extremely minute doses used in homeopathic medicine; studies have shown it can damage the heart if taken improperly.

Artemisia absinthium

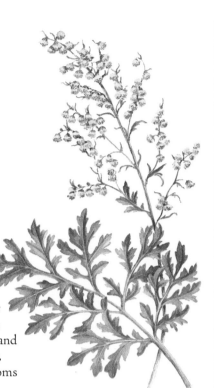

COMMON NAMES
Wormwood, Artemisia

LATIN NAME
Artemisia absinthium

FAMILY Asteraceae

PART USED
Whole herb

DESCRIPTION
Reaching one to four feet high, the branched, fast-growing stems of this perennial bear deeply serrated silver-green leaves. Wormwood's stems and leaves are covered with fine, silky hairs. Its yellow blossoms appear in clusters of small, round, drooping flower heads.

HABITAT
Indigenous to Eurasia and North Africa, wormwood can also be found in eastern North America. The herb grows wild on rocky hillsides and wastelands and is cultivated in temperate regions worldwide.

FOLKLORE AND TRADITIONAL USES
The name "wormwood" probably came from this herb's use in ancient times in eliminating intestinal worms. Another theory is that "worm" is derived from the Teutonic *wer* (man) and "wood" from *mod* (courage) —meaning "man's courage," in reference to the herb's alleged aphrodisiacal and healing properties. In the Mexican festival for the goddess of salt, women wear garlands of wormwood on their heads as they perform a celebratory dance. Absinthe, a hallucinogenic liqueur made from wormwood that was eventually deemed toxic and outlawed in the early 20th century, was extremely popular among the Impressionists. Used in gardens as a companion plant, wormwood acts as a deterrent against several insect pests, thus serving as a repellent and an insecticide.

MEDICINAL USES
Native American tribes use this plant as a vermifuge, as well as to treat strained muscles, head and chest colds, stomach ailments, broken limbs, tuberculosis, and venereal diseases. Wormwood contains a number of bitter constituents that stimulate the secretion of digestive fluids. It improves the absorption of nutrients, eases gas and bloating, and strengthens the digestive system. One constituent of wormwood is thujone, which is toxic if taken in improper doses. The USFDA lists it as an unsafe herb.

Aspilia mossambicensis

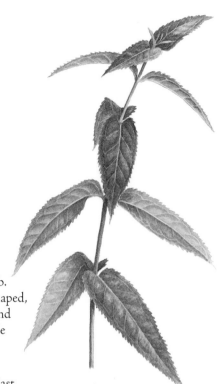

COMMON NAMES
Aspilia, Wild sunflower

LATIN NAMES
Aspilia mossambicensis,
A. africana

FAMILY Asteraceae

PART USED
Leaf

DESCRIPTION
A perennial, aspilia is a semi-woody herb or shrub. Leaves are rough, lance shaped, creased accordion-style, and covered with short, flexible hairs called trichomes.

HABITAT
Aspilia is indigenous to East Africa and grows throughout tropical Africa.

FOLKLORE AND TRADITIONAL USES
In African countries people who use aspilia call it a variety of names. In Nigeria, where it is known as "headband," "friend of pepper," and "to draw out mucus," aspilia is grazed by cattle and sheep. It is traditionally seen as a male plant and tied around the head or hidden in the house to attract notice of the opposite sex. A decoction of aspilia is used as a wash for horses, as a dye, and as an ingredient in plaster.

MEDICINAL USES
Aspilia came to the recognition of modern research because of its use by chimpanzees in Gombe National Park and Mahale Mountains National Park of Tanzania. Chimps swallow the leaves whole and then defecate them intact. The leaves show no visible evidence of having passed through the digestive tract. In one study, more than 20 worms and 56 leaves were expelled in a single instance of defecation. Short flexible hairs on the leaves' surfaces have a "velcro effect," attaching to and expelling worms as they travel through the intestine. This action is enhanced by the release of chemicals that may inhibit the parasites' ability to adhere to intestinal walls. Aspilia is not only a powerful antiparasitic but also an effective antibiotic. Scientists have found traces, in the root of this plant, of thiarubrine A, a red oil that kills parasites, viruses, fungi, and bacteria. It has also been found to kill cancer cells in solid tumors, such as those found in the lung and breast. Africans use aspilia for many illnesses, including lumbago, sciatica, scurvy, malaria, rheumatism, tuberculosis, and gonorrhea.

Astragalus membranaceus

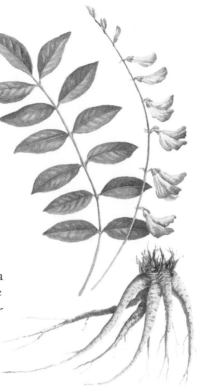

COMMON NAMES
Astragalus, Huang qi,
Milk vetch

LATIN NAME
Astragalus membranaceus

FAMILY Leguminosae

PART USED
Root

DESCRIPTION
A perennial herb, astragalus grows up to a foot tall, with a tough, fibrous root and some branches. The bark is brownish yellow, irregular, and wrinkled or furrowed. The flowers are yellowish white. Its leaves are divided into 12 to 18 pairs of leaflets.

HABITAT
Astragalus is indigenous to northern China. It is also cultivated in other parts of Asia. This herb thrives in sandy, well-drained soil that receives ample sun.

**FOLKLORE
AND TRADITIONAL USES**
The Chinese characters used to represent "huang qi" have many levels of meaning. The character *huang* means "yellow," which alludes to both its yellow interior and what the Chinese consider to be the color of life-giving earth. The character *qi* means "venerable," which alludes to its superior status in Chinese medicine. When pronounced with different inflections, *qi* also means "vital force," "to eat," and "addiction to sensual pleasures."

MEDICINAL USES
Astragalus has been used for more than 2,000 years in traditional Chinese medicine as a diuretic and as an immunostimulant. It is commonly employed to treat diabetes and nephritis. In the United States it is used to strengthen immune function after cancer chemotherapy. Studies have shown that huang qi encourages bone marrow to produce more phagocytes, cells that destroy bacteria and viruses. These actions are attributed to huang qi's active constituents—glycans, which stimulate the action of phagocytes; polysaccharides, which enhance immune function; and saponins, which stimulate the growth of lymphocytes. Some believe that huang qi has the potential to treat HIV infection; further study is needed.

Atropa belladonna

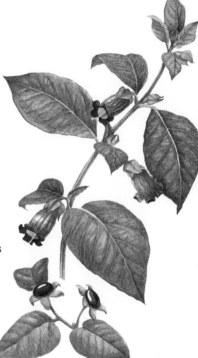

COMMON NAMES
Belladonna, Deadly nightshade, Dwale

LATIN NAME
Atropa belladonna

FAMILY Solanaceae

PARTS USED
Root, leaf

DESCRIPTION
A perennial, belladonna stands between two and six feet in height, with two or three branches and a purplish stem. Leaves are dark green and three to ten inches long. Bell-shaped flowers are dark purple. When crushed, the plant gives off a strong odor. All parts are poisonous in the extreme.

HABITAT
Belladonna grows in Europe, Asia, and North America. It thrives in chalky soil.

**FOLKLORE
AND TRADITIONAL USES**
The name "belladonna," or "beautiful woman," is said to come from a superstition that the plant could become a beautiful enchantress upon whom it is dangerous to look. Others say it refers to the cosmetic practice of Mediterranean women who dropped the sap of the plant into their eyes to enlarge their pupils and give them a dreamy effect. The Latin *atropa* is derived from the Greek *Atropos*, the Fate who cuts the thread of human life. In old English legends, belladonna belongs to the devil, who leisurely tends it except on the witches' sabbath. A Scottish tale relates how Macbeth's soldiers slipped it to invading Danes in a truce drink, then murdered them in their drug-induced slumber.

MEDICINAL USES
Belladonna contains tropane alkaloids, atropine, hyoscamine, and scopalamine, all of which have sedative, antispasmodic, and narcotic (sleep-inducing or addictive) effects. Doctors use atropine to treat eye disorders and to dilate pupils for eye exams and surgery. Since it numbs nerve endings, belladonna lessens pain when applied locally. Samuel Hahnemann, the founder of the medical system called homeopathy, treated scarlet fever with small doses of belladonna. The therapeutic dose of the plant is very close to the toxic amount.

Barosma betulina

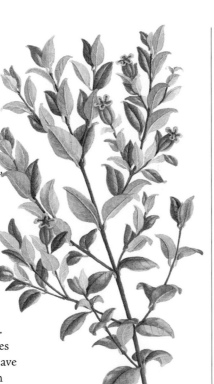

COMMON NAME
Buchu

LATIN NAMES
Barosma betulina (short leaves),
B. crenulata (oval leaves),
B. serratifolia (long leaves)

FAMILY Rutaceae

PART USED
Leaf

DESCRIPTION
These woody shrubs grow
as tall as six feet, with red-
brown or violet-brown bark.
Their leathery, lustrous leaves
are dotted with oil glands, have
jagged margins, and range in
color from yellow-green to
brown. The flowers are small
and star-shaped.

HABITAT
Drought resistant, buchu is
native to southern Africa,
within the Cape region.

**FOLKLORE
AND TRADITIONAL USES**
Indigenous peoples of southern Africa have prized buchu
so much that, it is said, a small
amount was worth a lamb.
In the 19th century, New York
entrepreneur Henry T.
Hembold practiced a lucrative
trade with buchu to treat venereal diseases, kidney stones,
and urinary problems. He was
so widely successful in intro-
ducing the plant to the American public that he called
himself Hembold, the Buchu
King. In the 20th century, the
"sleeping prophet," psychic
Edgar Cayc, prescribed it for
his clients. Buchu water is
now marketed as a mineral
water in parts of the world.

MEDICINAL USES
The native peoples of southern
Africa, most prominently the
Khoi San of the western Cape
region, pioneered the medicinal use of buchu, employing it
to treat urinary problems long
before Europeans arrived.
Dutch Afrikaner settlers
adopted the plant in treating
kidney stones, arthritis,
cholera, muscle aches, and urinary infections when they colonized the Cape region in the
17th century. English who settled there later claimed it had
been used to treat nearly every
human affliction. Although
buchu contains volatile oils
that may give it mild diuretic
and antiseptic properties, its
efficacy in treating sexually
transmitted diseases is unsub-
stantiated. Fluidex and
Odrinil, two prescription
drugs that relieve premenstrual
bloating, both contain buchu.

Bertholletia excelsa

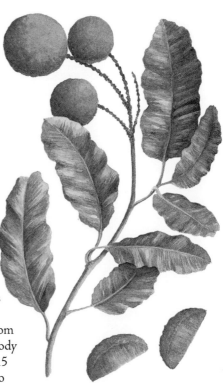

COMMON NAMES
Brazil nut, *Castanheiro
do para* (Brazilian name),
Creamnut

LATIN NAME
Bertholletia excelsa

FAMILY Lecythidaceae

PARTS USED
Nut, seedpod, bark

DESCRIPTION
This enormous evergreen
tree often grows to heights
of 150 feet or above, with
branches emerging only from
its top. Its fruit, a large woody
seedpod containing from 15
to 25 nuts, usually grows to
the size of a large grapefruit
or melon.

HABITAT
The Brazil nut tree grows
throughout forests of the
Amazon River basin of South
America. The tree is harvested
wild and is rarely cultivated
because of its extremely slow
growth rate.

**FOLKLORE
AND TRADITIONAL USES**
For centuries the Brazil nut
has remained a dietary staple
and a trade commodity of the
indigenous tribes of the Amazon rain forests. Peoples of the
rain forests use the empty
seedpods for drinking cups
and to hold small smoky fires
for repelling black flies. Oil
extracted from the nuts is
employed as cooking oil, in
high-precision machinery
lubrication, and livestock feed.
Also popular in other countries, the nuts are usually
found in food markets in winter. Brazil nut oil is used to
make hair-conditioning products, soaps, and skin creams;
it has both detergent and
moisturizing properties.

MEDICINAL USES
Tribes of the Amazon rain forest drink tea prepared from the
bark of the Brazil nut tree as a
remedy for liver ailments. In
Brazilian folk medicine, the
husks of the seedpods are also
administered in the form of tea
to treat stomachaches. Brazil
nuts are rich in protein and
Vitamin E, an important
antioxidant, and in mono-
unsaturated fats, which can
counteract some forms of heart
disease. Additionally the nuts
are an extraordinary source of
selenium, another antioxidant;
one Brazil nut contains
approximately 2,500 times as
much selenium as other nuts.
This nonmetallic element has
been shown to improve mood
as well as mental functioning
and to increase blood flow to
the brain.

Bryonia alba

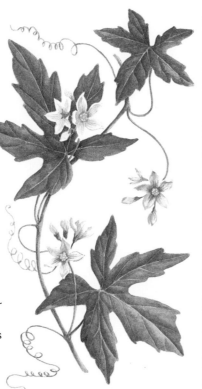

COMMON NAMES
White bryony, Wild hops, English mandrake, Wild vine, Ladies' seal

LATIN NAMES
Bryonia alba,
B. excelsa

FAMILY Cucurbitaceae

PART USED
Root

DESCRIPTION
Bryony, a fast-growing perennial with a thick root and angular, branching stems, has yellow-white flowers with green veins. The plant bears one or two seeded, thin-skinned black berries.

HABITAT
Bryony is commonly found in southern England, as well as in eastern and southeastern Europe.

FOLKLORE
AND TRADITIONAL USES
Augustus Caesar, adopted son and successor to Julius Caesar, wore a wreath of bryony to protect himself from lightning during thunderstorms. John Gerard, 16th-century botanist and chief secretary of state to Queen Elizabeth I, recommended its use for leather tanning. Because bryony's root resembles a person, as does the mandrake root, people associated bryony with that plant and thought it brought bad luck. William Withering, 18th-century botanist and physician famous for his work with digitalis, advocated bryony's use in veterinary medicine.

MEDICINAL USES
Used in the 14th century as a treatment for leprosy, bryony was a popular herbal medicine among the ancient Greeks and Romans and was prescribed by Galen and Dioscorides. It is currently used to treat gastrointestinal, respiratory, and rheumatic disorders. Bryony acts as an irritant and often causes inflammation where it is applied. Various extracts display an antitumoral effect. Bryony is toxic; ingestion can cause vomiting, kidney damage, convulsions, and abortion. Because of these risks, it is prescribed mainly by homeopathic practitioners to be taken in extremely small doses. Homeopathically, it treats fevers that are accompanied by dry mouth and extreme thirst.

Camellia sinensis

COMMON NAMES
Tea, Green tea, Black tea

LATIN NAMES
Camellia sinensis, Thea sinensis

FAMILY Theaceae

PARTS USED
Leaf, bud

DESCRIPTION
An evergreen tree that grows to about eight feet, tea has white flowers. The leaves are oblong with jagged edges. The fruit, a brown capsule with three seeds, is less than an inch in diameter.

HABITAT
Tea has been cultivated for millennia in China and now grows throughout Asia and India. This tree thrives in moist, well-drained, slightly acidic soils and prefers partial shade.

FOLKLORE
AND TRADITIONAL USES
Tea is the second most popular drink worldwide, after water. The English word comes from *t'e* in the Chinese Amoy dialect. According to Chinese legend, it was discovered in 2737 B.C. when a tea leaf accidentally fell into Emperor Shen Nung's cup of hot water. Pleased with the aroma and taste, he believed it came from heaven. One Chinese proverb states, "The wisdom of 10,000 universes can be found in a cup of tea." Japanese Zen monks drank tea to keep themselves awake during long sessions of meditation. Outraged by a price increase by the British Empire in 1773, the American colonists, protesting "taxation without representation," dumped green tea into the harbor, a revolutionary incident now called the Boston Tea Party, which helped solidify the American Colonies in their rebellion against the British.

MEDICINAL USES
Green tea, unlike black and oolong tea, is not fermented, so the active constituents remain unaltered. Tea contains a large number of strong antioxidants called catechins. An antioxidant reduces oxidation, a process in cellular tissue whereby electrons are stripped from molecules, leaving cells vulnerable to cancer. Green tea has been shown in studies to have a wide variety of medicinal effects. It has antibacterial properties, even against the bacteria that cause dental caries, and has been shown to lower certain types of cholesterol. Tea can also aid in the treatment of digestive tract problems ranging from diarrhea to cancer.

Camptotheca acuminata

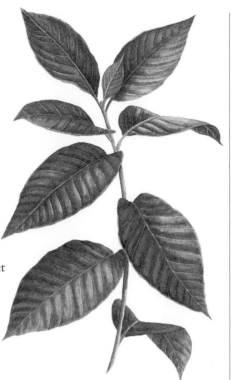

COMMON NAMES
Xi shu, Tree of joy,
Happy tree, Cancer tree

LATIN NAME
Camptotheca acuminata

FAMILY Nyssaceae

PARTS USED
Wood, bark, leaf, fruit

DESCRIPTION
Xi shu grows up to 80 feet tall with slender reddish brown bark and a few branches near the top.

HABITAT
Xi shu, indigenous to China and Tibet, grows best in warm zones.

FOLKLORE AND TRADITIONAL USES
Camptotheca goes by many names in its native lands. *Xi shu* translates as "happy tree" and has been called this by people whom it cured of colds and other illnesses. Its other names include *long shu* (dragon tree), *jia shu* (fine tree), and *tian zi shu* (heaven wood tree). The Chinese have also used this tree for firewood and as an ornamental plant. All American specimens of the *Camptotheca* are descendants of two trees germinated from seeds brought from China in the 1930s.

MEDICINAL USES
The Chinese have used *xi shu* for traditional drug purposes for hundreds, and possibly thousands, of years. They have employed this plant against psoriasis and in the treatment of diseases of the liver, gall-bladder, spleen, and stomach. It has also been used to treat leukemia. In fact, one common name for *Camptotheca* is the "cancer tree." For treating cancer its primary constituent is camptothecin, which inhibits topoisomerase I, an enzyme linked with cell division and DNA replication. By inhibiting this enzyme, camptothecin appears to stunt tumor growth. A host of other anticancer drugs have been modified from camptothecin, two of which are approved by the U.S. Food and Drug Administration. Topotecan is used to treat ovarian and small lung cancers. Irinotecan is used to treat metastatic colorectal cancer, the second leading cause of cancer deaths in the United States. Other camptothecin-related drugs are no longer in use because of their severe toxicity.

Cannabis sativa

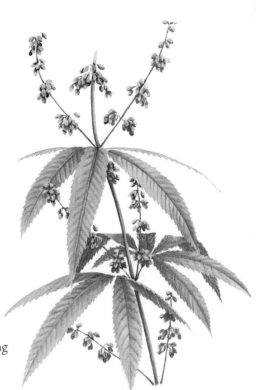

COMMON NAMES
Marijuana, Cannabis, Hemp, Hashish

LATIN NAME
Cannabis sativa

FAMILY Cannabaceae

PARTS USED
Flower, leaf, seed, resin

DESCRIPTION
Marijuana, an annual or biennial plant, can reach heights of over ten feet. Leaves grow in groups of three to seven and are long and thin, with slightly serrated margins. The male and female flowers, borne on separate plants, are small and greenish.

HABITAT
Marijuana probably came from Asia and the Middle East, but it now grows worldwide in temperate and tropical regions.

FOLKLORE AND TRADITIONAL USES
The use of marijuana dates back 4,000 years. Archaeologists believe that by 1000 B.C. nomadic Middle Eastern tribes introduced it to India, China, Europe, and Africa. Under Queen Elizabeth I, it was lawful in England to grow marijuana on a certain amount of one's own land. According to a Hindu legend, Lord Siva brought marijuana down from the Himalaya for people's enjoyment. In Africa, cults formed around the herb in the belief that it came from the gods. In the West in the 1930s, concerns about addiction resulted in restrictions on the use of marijuana; later it became illegal in some countries, including the United States. Hemp fiber has been used in making many things, from ropes to fishing nets. It was the original fabric for blue jeans. The oldest existing paper made of hemp was discovered in a Chinese grave dating from before the early Han Dynasty.

MEDICINAL USES
Thousands of years ago, the Chinese described using marijuana medicinally for treating malaria, gout, rheumatism, absentmindedness, and female disorders. Until the early 20th century, Europeans used it as a painkiller for migraines and to relieve anxiety. Marijuana is the only plant known to contain the psychoactive constituent tetrahydrocannabinol, or THC. When smoked or eaten, marijuana relieves nausea, moderates chronic pain, increases appetite, and reduces muscle spasms.

Capsicum annuum

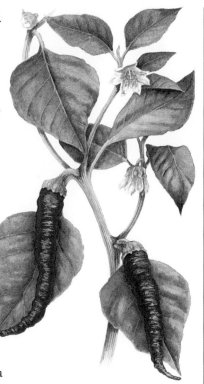

COMMON NAMES
Cayenne pepper, Red pepper

LATIN NAME
Capsicum annuum

FAMILY Solanaceae

PART USED
Fruit

DESCRIPTION
An annual or biennial, cayenne pepper grows between two and six feet tall and has an angular, erect stem. Leaves are oval and long-stemmed. Flowers are usually solitary. The red, yellowish green, or brownish fruit has a leathery skin and is up to two inches long and one inch thick. Seeds are yellowish white.

HABITAT
Cayenne pepper is indigenous to Mexico, Central America, and South America. It is also cultivated in most tropical and subtropical countries, especially Zanzibar, a part of Tanzania.

**FOLKLORE
AND TRADITIONAL USES**
South American natives once believed eating six cayenne peppers daily for eight days would make them excellent blowgunners. Deriving its name from the Greek word meaning "to bite," cayenne pepper is hot and pungent. The Latin name *capsicum* refers to the hot, pungent taste. It is commonly used to spice foods, especially in the form of pepper sauce. One of its common names, Tabasco sauce, comes from the Mexican state of Tabasco. In Mexico cayenne pepper is used even to flavor ice cream. Manufacturers of self-defense tear-gas sprays employ cayenne pepper in their products.

MEDICINAL USES
The Aztec used cayenne pepper to treat toothaches and scabies. Since the 18th century it has been considered a powerful stimulant and has proved useful in treating many gastrointestinal and circulatory ailments, especially indigestion. Cayenne pepper's active constituent, capsaicin, the substance that produces the heat sensation, is used to treat pain caused by herpes, shingles, arthritis, rheumatism, and other neuralgias by desensitizing the neurons that transmit pain. Capsaicin has been employed to treat overactive bladders by desensitizing the neurons that trigger excess activity. Cayenne may stimulate the release of opiatelike endorphins and contain aspirinlike salicylates.

Caulophyllum thalictroides

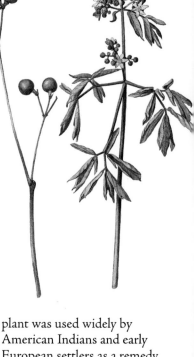

COMMON NAMES
Blue cohosh, Papoose root, Squawroot

LATIN NAME
Caulophyllum thalictroides

FAMILY Berberidaceae

PARTS USED
Root, rhizome

DESCRIPTION
This leafy perennial plant, which grows two-to-three feet tall, has a gray-brown, four-inch-long rhizome. Blue cohosh bears yellow-green or green-purple flowers and dark blue seeds the size of large pears.

HABITAT
This plant is found in the damp, rich woodlands of the eastern part of North America.

**FOLKLORE
AND TRADITIONAL USES**
The "blue" in this herb's name refers to its paired blue seeds. The "cohosh" is probably derived from the Algonquian word *kóshki*, meaning "it is rough." When roasted and ground, the seeds have been used as a coffee substitute. This herb was included in the *Pharmacopoeia of the United States* until 1905. Blue cohosh should not be confused with black cohosh, *Cimicifuga racemosa*, and white cohosh, *Acataea alba*.

MEDICINAL USES
Native American women brewed bitter blue cohosh to ease childbirth pains and to relieve cramps. The root was taken as a contraceptive and was used by both sexes to treat genitourinary conditions. The plant was used widely by American Indians and early European settlers as a remedy for rheumatism, anxiety, bronchitis, colic, sore throat and a range of other ailments. It is still used in India for a variety of purposes, including as a treatment for gynecological disorders. In 20th century Western medicine, blue cohosh has treated worm infestation, dehydration, and cramps. It has also been used to assist the labor of childbirth. The plant is known to stimulate smooth muscle contraction and increase blood pressure. Researchers have isolated the alkaloid methylcytisine, which, like nicotine, stimulates intestinal activity and raises respiration. Methylcytisine is considered toxic, and may interfere with normal cell division. Blue cohosh should not be ingested during pregnancy.

Chondrodendron tomentosum

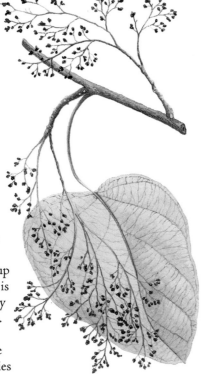

COMMON NAMES
Curare, Pareira

LATIN NAME
Chondrodendron tomentosum

FAMILY Menispermaceae

PARTS USED
Root, bark, leaf

DESCRIPTION
A woody vine often found in trees, pareira has a velvety appearance and may extend up to a foot in length. The stem is gray and furrowed, and it may be partly covered with lichen. Roots are blackish brown, tough, heavy, and knotty. The inside is reddish yellow. Berries are black or scarlet.

HABITAT
Pareira is confined mainly to the Guianas and the Amazon basin. It is also found in the West Indies and other regions of South America. This plant requires a tropical or a sub-tropical climate.

FOLKLORE AND TRADITIONAL USES
Pareira is a popular source of curare, the deadly arrow poison used by Amazonian tribes. Many European explorers, including Christopher Columbus and Sir Walter Raleigh, returned from South America with tales of men killed by these "evyll frutes." A silent killer, curare gave the native peoples an almost supernatural superiority over their gun-bearing adversaries. Tubocurarine, a derivative of pareira, has been administered as a lethal injection in capital punishment and euthanasia in countries such as the United States and the Netherlands. It is subject to restrictions in some countries.

MEDICINAL USES
Pareira is the only known source of the not-yet-synthesized alkaloid delta-tubocurarine, first isolated in 1935. D-tubocurarine is given in small quantities with general anesthesia to produce muscle paralysis; it interferes with nerve impulse transmission at the receptor sites of skeletal muscles. It is also used in shock therapy and in the setting of fractures. Some consider pareira a diuretic and a uterine stimulant, including the Brazilians, who also use it to treat poisonous snakebite.

Cinchona pubescens

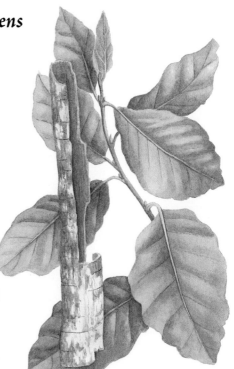

COMMON NAME
Cinchona

LATIN NAME
Cinchona pubescens

FAMILY Rubiaceae

PART USED
Bark

DESCRIPTION
An evergreen tree, growing to between 50 and 100 feet, cinchona has leaves that are flat and broad, with a shiny green surface and large veins. The flower is white and elongated, covered thickly with silky hairs.

HABITAT
Cinchona, native to Central and South America, is culti-vated in many tropical areas.

FOLKLORE AND TRADITIONAL USES
Cinchona was reputedly named for the Spanish Count-ess Chinchon, who recovered from a fever by using the bark. The countess had it sent to Europe, where it became known by her name. When Jesuits visited Peru in the 17th century, they discovered that the native people chewed on cinchona bark to prevent the shaking and chills they suf-fered after working in icy streams for the Spanish mines. Linking the shaking from cold to the shaking during a malar-ial fever, the Jesuits tried chew-ing the bark to treat malaria. Because some strains of the bark are less potent, it did not always cure malaria, which led to the distrust and persecution of many Jesuits in Europe.

MEDICINAL USES
French chemists J. B. Caventou and P. J. Pelletier isolated the alkaloid quinine from the cin-chona bark in 1820. And in 1944 American scientists syn-thesized quinine in the labora-tory. From this came various quinine-based drugs, such as chloroquine and primaquine, for the treatment of malaria. Recently certain resistant strains of malaria pathogens have been identified, sparking debate about the effectiveness of the whole plant over a syn-thetic chemical. People around the world still use the natural bark in herbal remedies. In Brazil, it is considered an appetite stimulant and a cure for fatigue. In Venezuela peo-ple use the bark as a remedy for cancers. Cinchona bark is also the source of the drug quinidine, used to treat cardiac arrhythmias.

Cinnamomum aromaticum

COMMON NAME
Cinnamon

LATIN NAMES
Cinnamomum aromaticum,
C. verum

FAMILY Lauraceae

PARTS USED
Bark, flower, twig

DESCRIPTION
An evergreen tree, cinnamon can grow more than 25 feet tall, with angular branches. The bark is reddish brown, thick, aromatic, and scabrous. Oval, or lance-shaped, leaves are green on top and brown underneath, large, downy, and leathery when mature. Flowers are small and white or yellow. The fruit is berrylike and bluish with white spots when ripe.

HABITAT
Cinnamon is indigenous to Asia. Other species are found in South America and the Caribbean.

**FOLKLORE
AND TRADITIONAL USES**
Historically a trade item, cinnamon has been long valued for its aromatic, medicinal, and preservative properties. The ancient Egyptians used cinnamon as a holy offering and an embalming oil, and the ancient Arabians monopolized its trade by concocting magical tales about its harvesting. After murdering his wife, the emperor Nero is reported to have buried her in a year's worth of Rome's imported cinnamon. It was considered the tree of life by the ancient Chinese, and Europeans once thought it originated in the Garden of Eden. Previously expensive, cinnamon is now commonly enjoyed as a cooking spice, an incense, and a flavoring in toothpastes and mouthwash. Most cinnamon in the U.S. spice market is actually the bark of the cassia tree, containing some of the same aromatic oil components and thus having a similar flavor. It is more abundant and therefore less expensive than true cinnamon.

MEDICINAL USES
Cinnamon is an ancient herbal medicine, long used to treat gastrointestinal disorders. It increases intestinal movement, heart rate, and perspiration by stimulating the vasomotor center. Taken in the correct dosage, cinnamon is believed to improve circulation. The astringent tannins in cinnamon treat diarrhea; the catechins treat nausea. Its essential oils are considered analgesic, antifungal, and germicidal.

Colchicum autumnale

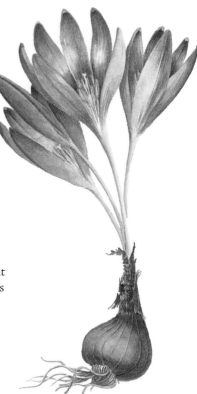

COMMON NAMES
Autumn crocus,
Meadow saffron

LATIN NAME
Colchicum autumnale

FAMILY Liliaceae

PARTS USED
Corm, seed, flower

DESCRIPTION
This foot-high perennial plant has dark green, tuliplike leaves that grow out of a corm, a fleshy, bulblike base. Crocus flowers are light purple or white.

HABITAT
Indigenous to Europe, the autumn crocus is widely cultivated as an ornamental plant.

**FOLKLORE
AND TRADITIONAL USES**
According to legends, the crocus indicates either the place where the gods Jove and Juno lay together or the place where the enchantress Medea spilled an elixir of life. Related species produce saffron, used since antiquity as a spice and dye. The crocus's corm, an underground bulblike organ, has been used historically as a potent poison, ground into a powder, and was often administered in wine. According to the Greek naturalist Theophrastus, slaves ate small pieces of the corm when they were angry with their masters to make themselves ill and unable to work. Scientists use colchicine, the plant's principal alkaloid, to develop strains of crops that produce larger fruits and vegetables and are more disease resistant.

MEDICINAL USES
The autumn crocus's main active principle is the alkaline substance colchicine, which is used today as one of the principal drugs in gout therapy, as it may have been 4,000 years ago by the ancient Egyptians. The plant has been used to treat rheumatism, dropsy, and prostate enlargement. With colchicine, Egyptian and Israeli doctors have treated familial Mediterranean fever, which is fever accompanied by abdominal, joint, and chest pain. Because colchicine has been shown to stop cell division, scientists have researched its use as an anticancer agent, but it is currently regarded as too toxic for cancer treatment. Research is now being done on colchicine's effectiveness as a treatment for chronic hepatitis and cirrhosis.

Coleus forskohlii

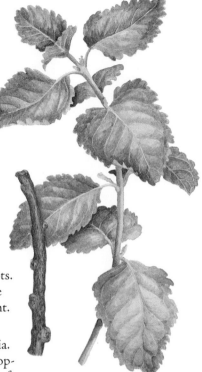

COMMON NAME
Coleus forkolil

LATIN NAME
Coleus forskohlii

FAMILY Labiatae

PARTS USED
Root, leaf

DESCRIPTION
A perennial, coleus grows up to two feet tall, with an erect stem and tuberlike roots. Leaves are colorful and large and have a camphorlike scent.

HABITAT
Coleus is indigenous to India. It is also cultivated in the tropical and subtropical regions of Asia and eastern Africa. It flourishes in well-drained soil in sun or partial shade.

FOLKLORE AND TRADITIONAL USES
Large colorful leaves make coleus a popular ornamental plant that is displayed both in the home and garden. Coleus is also cultivated in some parts of India for use in pickles and salads. In parts of Asia, species such as *C. edulis* and *C. parvifloris* provide edible tubers. Some people have attempted to use the leaves as a mild hallucinogen. In studies, coleus is often used to test such varied topics as the ability of plants to perceive stress and the effects of fluoride on them.

MEDICINAL USES
Coleus is part of traditional Indian folk medicine as a digestive remedy for flatulence, bloating, and abdominal discomfort and as an aid against vaginal and urinary infections. Coleus's principal constituent, the diterpene forskolin, first isolated in the 1970s, is a cardiotonic and an inhibitor of platelet aggregation. Forskolin is used for circulatory problems like heart failure and high blood pressure and for respiratory problems such as bronchial asthma. It has also been shown to relieve pressure within the eye, a major symptom of glaucoma. *Coleus forskohlii* is the only source of forskolin.

Crataegus oxyacantha

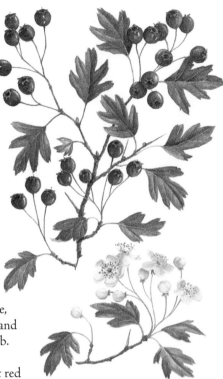

COMMON NAMES
Hawthorn, Maybush, Mayhaw, Whitethorn, Mother-die, Bread and cheese

LATIN NAMES
Crataegus oxyacantha, *C. monogyna*

FAMILY Rosaceae

PARTS USED
Leaf, flower, berry

DESCRIPTION
Hawthorn, a deciduous tree, can reach 30 feet in height and can also be grown as a shrub. Clusters of white flowers bloom in spring, and bright red berries, called haws, form in the fall.

HABITAT
This tree grows in temperate regions in Europe, North Africa, India, and North America.

FOLKLORE AND TRADITIONAL USES
Hawthorn's name comes from "haw," derived from the Old English *haga*, which also meant "hedge," because its thorns and sturdy twigs made it a perfect barrier for cattle and pigs. It earned its former nickname "bread and cheese" when people ate the leaves during hard times. The branches were used in Maypole ceremonies to symbolize renewed life, fertility, and spring. Romans attached hawthorn sprigs to the cradle of a newborn baby to protect it against illnesses and evil influences. This was reputedly the plant used in Christ's crown of thorns. For centuries, people believed that lightning, the work of the devil, would never strike a hawthorn tree, because this plant had rested upon the forehead of Christ.

MEDICINAL USES
Historically hawthorn was used as a diuretic and to treat kidney stones. By the late 19th century, doctors understood the connection between hawthorn and the heart. An extract of the flowers and leaves improves cardiac output and the contractility of the heart muscle itself. Flavonoids in hawthorn have been shown to increase blood flow in the heart by dilating blood vessels in coronary arteries. Hawthorn has lowered cholesterol in animal studies, probably due to its oligomeric procyanidins (OPC), a type of bioflavonoids similar to that found in the extracts of grape seed and grape skin.

Cucurbita pepo

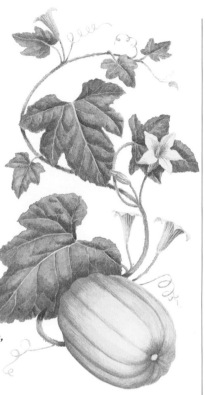

COMMON NAMES
Pumpkin, Vegetable marrow

LATIN NAME
Cucurbita pepo

FAMILY Cucurbitaceae

PART USED
Seed

DESCRIPTION
An annual fruit, pumpkin has vines that grow up to 26 feet long. The leaves are large and bristly; the flowers are big, yellow, and solitary. The fruit is large, greenish to orange, and fibrous. Its many seeds have flat, shallow grooves.

HABITAT
Pumpkin is indigenous to North America. It is also cultivated widely, especially in temperate climates.

**FOLKLORE
AND TRADITIONAL USES**
According to archaeological records in Mexico (8750 B.C.), *C. pepo* appears to be one of the first domesticated plant species. Pumpkins and other species of squash, along with beans and corn, were considered the "three sisters" by Native Americans, who planted them together. The bean vines used the cornstalks as supports and fixed nitrogen in the soil. And for all of them, the large squash leaves shaded the soil and helped hold moisture in it. In the Grimms' fairy tale *Cinderella*, the heroine's fairy godmother turned a pumpkin into a magical golden coach. During Halloween, the pumpkin is made into jack-o'-lanterns and pumpkin cakes and pies; and it is represented in trick-or-treat costumes and decorations.

MEDICINAL USES
Pumpkin was used in folk medicine to treat kidney inflammation and intestinal parasites and was once listed as one of the Four Greater Cold Seeds in an 18th century list of medicines. Today pumpkin is employed to treat irritable bladder and prostate complaints, namely benign prostatic hyperplasia (BPH). The fatty oil in pumpkin seeds is mildly diuretic, and the seeds' principal constituent, cucurbitacins, appears to inhibit the conversion of testosterone into dihydrotesterone. The presence of zinc and amino acids further treat BPH. Pumpkin does not reduce prostate enlargement—it relieves symptoms only. Pumpkin seeds are also thought to help relieve dizziness.

Curcuma longa

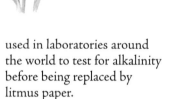

COMMON NAMES
Turmeric, Haldi, Jiang huang

LATIN NAME
Curcuma longa

FAMILY Zingiberaceae

PART USED
Rhizome

DESCRIPTION
A perennial, turmeric grows up to five feet tall, with a short stem. The rhizome is thick, knobby, and yellowish orange inside. Leaves are large and oblong with maroon bands on both sides of the midrib. Flowers are yellowish white with pink bracts.

HABITAT
Turmeric is indigenous to India and southern Asia and is cultivated throughout Asia. It needs well-drained soil and a humid climate.

**FOLKLORE
AND TRADITIONAL USES**
Turmeric features in many ancient Malaysian myths and Indian ceremonies. One tale indicates it has the power to repel crocodiles. Mentioned in the Bible, turmeric is a popular culinary spice and is the principal ingredient used to flavor and color curries and some prepared mustards. It is often recommended as a substitute for saffron, a more expensive spice, and its oil is sometimes used to manufacture perfume. Turmeric has long served as orange-yellow textile dye in East Asia. During the late 19th century, "turmeric paper" was used in laboratories around the world to test for alkalinity before being replaced by litmus paper.

MEDICINAL USES
Turmeric is highly regarded in Ayurvedic medicine, especially as a remedy for jaundice and digestive problems. In recent decades, scientific studies have confirmed these historic uses. Turmeric has been shown to lower cholesterol and to thin blood. Its principal constituent, curcumin, helps protect the liver against a number of toxic substances by inhibiting cytochrome 4501A, a type of enzyme involved in the activation of several toxins. Curcumin also increases bile flow, relieves indigestion, and helps prevent the formation of cholesterol gallstones in the gastrointestinal tract. Turmeric can be used in a paste externally to treat psoriasis and athlete's foot.

Daucus carota

COMMON NAMES
Carrot, Bird's nest,
Bee's nest, Queen Anne's lace
(wild carrot)

LATIN NAME
Daucus carota

FAMILY Umbelliferae

PARTS USED
Root, leaf, seed

DESCRIPTION
This two- to four-foot herb
is usually biennial. Its root,
while commonly orange, can
also be purple, red, yellow,
or white.

HABITAT
Indigenous to Afghanistan and
surrounding areas, it is now
cultivated in temperate areas
worldwide.

**FOLKLORE
AND TRADITIONAL USES**
Associated with rabbits from
Peter Rabbit to Bugs Bunny,
the carrot is a popular food.
The British have made wine
with carrots. The Germans
used the carrot as a coffee substitute, and the French and the
Germans made liquor from it.
The plant has also been
employed as a dye and a flavoring agent for butter. During a
Latin grammar lesson in
The Merry Wives of Windsor,
Shakespeare makes a pun of
caret, Latin for "is wanting,"
and "carrot." He quips, "And
that's a good root!" In England
in the 17th century, fashion-
able ladies wore feathery carrot
leaves in their headdresses.

MEDICINAL USES
The carrot is an ancient remedy mentioned in the writings
of Pliny. Studies completed
recently show that increasing
daily consumption of carrots
as a good source of beta-
carotene can significantly
reduce the risk of heart attacks
and strokes in women. According to another study, stroke
patients are more likely to survive and recover if they have
significant levels of beta-
carotene in their bloodstream.
Regular consumption of carrots may also reduce the risk of
lung and larynx cancer, even in
former smokers. The carrot
has been used to treat intestinal parasites, diarrhea, digestive problems, and high
cholesterol. Perhaps its most
famous use, to help eyesight,
has been confirmed by science:
Carrots contain Vitamin A, a
source of retinal, a compound
that in combination with proteins forms the visual pigments
of the retinal rods and cones.

Delphinium staphisagria

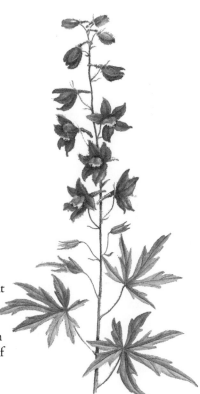

COMMON NAMES
Delphinium, Stavesacre,
Lousewort

LATIN NAME
Delphinium staphisagria

FAMILY Ranunculaceae

PART USED
Seed

DESCRIPTION
Delphinium is an annual or
biennial with a stout stem that
reaches a height of three
feet or more. Bluish or
purple flowers narrow to form
a loose spike toward the top of
the stalk with quadrangular
gray-black, wrinkled seeds.

HABITAT
Delphinium is indigenous to
southern Europe and Asia
Minor.

**FOLKLORE
AND TRADITIONAL USES**
The name "delphinium" comes
from the resemblance of this
plant's buds to a dolphin. In
Victorian times lovers gave
each other a related species,
larkspur, to signify fidelity.
The nickname "lousewort"
comes from its long-standing
use for destroying lice and nits
in the hair. Pliny the Elder,
first century Roman encyclo-
pedist and naturalist, mentioned this use in his writings,
and the plant continues to
serve this purpose.

MEDICINAL USES
Delphinium was employed by
the Greeks and the Romans.
Dioscorides, a first-century
Greek physician famous for his
writings on medicines, mentions it. Delphinine, the plant's
main alkaloid, has effects similar to those of aconitine, the
main alkaloid of aconite. Delphinine has been employed to
treat neuralgia, rheumatism,
and asthma. Because improper
dosage and administration can
prove fatal, internal administration is almost exclusively
given in homeopathic remedies, which are extreme dilutions of the original active
substance. Homeopaths give
delphinium to patients with a
variety of symptoms, ranging
from bleeding gums to
masochism. In homeopathy, it
can also treat patients recover-
ing from pelvic or genital
surgery. In addition, delphinium is used to expel
worms and other intestinal
parasites. However, scientific
efficacy is not well established,
and delphinium may cause cardiac problems. For this reason,
it is not recommended by
Germany's herbal experts,
Commission E.

Digitalis purpurea

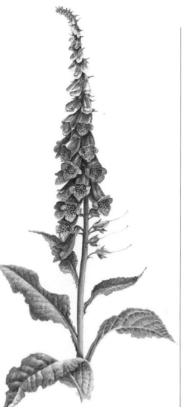

COMMON NAMES
Foxglove, Fairy's glove, Folk's glove

LATIN NAME
Digitalis purpurea

FAMILY Scrophulariaceae

PART USED
Leaf

DESCRIPTION
Foxglove is a biennial that can grow to six feet tall, with a straight, unbranched stem. The flowers hang in bunches and are dull pink or purple, often with white spots. Leaves are large with prominent veins.

HABITAT
Primarily an English plant, foxglove also grows widely throughout Europe and North America. It usually occurs in rocky terrain, but it does best in loose, well-drained, cultivated soil.

FOLKLORE AND TRADITIONAL USES
Foxglove has been called by many names. The Irish called it "dead man's thimbles" in reference to the secretion of its harmful juice. An English variant, "folks glove," referred to the fairy folk who lived in woody areas where the plant grows. Spots on the flowers were said to mark the places where elves put their fingers, warning of the plant's poison. To Norwegians it was *Revbielde*, or "fox bell," from the legend that bad fairies gave the plant to the fox so he could quiet his footsteps with the blossoms while hunting around chicken roosts. People in North Wales used the leaves to give their stone floors a mosaic-like appearance.

MEDICINAL USES
Originally employed as a healing herb in Ireland, foxglove was used to treat boils, ulcers, headaches, and paralysis. Foxglove contains the glycoside digitoxin, which scientists have isolated and now use as a drug, called digitalis, for congestive heart failure and congenital heart defects. Digitoxin strengthens cardiac muscle contractions and slows the beat of the heart. Another glycoside in foxglove, digoxin, acts as a diuretic on the kidneys. Any of foxglove's constituents are extremely dangerous in high doses; cardiac rhythm disorders, depression, heart failure, or asphyxiation may occur.

Dioscorea villosa

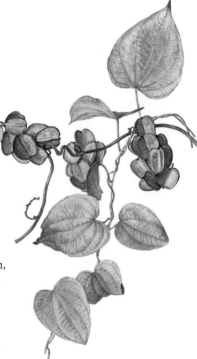

COMMON NAME
Wild yam

LATIN NAMES
Dioscorea villosa,
D. barbasco (Mexican wild yam)

FAMILY Dioscoreaceae

PARTS USED
Rhizome, root

DESCRIPTION
A perennial vine with smooth, alternate, heart-shaped leaves and small, greenish yellow to white flowers, wild yam vines grow up to 40 feet long. Pale-brown rhizomes are tuberous and potatolike, and the roots are long and woody, with knotted rootstocks.

HABITAT
Wild yam is indigenous to the southern U.S. and Canada. It is also widely cultivated in tropical, subtropical, and temperate regions, including Latin America and Asia. It thrives in sunny conditions and rich soil.

FOLKLORE AND TRADITIONAL USES
Yams are a staple part of the diet in many parts of the world and figure large in myth and ritual. To promote a good harvest, families in New Caledonia collected stones of shapes and colors representing the various species of yams, placed them beside ancestral skulls, then buried the stones in the yam fields. In Australia temporary camps where yams were dug date back thousands of years. For centuries, in Mexico the grated root of the wild yam has been used to stun fish before netting them. What many Americans think of as yams are really the unrelated sweet potato.

MEDICINAL USES
The Aztec and Native Americans used wild yam as a pain reliever and to aid in the labor of childbirth. The Chinese used it for ailments of the stomach and spleen. In the 1930s Japanese scientists identified the wild yam's main constituent, diosgenin, the principal ingredient in the progesterone-containing oral contraceptive commonly known as the pill. Diosgenin, now totally synthetic, is still used to manufacture cortisone, progesterone, and other steroids. Wild yam is also a source of synthetic DHEA, a hormone that inhibits the production of excess fatty acids and cholesterol. For its anti-cancer, expectorant, and diuretic properties, wild yam is used in homeopathic remedies.

Echinacea angustifolia

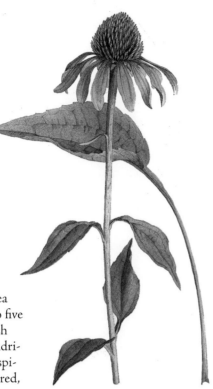

COMMON NAMES
Echinacea, Coneflower, Narrow-leaved purple coneflower, Rudbeckia

LATIN NAMES
Echinacea angustifolia, E. purpurea

FAMILY Asteraceae

PART USED
Root

DESCRIPTION
A hairy perennial, echinacea may grow as high as two to five feet. It has a sturdy, purplish green stem. Roots are cylindrical, furrowed, and slightly spiral. Leaves are narrow, tapered, and hairy, with three to five veins. Flowers are mainly purple, singular, and long stalked, with down-turned ray florets seated around a high cone.

HABITAT
Echinacea is indigenous to the central plains of North America. It is also cultivated in other parts of the world.

FOLKLORE AND TRADITIONAL USES
Part of the plant's Latin name *echinacea* means "prickly" and derives from the Greek word for "hedgehog." It refers to the coneflower's black spiny seed heads. The Native American Plains tribe held echinacea in high esteem. Magicianlike shamans washed their hands with its juice before plunging them into scalding water as a ritual act.

MEDICINAL USES
Native Americans used echinacea to treat snakebites, insect bites, toothaches, burns, enlarged glands, colds, headaches, and throat infections. During the 19th century it was employed as an antiseptic and blood cleanser. Today it is a proven antiviral agent and wound-healer, and it is considered a nonspecific immune system stimulant. No single compound has been identified as responsible for these actions. Chicoric acid may inhibit the enzyme integrase to decrease viral reproduction. Or the herb's polysaccharides may stimulate white blood cell activity, increasing phagocytosis, the collection of bacterial, viral, and cellular debris. One hypothesis is that the root extract acts like interferon, the body's own antiviral compound. In any case, echinacea is effective against a plethora of ailments, including flu, yeast infections, herpes sores, and inflammatory diseases. In Germany it is used in more than 200 preparations.

Ephedra sinica

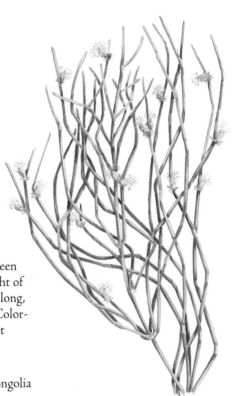

COMMON NAMES
Ma huang, Ephedra

LATIN NAME
Ephedra sinica

FAMILY Ephedraceae

PART USED
Stem

DESCRIPTION
Ephedra is a spiky evergreen shrub that reaches a height of 20 inches. The stems are long, narrow, and cylindrical. Coloring is gray-green to bright green.

HABITAT
Northern China and Mongolia

FOLKLORE AND TRADITIONAL USES
Ephedra has been used in a variety of ways throughout history. In Pakistan, it is mixed with chewing tobacco. American species, which are believed to be alkaloid-free, were made into beverages, both by settlers and Native Americans. The tea was believed to be effective in treating gonorrhea and was formerly served in brothels in some parts of the Old West, giving it its name "whore house tea." The mashed fibers of this plant provided material for mats, and the wood was used to produce charcoal for tattoos and dyes.

MEDICINAL USES
The Chinese have employed ma huang for more than 2,000 years to treat asthma, coughs, and flu. Southwestern American Indians in western Texas and northern Mexico used other species of ephedra to treat urogenital diseases and as a poultice. The alkaloids ephedrine and pseudoephedrine were isolated at the turn of the 20th century. Both stimulate the central nervous system, increase blood pressure and heart rate, and have effects similar to adrenaline in the body. Western medicine primarily uses the alkaloid drugs derived from ephedra to treat asthma and hay fever. Recent use in a weight-loss product has stimulated controversy about safety, because ephedra in too high a dose can elevate blood pressure and even cause angina.

Erythroxylum coca

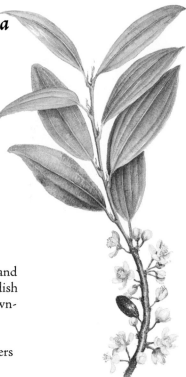

COMMON NAME
Coca

LATIN NAME
Erythroxylum coca

FAMILY Erythroxylaceae

PART USED
Leaf

DESCRIPTION
A shrubby tree, coca grows between 6 feet (cultivated) and 18 feet (wild) tall, with reddish brown bark. Leaves are brownish green, stiff, and bitter tasting, with two faint lines parallel to the midrib. Flowers are small, greenish white, and clustered. Fruits are red berries.

HABITAT
Coca is indigenous to the Andes region of South America, especially Bolivia and Peru. It is also cultivated in many parts of Asia. Coca requires moisture and an equatorial habitat.

**FOLKLORE
AND TRADITIONAL USES**
Coca has been cultivated for centuries since the time of the Inca Empire. It was used in religious rituals to show respect for the Earth god. Pope Leo XII, Sarah Bernhardt, Thomas Edison, and Ulysses S. Grant enjoyed coca mixed with wine, a drink called "Vin Mariani." During the 1880s physicians claimed that coca's alkaloid, cocaine, could cure everything from stomach pain to opium addiction. A nonaddictive coca leaf extract took many forms, including candies, over-the-counter injections, and soft drinks such as the original Coca-Cola.

MEDICINAL USES
Coca's principal tropane alkaloid is cocaine, first extracted in 1860. A powerful topical anesthetic, cocaine paralyzes the sensory nerve fibers and is commonly employed in eye, nose, and throat surgery, as well as in upper respiratory and digestive tract examinations. Chewed coca leaves are high in valuable nutrients, containing calcium, iron, phosphorus, and Vitamins A, B_2, and E. Peruvian and Bolivian tribes use coca leaves to treat dietary inadequacies, gastrointestinal disorders, nausea, headaches, and altitude sickness. In concentrated forms, coca is highly addictive and dangerous.

Eucalyptus globulus

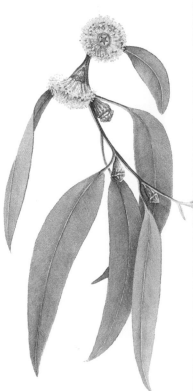

COMMON NAMES
Eucalyptus, Blue gum tree

LATIN NAME
Eucalyptus globulus

FAMILY Myrtaceae

PART USED
Leaf

DESCRIPTION
An evergreen, the eucalyptus tree reaches up to about 400 feet in height. The trunk is twisted, with silver gray bark. Mature leaves are bluish green and have a tough, leathery texture. Glands containing volatile oil are on the leaf surface.

HABITAT
The eucalyptus is native to Tasmania and southeastern Australia. It grows in tropical, subtropical, and temperate regions of the world.

**FOLKLORE
AND TRADITIONAL USES**
Australian Aborigines in the dry outback chew eucalyptus roots for water. Europeans thought that eucalyptus might cure malarial fevers, and by the 1860s they were shipping the leaves and oil around the Mediterranean. Although eucalyptus does not cure malaria, the trees the Europeans planted around the swamps drew up much of the water and reduced the breeding area of malarial mosquitoes, thus reducing their numbers. Eucalyptus is the sole food source for the koala, an Australian marsupial. In addition to being a source of paper pulp and fuel, this tree has proved to be an important lumber species. For example, it is used to build parts of ships.

MEDICINAL USES
In folk medicine eucalyptus is used to treat asthma, gastric complaints, incipient scarlet fever, and worm infestation. The oil from eucalyptus leaves contains eucalyptol, a chemical that makes it a very powerful antiseptic. Studies show that eucalyptol can kill some influenza viruses. It is approved by the U.S. Food and Drug Administration (FDA) as a cold and flu remedy. Other studies show that this chemical kills some kinds of bacteria, making it a treatment for bronchitis. Since eucalyptol loosens phlegm in the chest, it is an effective and popular ingredient in many lozenges.

Foeniculum vulgare

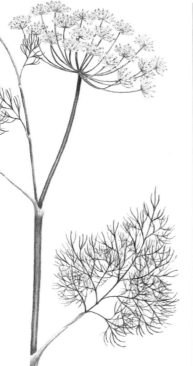

COMMON NAME
Fennel

LATIN NAME
Foeniculum vulgare

FAMILY Umbelliferae

PARTS USED
Fruit, seed

DESCRIPTION
Fennel is a perennial or biennial that grows to about five feet in height. The stem is round and straight with long, feathery leaves and umbels of small yellow flowers. Fennel is dark green and has a strong scent.

HABITAT
Indigenous to the Mediterranean, fennel now grows in temperate regions worldwide. It thrives in sunny areas with well-drained, loamy soil.

FOLKLORE AND TRADITIONAL USES
The name, *Foeniculum*, comes from the Latin for either "fragrant hay" or "product of the meadow." In Greek legend, knowledge came to humans from Mount Olympus in the form of a burning coal inside a fennel stalk. Europeans in the early Middle Ages positioned the plant over doors to ward off the possible ill effects of witchcraft. In England people put sprigs of fennel in horses' harnesses to keep flies away. It was also very popular as a seasoning and as an appetite suppressant.

MEDICINAL USES
Fennel oil contains anethole and fenchone, which reduce bloating and, in higher concentrations, act as antispasmodics. An infusion of the seeds relieves sore throats and coughs and acts as a mild expectorant. People use crushed fennel seeds effectively as an eyewash for conjunctivitis. The plant has been employed to treat menstrual problems, promote lactation, and facilitate birth. Researchers have documented the validity of these traditional treatments by finding that an extract of the seeds has had an estrogenic effect on laboratory rats. Caution should be exercised because excess dosage of the oil can lead to seizures and greater sensitivity of the skin to sunlight.

Galega officinalis

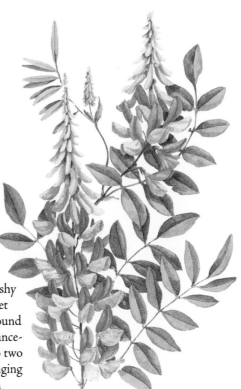

COMMON NAMES
Goat's rue, French lilac

LATIN NAME
Galega officinalis

FAMILIES Leguminosae, Fabaceae

PARTS USED
Flower, leaf, stem, seed

DESCRIPTION
The erect, smooth, hollow, branching stems of this bushy perennial may reach five feet tall. Its bright green compound leaves consist of 13 to 17 lance-shaped leaflets, each one to two inches long. Its flowers, ranging from white to lilac, grow in spikes and bear red-brown seedpods in autumn that hold two to six kidney-shaped seeds.

HABITAT
Indigenous to central and southern Europe, Russia, Japan, and Asia Minor, goat's rue is naturalized and widely cultivated in Britain. It grows in damp meadows and on river banks, as well as in other low, moist areas.

FOLKLORE AND TRADITIONAL USES
Dried flowers of goat's rue were used to help female goats increase their milk supply. The meaning of its Latin name, *Galega*, derives from the Greek *gala*, or milk, which reflects this use. Goat's rue was also known in parts of England as "cheese rennet" because juice pressed from the green parts of the plant can be used to clot milk and make cheese. Goat's rue has been widely cultivated as cattle feed. Reported deaths of sheep that grazed on goat's rue brought the plant's toxicity to the attention of researchers.

MEDICINAL USES
This hardy herb was once employed as a treatment for the plague, intestinal worms, fevers, and snakebites. The herb has since been shown in some cases to increase the production of milk in lactating mothers up to 50 percent. Some doctors do not recommend this use of the plant, however, because its effect on infants is not known. Galegin, an alkaloid isolated from goat's rue, lowers blood sugar levels and could therefore potentially treat diabetes mellitus. A synthetic drug based on guanidine was introduced in France during the late 1950s, and it was approved by the FDA in 1995.

Gelsemium sempervirens

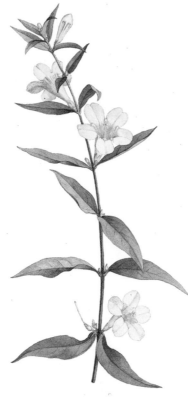

COMMON NAMES
Yellow jessamine, Yellow jasmine, False jasmine, Woodbine

LATIN NAME
Gelsemium sempervirens

FAMILY Loganiaceae

PARTS USED
Rhizome, root

DESCRIPTION
This perennial evergreen twines in vines that can grow up to 40 feet long, depending on their support system. Jessamine's glossy green leaves, two to four inches long, grow along its stem in opposite pairs. Clusters of fragrant funnel-shaped yellow flowers bloom in early spring.

HABITAT
Yellow jessamine is native to North America, growing in moist rich soils along the East Coast from Virginia down to Florida and into Mexico. It also grows in forests of the southeastern United States.

FOLKLORE AND TRADITIONAL USES
Yellow jessamine is the state flower of South Carolina. In 1924, the South Carolina General Assembly adopted it in the hope that its consistent reemergence at the end of winter would send a message of loyalty and patriotism. A South Carolina native wrote in "Legend of the Yellow Jessamine," a turn of the century poem, "No flower that blooms holds such perfume/As kindness and sympathy won.

Wherever there grows the sheltering pine/Is clinging a yellow jessamine vine."

MEDICINAL USES
Native Americans used yellow jessamine as a blood purifier. More recently, a Mississippi farmer brought yellow jessamine's medicinal properties to light by accidentally mistaking its root for that of another medicinal plant and curing his fever with it. Yellow jessamine root is extremely toxic. Only one teaspoon of the root can cause vertigo, weakness, and death from paralysis of respiratory muscles. Yellow jessamine contains substances that depress the nervous system, an action that makes it effective as a sedative, painkiller, and antispasmodic. Currently it is used only in homeopathic remedies to treat fever, convulsive coughing, and severe phobias.

Ginkgo biloba

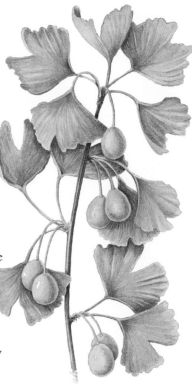

COMMON NAMES
Ginkgo, Gingko, Kew tree, Maidenhair tree

LATIN NAME
Ginkgo biloba

FAMILY Ginkgoaceae

PART USED
Leaf

DESCRIPTION
The ginkgo is a deciduous tree that grows to a hundred feet or more, with a trunk eight feet in diameter. Its bark is gray and fissured. The distinctive fan-shaped light-green leaves turn bright yellow in the autumn, have two lobes, and are about two to three inches across with a notch in the middle. The ginkgo bears flowers when it is 20 to 30 years old.

HABITAT
The ginkgo is native to Japan, China, and Korea. Now it is grown in moist, fertile urban areas in many parts of the world.

FOLKLORE AND TRADITIONAL USES
Considered a living fossil, ginkgo is the world's oldest living tree species. It can be traced back more than 200 million years. Individual trees may live as long as a thousand years. The word "ginkgo" comes from the Japanese *ginkyo* and the Chinese *yinhsing*, which means "silver apricot." Ginkgo leaves resemble the leaflets of the maidenhair fern, and some botanists believe that this tree species is the missing link between seed-bearing plants and ferns.

MEDICINAL USES
Scientists have clinically established that a concentrated extract of ginkgo leaf increases memory performance and learning capacity, inactivates toxic radicals, and improves blood flow. Scientists have reported that Alzheimer patients receiving doses of ginkgo had delayed mental deterioration in the early stages of the disease. Clinical trials have also shown ginkgo to improve airway passages of asthma patients and to help relieve symptoms of vertigo and tinnitus. A concentrated, standardized extract from the leaf can treat circulatory problems such as arteriosclerosis and high blood pressure.

Glycine max

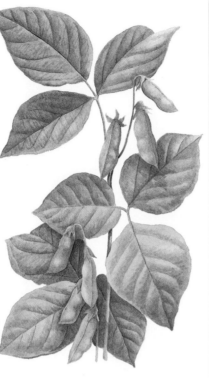

COMMON NAMES
Soy, Soybean, Soya

LATIN NAME
Glycine max

FAMILY Leguminosae

PARTS USED
Seed, bean

DESCRIPTION
An annual, soy grows up to five feet tall. It has an erect, semi-trailing stem and trifoliate leaves that are covered in fine, downy hair. Flowers are white or purple, and the oblong pods contain up to four yellow to brownish seeds.

HABITAT
Indigenous to east Asia, soy is now cultivated in the United States and Europe.

FOLKLORE AND TRADITIONAL USES
Known as the "cow of China," soy has been cultivated in China since at least the 11th century B.C. In Japan during the annual *Setsubun*—beginning of Spring—festival, celebrants scatter lucky roasted soybeans at home to ward off evil and to welcome in the new year with happiness. These soybeans are then eaten in a quantity equivalent to one's age to guarantee good health for the coming year. Soy-based products include glycerine, soaps, paint, linoleum, varnishes, enamel, rubber substitutes, artificial petroleum, and ink.

MEDICINAL USES
Soy's principal constituents, isoflavones, bind at estrogen receptor sites. These phyto-estrogens, or plant estrogens, are used to treat menopausal symptoms, especially hot flashes, and to help prevent osteoporosis. Soy is also used to inhibit hormone-dependent—especially estrogen-dependent—cancers, such as breast, ovarian, and prostate malignancies. The isoflavones genistein and daidzein block natural estrogen and its potentially harmful effects, while simultaneously giving the benefits of increased estrogen. Products containing 6.25 grams per serving of soy protein are approved by the Food and Drug Administration to help prevent heart disease and lower cholesterol levels. Soybeans are high in nutritional value. They are rich in protein, fiber, and minerals. Soy treats intestinal problems, including constipation and bowel disease, due to its high cellulose content.

Glycyrrhiza glabra

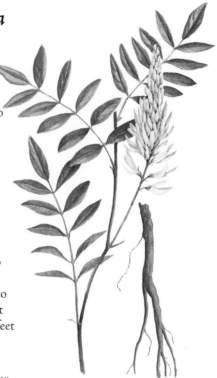

COMMON NAMES
Licorice, Sweetroot, Gan cao

LATIN NAME
Glycyrrhiza glabra

FAMILIES Leguminosae, Fabaceae

PARTS USED
Root, rhizome

DESCRIPTION
Licorice is a perennial shrub that grows up to four or five feet tall. It has small bluish to pale violet flowers and a root system that reaches several feet below the soil's surface.

HABITAT
Licorice grows in the Mediterranean and in parts of Eastern Europe and Asia.

FOLKLORE AND TRADITIONAL USES
Archaeologists discovered a bundle of licorice sticks among the treasures of King Tut's tomb. The miller in Chaucer's *Canterbury Tales* chewed licorice to make his breath sweet before meeting a possible lover. This herb is used in chewing tobacco and some cigarettes as flavoring. What is thought of as "licorice" flavor is actually anise; licorice itself tastes very sweet and musty. Licorice's value as a comestible and as a medicine dates back hundreds of years. Sixteenth-century herbal writer John Gerard describes a candy that he calls "ginger bread" containing "the juice of licorice, ginger, and other spices" that is "verie good against the cough." This flip-flopping of licorice from confection to medicine has been its story throughout history.

MEDICINAL USES
The Chinese consider a similar species, *G. uralensis*, which they call by the common name of *gan cao*, a "drug of first class" and believe that it lengthens life. Romans and others in antiquity used it to remedy gastric irritation and as an expectorant. Glycyrrhizic acid, from the species illustrated on this page, is 50 times sweeter than sugar and can accelerate the healing of gastric ulcers. Licorice treats such respiratory ailments as bronchitis and asthma and is an ingredient in herbal cough medicines. Glabridin inhibits inflammation of skin and the creation of melanin. In 1985 Japanese researchers showed that glycoside glycyrrhizin was effective in the treatment of chronic hepatitis and liver cirrhosis. High doses should be avoided, as they could eventually result in high blood pressure and possibly cardiac arrhythmia.

Guaiacum officinale

COMMON NAMES
Guaiacum, Guaiac, Guajacum, Lignum vitae

LATIN NAME
Guaiacum officinale

FAMILY Zygophyllaceae

PARTS USED
Wood, bark, resin

DESCRIPTION
This slow-growing evergreen tree, which can reach to 60 feet in height, usually has a twisted trunk. It bears opposite, oval, compound leaves and produces blue star-shaped flowers. Its laxative greenish-brown heart-wood should not be confused with other hardwoods of Australasia that also have the name "lignum vitae."

HABITAT
Lignum vitae is indigenous to South America, Central America, the Caribbean, and southern Florida. Preferring moist soil and partial sun, the tree is cultivated as an ornamental in Florida and California.

FOLKLORE AND TRADITIONAL USES
The tree's name, lignum vitae, meaning "wood of life," probably derives from the tree's medicinal properties. Christopher Columbus found lignum vitae, or guaiacum, upon his arrival to the New World. Europeans perceived it as a miracle cure for syphilis and hung pieces of the tree's bark in churches as objects of devotion. The tree's wood is so rich with fat and resins that objects made from it are self-lubricating and nearly impervious to water. Until the introduction of

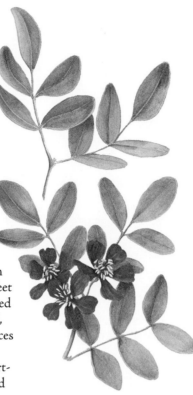

high-quality plastics, lignum vitae wood was used in pulley sheaves, machine bushings, and propeller shafts for steamships. It has also been used to make bowling balls, axles, mallets, and other objects that must absorb tremendous stress.

MEDICINAL USES
Native Americans used lignum vitae to treat tropical diseases. From the mid- to late 16th century in Europe, the bark became popular as a treatment for syphilis. It is a traditional British treatment for rheumatoid arthritis and gout. In folk medicine, people used guaiac resin to treat respiratory problems and skin disorders. A derivative has been used in cough medicines. Guaiacum also has served as an anti-inflammatory, a local anesthetic, and a help for herpes. Lignum vitae is subject to legal restrictions in some countries.

Hamamelis virginiana

COMMON NAMES
Witch hazel, Hamamelis, Winterbloom, Tobacco wood

LATIN NAME
Hamamelis virginiana

FAMILY Hamamelidaceae

PARTS USED
Bark, leaf, root

DESCRIPTION
This deciduous shrub or small tree, which may reach a height of 20 feet, has smooth brown bark. Its leaves are broad and oval with blunt indentations. It bears golden yellow flowers after the leaves drop off in autumn. Each of its woody fruit capsules ejects two seeds up to 13 feet away.

HABITAT
Witch hazel is indigenous to the deciduous forests of the eastern United States and Canada. It is cultivated in Europe and can be found throughout North America.

FOLKLORE AND TRADITIONAL USES
Native Americans used witch hazel branches as dousing rods to locate buried treasures or underground water and to make bows. "Witch" most likely comes from the Anglo-Saxon *wych*, meaning "a tree with bendable branches." Witch hazel is a common home remedy in the United States, used in products ranging from aftershave lotions to astringents.

MEDICINAL USES
Several Native American tribes employed witch hazel extensively for treating more than 30 different ailments, including colds, skin problems, tumors, tuberculosis, bloody dysentery, arthritis, sore eyes, hemorrhage after childbirth, and heart problems. Witch hazel is a rich source of tannins, which tighten skin proteins to provide increased resistance to inflammation, assist the healing of broken skin, and help repair damaged blood vessels. For these reasons witch hazel is useful for a variety of skin conditions, as well as for varicose veins, hemorrhoids, bruises, and cysts or tumors. Witch hazel water is available commercially, approved by the FDA as an over-the-counter drug.

Humulus lupulus

COMMON NAME
Hop

LATIN NAME
Humulus lupulus

FAMILY Cannabaceae

PART USED
Strobile

DESCRIPTION
A perennial, the hop grows as tall as 25 feet and has a stout root. Stems are green, pencil-thin, twining, and flexible, yet tough. Leaves are dark green and heart-shaped, with finetoothed edges. The flowers are yellow-ish green, with loose male flowers and strobite female flowers. The fruits, found inside the female flower, are yellow.

HABITAT
The hop is indigenous to Europe. It is also cultivated in Asia, the United States, and elsewhere. Hops grow best in deep, rich soil, with free air circulation.

**FOLKLORE
AND TRADITIONAL USES**
Hops, now famous as a beer ingredient, were first used in Dutch and German breweries during the early 14th century, and in English breweries during the 16th century. Unlike the malt fermentation technique used to make ale, beer's precursor, the technique used in making beer involves oxidizing hops' bitter principle, humulene, obtained from the fruit. Initially opposed by the British Parliament, the hop was labeled "a wicked weed that would spoil…and endanger the people." Today hops beer is common throughout the world. The hop is also used in cloth, paper, and brown dye.

MEDICINAL USES
A number of the hop's constituents, including valerianic acid, have a sedative effect. During the 1600s the plant was considered a remedy for melancholy. It is now used to treat insomnia, restlessness, and anxiety. Its bitter principles, humulon and lupulon, are gastrointestinal stimulants used to treat indigestion and loss of appetite. These bitter acids also have antibacterial and antimicrobial properties. The hop is believed to contain chemicals that promote menstruation, and certain flavonoids have shown potential chemopreventive activity against breast and ovarian cancer.

Hydnocarpus kurzii

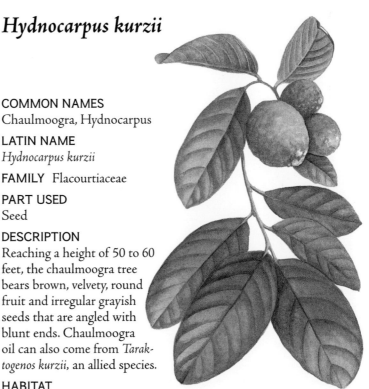

COMMON NAMES
Chaulmoogra, Hydnocarpus

LATIN NAME
Hydnocarpus kurzii

FAMILY Flacourtiaceae

PART USED
Seed

DESCRIPTION
Reaching a height of 50 to 60 feet, the chaulmoogra tree bears brown, velvety, round fruit and irregular grayish seeds that are angled with blunt ends. Chaulmoogra oil can also come from *Taraktogenos kurzii*, an allied species.

HABITAT
Chaulmoogra is native to the tropical areas of Malaysia and the Indian subcontinent.

**FOLKLORE
AND TRADITIONAL USES**
According to a pre-Buddhist legend, a Burmese king stricken with leprosy voluntarily exiled himself to the jungle. There, he chose to reside in a hollow tree and heal himself by eating the fruit and leaves of *Taraktogenos kurzii*, or the "Kalaw" tree. This tree was later identified as a source of chaulmoogra oil, an age-old leprosy treatment.

MEDICINAL USES
A physician is reported to have used chaulmoogra oil in ancient Egypt. Another early reference to the oil was made in the writings of the *Sushrata Samhitas*, dating back to 600 B.C. in India. The oil has long been widely employed as an accepted treatment for leprosy in China and India. Americans sought out chaulmoogra in the early 20th century until the development of a synthetic anti-leprosy drug in 1941. Botanist Joseph F. Rock brought the oil to the United States when he returned from an expedition in the hinterlands of the East that had been sponsored by the U.S. Department of Agriculture. In recent times, the efficacy of chaulmoogra in treating leprosy has been challenged.

Hydrastis canadensis

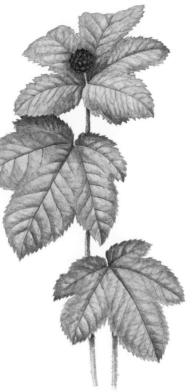

COMMON NAMES
Goldenseal, Indian dye

LATIN NAME
Hydrastis canadensis

FAMILY Ranunculaceae

PARTS USED
Root, rhizome

DESCRIPTION
A perennial woodland herb, goldenseal has a bright yellow, knotted rootstock, out of which grow small, hairy roots. In spring it sprouts an erect, hairy stem that grows up to one foot tall, with yellowish brown scales at the base. Leaves are dark green, downy, palmate, and ribbed. Flowers are greenish white. Fruits are dark red berries.

HABITAT
Goldenseal is indigenous to North America. It requires a well-drained, humus-rich soil.

FOLKLORE AND TRADITIONAL USES
The name "goldenseal" is derived from the plant's root scars, which resemble the old seal or stamp used on envelopes. Native Americans considered goldenseal sacred and used it for healing and as a body paint or dye for war dances. Early settlers believed that if they destroyed all goldenseal, Native Americans would not attack them because they would be unable to prepare their bodies with war paint. Since 1991 goldenseal's popularity as an herbal remedy has rendered this plant an endangered species. Ironically, so many people's desire to use goldenseal as a healing herb may do it more harm as a species than the early settlers' efforts to eradicate it.

MEDICINAL USES
Goldenseal contains the alkaloid berberine, which has proven antibiotic, antibacterial, and antifungal properties. Native Americans used it to treat a number of ailments, including whooping cough, liver problems, and eye sores. Berberine activates white blood cells called macrophages, which destroy viruses, bacteria, fungi, and tumor cells in a process known as phagocytosis. This alkaloid is also considered an immunostimulant, while another alkaloid, hydrastine, is also considered a potential gastric anti-inflammatory. Berberine does not appear to penetrate intestinal walls and get into the bloodstream; its actions are local to the gut.

Hypericum perforatum

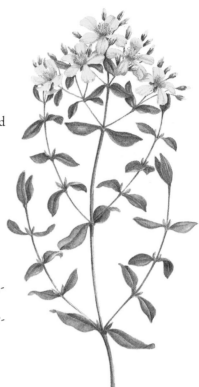

COMMON NAMES
St. John's wort, Klamath weed

LATIN NAME
Hypericum perforatum

FAMILY Hypericaceae

PARTS USED
Bud, flower, leaf

DESCRIPTION
An aromatic weed, St. John's wort generally reaches one to three feet high. This perennial bears yellow-green oval leaves and golden yellow flowers that are scattered with yellow or black dots of oil glands and lines.

HABITAT
Native to Europe, northern Africa, and western Asia, St. John's wort can be found around the world.

FOLKLORE AND TRADITIONAL USES
The ancient Greeks and Romans placed St. John's wort above statues of their gods and in their homes to protect them from evil spirits. Named by Christian mystics after John the Baptist, perhaps because the plant blooms around the time of the saint's feast day, June 24th, the plant was traditionally collected on that day and soaked in olive oil. After several days, the oil would turn blood-red, symbolizing the blood of the martyred Saint John. On the eve of his feast day, the plant was brought into houses and placed under pillows or was cast into bonfires to ward off evil spirits, to invoke the blessing of St. John, to prevent death, and to preserve crops.

MEDICINAL USES
St. John's wort has been used in herbal healing for more than two centuries. It was employed by Crusaders and Civil War soldiers to treat battle wounds. After Europeans introduced St. John's wort to America, Native Americans used it to treat minor cuts, premenstrual syndrome, rheumatism, diarrhea, fevers, snakebite, and skin disorders. Modern research has proved St. John's wort's effectiveness as an antidepressant in cases of mild-to-moderate depression. Hypericin, one of the plant's active constituents, has been investigated as an antiviral agent against HIV, but the research did not indicate its effectiveness.

Ignatia amara

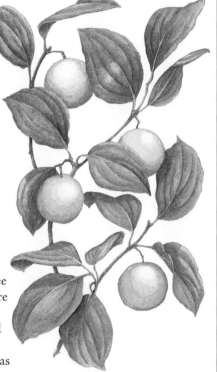

COMMON NAMES
Ignatius bean,
St. Ignatius bean

LATIN NAMES
Ignatia amara,
Strychnos ignatii

FAMILY Loganiaceae

PARTS USED
Seed, root

DESCRIPTION
St. Ignatius bean is a climbing shrub or small tree that reaches lengths of more than 60 feet. Its flowers are greenish white and covered with small silky hairs. The fruit, which grows as wide as five inches, contains yellow pulp and as many as 40 hard, oval seeds.

HABITAT
Ignatius beans are found throughout southeast Asia and are especially common in the Philippines and in Vietnam.

**FOLKLORE
AND TRADITIONAL USES**
Filipinos traditionally wore the seeds of the Ignatius bean as amulets to protect themselves from disease. Jesuits brought the plant from the Philippines to Europe in the 17th century and, it is believed, named it ignatia, or St. Ignatius bean, after the founder of the Jesuit order, Saint Ignatius of Loyola. The fruit has been called monkey apple because monkeys sometimes eat it. In Java and Malaysia the seeds were extracted and used as dart poisons for blowguns and in curare (see pareira).

MEDICINAL USES
Ignatius beans were frequently used as a cheap strychnine substitute for *Strychnos nux vomica,* because they have similar actions and alkaloidal composition. Once recommended as a remedy for cholera, the plant is used to treat fever and acute emotional and mental afflictions such as hysteria, insomnia, and depression. Ignatius beans are used chiefly as a homeopathic remedy, administered in very small doses because of extreme toxicity. Improper dosage—internal consumption of as little as a fraction of an ounce—can result in muscle spasms and painful convulsions and even death by asphyxiation.

Juniperus communis

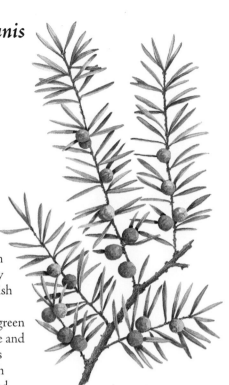

COMMON NAME
Common juniper

LATIN NAME
Juniperus communis

FAMILY Cupressaceae

PART USED
Berry cone

DESCRIPTION
An evergreen, the common juniper grows six to twenty feet tall with smooth reddish brown bark and tangled branches. Juniper has sea-green needles and yellowish male and greenish female flowers. Its pea-size berry cones, which vary in shades of blue or red, ripen in two to three years.

HABITAT
Juniper is found widely throughout temperate northern climates, including North Africa, northern Asia, Europe, and North America.

**FOLKLORE
AND TRADITIONAL USES**
It is customary in many parts of Wales to carefully preserve old juniper trees, because it is said that one who cuts down a juniper tree will die within a year. In the Middle Ages, Europeans believed that if they planted a juniper beside their front door, witches would be unable to enter unless they could correctly guess the number of needles on its branches. A Dutch pharmacist made an extract of juniper berries in alcohol to be used as a diuretic. In England the Dutch word for juniper, *ginevre,* was shortened to "gin." Some Native Americans in the U.S. used juniper in their religious ceremonies. Today it is used in perfumery, cosmetics, and seasoning for cooking.

MEDICINAL USES
Juniper has been used medicinally for centuries. Even sheep are said to eat it to prevent dropsy, although scientists are skeptical about this assertion. The ancient Egyptians and the ancient Greeks used juniper to ward off infection. Juniper has been administered in traditional Swedish medicine to treat inflammatory diseases and wounds. Native Americans treated a wide variety of complaints with it, from eye problems to wounds. Modern herbalists prescribe juniper as a diuretic as well as for bladder infections, arthritis, bronchitis, gout, and intestinal cramps. Pregnant women should not ingest juniper berries because the berries can stimulate uterine contractions.

Laminaria digitata

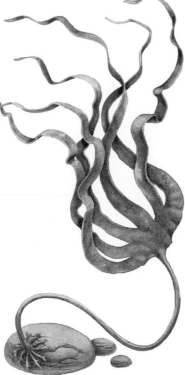

COMMON NAMES
Kelp, Tangleweed

LATIN NAMES
Laminaria digitata,
L. versiculosus

FAMILIES Fucaceae,
Laminariacea

PART USED
Blade

DESCRIPTION
Kelp varies in size from one foot in length to more than 200. There are three main parts: the holdfast, stipe, and blade. The bright green blades are long and leaflike.

HABITAT
Kelp grows in the rocky bottoms of offshore beds in ocean water. It requires large amounts of sunlight. Where kelp is abundant, it supports hundreds of species of marine animals.

**FOLKLORE
AND TRADITIONAL USES**
Ancient European seafarers learned to make use of the massive kelp beds that entangled their boats. They burned kelp as fuel and used it to wrap fish for baking. In the 19th century, both the English and the French, noting that kelp was a good source of iodine, harvested it at low tide. The cutting of the exposed fronds led to the plant's nickname, "cut weed." Kelp has a dominant place in Japanese sushi and other dishes. The pharmaceutical industry also uses it in products such as toothpaste, hand lotion, and skin cream.

MEDICINAL USES
Kelp's high iodine content was important in its early medicinal uses. Physicians first treated neck goiters, a condition caused by an iodine deficiency, with the plant. Because iodine stimulates the thyroid and speeds up the metabolism, kelp also gained a reputation for treating obesity. Its sodium alginate prevents the absorption of radioactive strontium 90, a toxic nuclear by-product that leads to cancer. Animal studies show that kelp may also help keep cholesterol and blood pressure low. However, because kelp is high in sodium, those who are sensitive to salt and tend toward high blood pressure should not consume large amounts of it.

Larrea tridentata

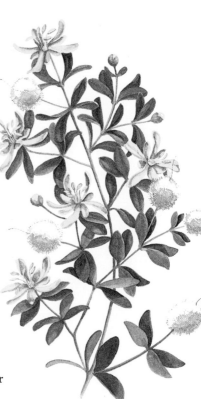

COMMON NAMES
Chaparral, Creosote bush,
Greasewood, Stinkweed

LATIN NAME
Larrea tridentata

FAMILY Zygophyllaceae

PARTS USED
Leaf, twig

DESCRIPTION
This evergreen shrub grows 6 to 13 feet tall and bears thick, resinous leaves on its numerous brittle branches. Its long, shallow roots, which require large amounts of oxygen to grow, emit repellents that deter the growth of most other plants near them. With a life span of approximately 9,000 to 12,000 years, chaparral may be among the longest-living organisms on Earth.

HABITAT
Drought-tolerant chaparral grows in large numbers in the arid regions of Mexico and the southwestern United States.

**FOLKLORE
AND TRADITIONAL USES**
According to Native American legend, chaparral was the first plant created by the Earth maker. The Papago used chaparral for a variety of purposes, including making arrows from its wood, preparing from it a permanent blue-green color for tattooing, and attaching handles made from its wood to gourd rattles. Chaparral earns the nickname "creosote bush" because after rare desert rains it emits a tarry smell reminiscent of creosote. For this reason Mexicans call it *hediondilla,* or little stinker.

MEDICINAL USES
Chaparral was extensively used in traditional Native American medicine as a treatment for diarrhea and stomach problems. A traditional folk remedy for respiratory distress, skin problems, and toothache, chaparral has also been used by herbalists against intestinal parasites, colds, and flu. Research indicates that chaparral mouthwash may reduce cavities by up to 75 percent. Products derived from extracts of chaparral are currently marketed as treatments for several forms of herpes. Chaparral tea has been proposed as a possible cancer treatment. Its efficacy has not been proved, however, and continued consumption of chaparral has been associated with hepatitis and irreversible liver damage in people with a prior history of liver disease.

Lavandula angustifolia

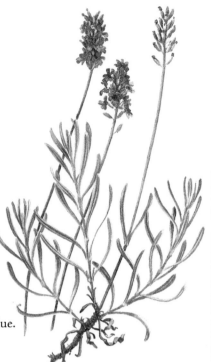

COMMON NAME
Lavender

LATIN NAME
Lavandula angustifolia

FAMILY Labiatae

PART USED
Flower

DESCRIPTION
Lavender is an evergreen ranging in height from 8 inches to 3 feet, depending on the species. It grows in clumps, with spiky flowers that are usually purple or blue.

HABITAT
Indigenous to the Mediterranean region, lavender is now found in temperate areas everywhere.

**FOLKLORE
AND TRADITIONAL USES**
The name "lavender" probably derived from the Medieval Latin for the species *livendula,* from *livere* (to make bluish) combined with *lavare* (to wash). Pedanius Dioscorides praised its fragrance as surpassing all other perfumes, and it is still used as a fragrance in sachets and potpourri. The Virgin Mary is reputed to have been fond of lavender because it protected clothes from insects and preserved chastity. During the Middle Ages and the Renaissance lavender covered the floors of houses and churches to keep out the plague. It is believed Queen Elizabeth I liked lavender conserve (prepared by mixing the flower with sugar) because it had a reputation as a mild tranquilizer.

MEDICINAL USES
Lavender has had a variety of uses throughout history. To Arabs it was an expectorant. Pilgrim settlers brought lavender to the New World and used its seeds to expel worms. The founder of aromatherapy, Maurice Gattefosse, accidentally burned his hand, put it in lavender oil, and found that it healed quickly. Research has since shown that some essential oils reduce the flow of nerve impulses. Perillyl alcohol, a compound distilled from lavender, may promote apoptosis—the ability of a cell to self-destruct when its DNA is damaged. One study compared the effects of smelling lavender oil with taking tranquilizers and found it worked as well against insomnia. Other studies suggest lavender may lower blood sugar. Germany's Commission E approves it as an antiflatulent and a treatment for mild stomach disorders.

Lentinula edodes

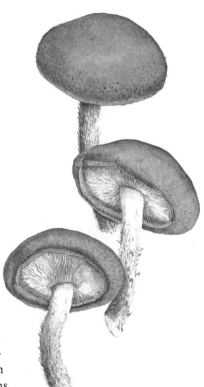

COMMON NAMES
Shiitake, Reishi

LATIN NAMES
Lentinula edodes (Shiitake),
Ganoderma lucidum (Reishi)

FAMILIES
Trichlomataceae (Shiitake),
Ganodermataceae (Reishi)

PART USED
Whole mushroom

DESCRIPTION
The main body of the mushroom consists of an underground network of filaments. The visible, fruiting part consists of a stalk and a cap. Both reishi and shiitake mushrooms have dark stalks and caps. Reishi's cap is somewhat rounded; shiitake's is flat.

HABITAT
Both species are native to Japan and China and grow best on logs or on organic waste in a moisture-rich environment.

**FOLKLORE
AND TRADITIONAL USES**
Once thought to be plants, mushrooms are now classified as fungi. "Mushroom" comes from the French *mousseron,* a derivative of the word for "moss," upon which they grow. In China, people worshiped the Reishi Goddess to bring health and eternal youth. Taoist monks have used reishi to help create a centered calmness. The British Isles had their fairy rings and Lewis Carroll's Alice used a mushroom to shrink and to grow. Spiritual or ritualistic practices using hallucinogenic mushrooms sprang up in various parts of the world, from Siberia to Mexico.

MEDICINAL USES
Shiitake and reishi mushrooms have a long history. Mushrooms are featured in the 2,000-year-old book *Shen Nong's Herbal Classic,* which describes them as having strong medicinal value. Scientists have discovered that the polysaccharide compound lentinan, found in shiitake mushrooms, possesses immunostimulant and antitumoral properties. Lentinan can also prevent platelet adhesion, which causes the clots responsible for coronary artery disease and strokes. Research shows that reishi mushrooms combat tumors, inhibit the body's production of cholesterol, and stimulate the immune system. Researchers are not yet certain as to which specific compounds are responsible for reishi's benefits. They have obtained results only by using the whole mushroom.

Leontodon utumnales

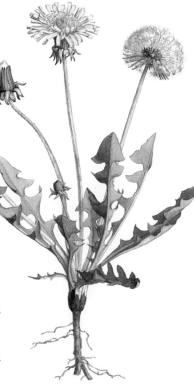

COMMON NAME
Dandelion

LATIN NAMES
Leontodon utumnales,
Taraxacum officinale

FAMILY Asteraceae

PARTS USED
Root, leaf, stem

DESCRIPTION
A perennial, the dandelion grows several inches tall, with a bright yellow head roughly an inch in diameter. The stem is thin and straight, with jagged leaves extending from the base. The root, leaves, and stem contain a milky fluid.

HABITAT
Dandelions grow throughout temperate regions of Europe, Asia, and North America.

**FOLKLORE
AND TRADITIONAL USES**
The dandelion's name derives from the French, *dent de lion* ("lion's tooth") because of the shape of its leaves. The English used dandelion flowers to make a wine thought to be good for the blood. Europeans made a coffee substitute from the roasted roots, using it to help the liver and kidneys. In parts of England and Canada, dandelion beer is still made, which is less intoxicating than regular beer. Children use the plumed seeds to make wishes, blowing them off the stem. In western Europe there was a widespread belief that picking the flowers or eating the greens led to nocturnal bed-wetting. Before clocks were common, in the country the dandelion was used to tell time; the flowers were said to open and close at certain times of the day. One of the common names for the dandelion in England is "priest's crown," because of its resemblance, after losing its seeds, to a medieval priest's shaved head.

MEDICINAL USES
Arabian physicians first mentioned dandelions in a medicinal capacity in the tenth century. Dandelions are a rich source of potassium and beta-carotene, a precursor to Vitamin A. Scientists performing studies on mice reported that the dandelion has a strong diuretic effect. It is a detoxifying herb, helping the gallbladder and liver remove waste from the body. The dandelion contains eudesmanolides, which cause its bitterness and make it an appetite stimulant. Chinese herbalists use the plant for various ailments, including tonsillitis, mastitis, colds, ulcers, and boils.

Ligustrum vulgare

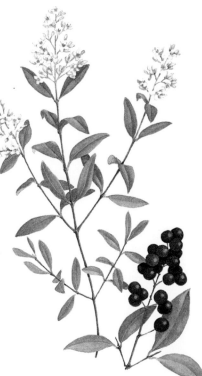

COMMON NAMES
Common privet, Prim

LATIN NAME
Ligustrum vulgare

FAMILY Oleaceae

PARTS USED
Berry, leaf, flower

DESCRIPTION
Common privet is a perennial shrub often used for hedges that can reach nine feet or more. It is an evergreen, with glossy dark green leaves, cream-colored flowers, and black berries.

HABITAT
Privet is native to Asia, North Africa, and Europe.

**FOLKLORE
AND TRADITIONAL USES**
Scholars are not sure of the origin of the name "privet"; some link it to "private" because the plant's use in hedges dates back to antiquity. Before the true nature of infection was understood, some people blamed flowers such as privet for the spread of disease and barred them from the house. Privet berries and bark make dyes; an unrelated species bearing the same name, Egyptian privet, or *Lawsonia inermis*, produces the popular dye henna. Privet is commonly used in topiary art by skilled gardeners to clip into animal shapes and other designs. The young branches are sometimes used in basketry, and the bark yields a yellow dye. The wood is a source of charcoal.

MEDICINAL USES
Privet was sometimes used in England for sore lips and the mumps and as an astringent in the form of gargles and mouthwashes. Settlers brought the plant to the U.S. where they devised medicinal uses for it. When placed on the head, the flowers relieved headaches. The berries were a strong laxative, and the leaves and flowers treated menstrual disorders. Asians use a related species as a tonic. Some herbalists consider privet an immune system strengthener. Tumors can suppress the ability of macrophages—cells that destroy bacteria and other debris—to function. Studies have shown that a combination of privet and astragalus may reverse this.

Linum usitatissimum

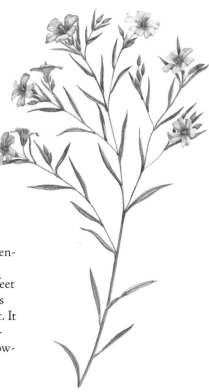

COMMON NAME
Flax

LATIN NAME
Linum usitatissimum

FAMILY Linaceae

PARTS USED
Seed, stem, oil

DESCRIPTION
An erect, slender annual, biennial, or perennial herb, flax usually grows one to three feet tall, with slender, wiry stems and a short, shallow taproot. It bears narrow, pointed, alternate leaves, blue to white flowers near the top of its stem, and globe-shaped seed capsules, each containing ten glossy, flattened brown seeds.

HABITAT
Native to Europe, Asia, and the Mediterranean region, flax was among the first plants cultivated in Europe. It is widely cultivated throughout temperate regions of the world.

**FOLKLORE
AND TRADITIONAL USES**
The use of flax dates back at least 10,000 years. One of the earliest records of writing consists of ancient Egyptian tax records that mention flax as payment. Linen shrouds in ancient Egypt and the ritual garments of Israel's high priests were made from it. According to the New Testament, Jesus wore material spun from flax when he was placed in the tomb by Joseph of Arimathea. In the Middle Ages, flax flowers were used as charms against sorcery. Pliny writes of it: "To think that here is a plant which brings Egypt to close proximity to Italy!" Today flax is employed in a variety of products—from flaxseed cakes, to cattle feed, to oilcloth and linoleum.

MEDICINAL USES
Flax has been used in herbal medicine since antiquity for a variety of purposes, including the removal of foreign materials from the eye and for colds, constipation, and urinary disorders. Studies using animals suggest that regular consumption of flaxseed can protect against certain types of tumors and reduce the risk of colon cancer. Flaxseed, also called linseed, has been shown in some studies to improve kidney function, lower LDL cholesterol levels, and increase bowel movements. A compound from flax is being investigated as a possible treatment for lupus.

Lobelia inflata

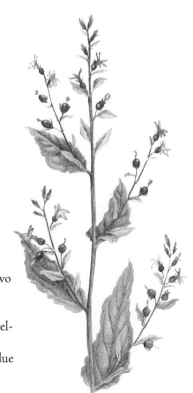

COMMON NAMES
Lobelia, Indian tobacco, Pukeweed, Bladderpod

LATIN NAME
Lobelia inflata

FAMILY Campanulaceae

PARTS USED
Flower, seed, root

DESCRIPTION
Growing as high as one to two feet, this annual or biennial hair-covered herb has an angled, branched stem and yellowish or light green leaves. The herb bears pale violet-blue spiky flowers and oval fruit with small brown seeds.

HABITAT
Indigenous to North America, lobelia is found along roadsides in the eastern United States, Canada, and Russia's Kamchatka Peninsula.

**FOLKLORE
AND TRADITIONAL USES**
Carl von Linné, the Swedish botanist known as Linnaeus, the father of modern botany, named this plant family after the Flemish botanist and private physician to King James I, Matthias de Lobel. Native Americans employed it ceremonially as they did tobacco to ward off storms, place on graves, or use in rain dances. Other groups made lobelia part of their love potions or used it as an antidote to such charms. Some burned it to smoke away gnats.

MEDICINAL USES
Native Americans treated dozens of ailments with lobelia, ranging from fevers and venereal diseases to earaches and stiff necks. American herbalist Samuel Thomson, whom most Westerners credit with discovering the medicinal uses of lobelia, created a controversial healing system centered around it, which he prescribed to induce vomiting. Containing relatively high levels of manganese, Vitamin A, and Vitamin C, lobelia is currently employed as a blood cleanser and used as a respiratory stimulant to treat bronchial and spasmodic asthma and chronic bronchitis. Lobeline, its principal alkaloid, stimulates deeper breathing. Applied externally, lobelia works as a muscle relaxant to treat sprains and certain back problems.

Lycopodium clavatum

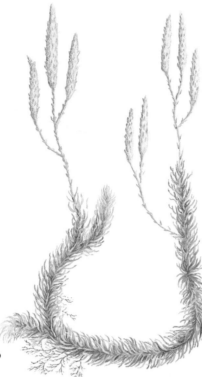

COMMON NAMES
Common club moss, Running club moss, Lycopodium, Wolf's claw, Ground pine

LATIN NAME
Lycopodium clavatum

FAMILY Lycopodiaceae

PART USED
Whole herb

DESCRIPTION
A low-growing evergreen, club moss has a three-foot stem that runs along the ground and dense spirals of yellow-green leaves. Two or three cylindrical yellow-green cones, which grow at the ends of six-inch stalks, carry many small yellow spores.

HABITAT
Common club moss is found throughout the world.

FOLKLORE AND TRADITIONAL USES
During the Carboniferous period, 360 million years ago, club mosses achieved dominance as a plant group, growing to the size of trees. Club mosses are not true mosses but, rather, primitive vascular plants. In China one variety was known as stone pine and grown ornamentally in pots. Because of their extreme resistance to water, club moss spores, in powder form, are employed not only as a coating for pharmaceutical pills to keep them from sticking to each other when placed together in a container but also to disguise their taste. Quite flammable, the spores were also used before the advent of electricity to produce special effects in theaters and in fireworks.

MEDICINAL USES
The whole plant was dried, chopped, and prepared as a tea in traditional medicine for kidney and bladder complaints. In the 17th century, spores began to be used alone to treat diarrhea, dysentery, hydrophobia, gout, scurvy, and rheumatism. Homeopathic remedies of this herb, called lycopodium, are prepared by triturating club moss in lactose until the seeds break up and release their oily contents. Homeopathic practitioners use it to treat constipation, chronic lung and bronchial disorders, aneurysms, and fever.

Matricaria chamomilla

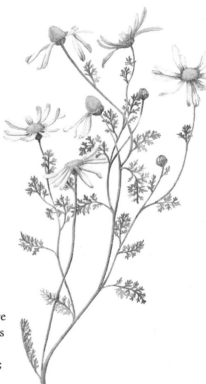

COMMON NAMES
Genuine chamomile (German), Common chamomile (English)

LATIN NAMES
Matricaria chamomilla (German), *Anthemis nobilis* (English)

FAMILY Asteraceae

PARTS USED
Flower, whole herb

DESCRIPTION
Both species of chamomile are gray-green plants with flowers about a foot tall. German chamomile is an erect annual; English chamomile is a slow-growing perennial. The stems branch often and have very thin leaves all along them. Flowers have white petals with yellow disks.

HABITAT
Chamomile is native to Europe and northwest Asia and is also cultivated in North America. Both types grow best in grassy areas with sandy soils.

FOLKLORE AND TRADITIONAL USES
The Egyptians called chamomile the "plant of the sun" and used it both as medicine for malarial fever and in dedications to their gods. The Greeks named it "ground-apple" for its scent. The Spaniards called it "little apple" and used it to flavor a light sherry. Gardeners in the Middle Ages believed it would heal plants growing in its vicinity. Chamomile is also employed in the manufacture of herb beers and to flavor cigarette tobacco.

MEDICINAL USES
Medicinally, the two species of chamomile are similar. Both produce an oil that contains the chemical azulene and turns blue when distilled. Several chemicals in this oil relax the smooth muscle in the digestive tract and have been shown in experiments to help heal ulcers. A German company markets a chamomile product that, in addition to helping prevent ulcers and indigestion, is used externally to treat wounds. In America, Eclectics—a 19th-century medical movement that ended in the 1930s—found that the oil in chamomile kills certain bacteria and reduces the time it takes burns to heal. British researchers have determined that chamomile stimulates the immune system.

Medicago sativa

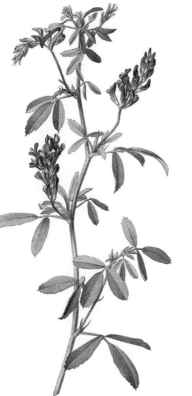

COMMON NAMES
Alfalfa, Lucern

LATIN NAME
Medicago sativa

FAMILY Leguminosae

PARTS USED
Whole flowering herb,
germinating seeds

DESCRIPTION
Usually reaching between 15
and 25 inches high, alfalfa's
erect stems are smooth, thin,
and branched. The roots of
this herbaceous perennial can
reach 30 feet deep, and its
alternate leaves usually have
three lobes and serrated tips.
It bears oblong, clover-like
flowers, which vary in color
from yellow to blue-violet, and
spiraling seedpods.

HABITAT
Alfalfa grows in meadows of
temperate areas and is indigenous to North Africa, Asia,
and Europe.

**FOLKLORE
AND TRADITIONAL USES**
Arabs discovered the herb and
named it *al-facl-facah*, or father
of all foods, which the Spanish
changed to "alfalfa." For centuries, the Arabs fed it to
horses in the belief that it
would make them strong and
swift. According to Pliny, King
Darius of Persia (550-486 B.C.)
brought alfalfa to Greece when
he attempted to conquer
Athens. The oldest forage crop
in the United States, it was
dubbed "the Queen of All For-
ages." The leaves and sprouted
seeds are eaten in salads or
blended into a health drink
valued by athletes. The leaves
are also a commercial source of
chlorophyll, and the seeds yield
yellow dye.

MEDICINAL USES
Because of its deep roots,
alfalfa is rich in nutrients and
minerals, including calcium,
potassium, iron, magnesium,
and zinc. A source of eight
essential amino acids, alfalfa is
used in China to treat fever, in
India to treat ulcers, in Iraq
and Turkey to treat arthritis,
and in the United States in
some natural therapies for cancer. It has also been employed
for urinary infections,
menopause, and fatigue, and as
an antibiotic and an anti-
asthmatic. Animal studies
indicate that eating alfalfa can
reduce the absorption of cholesterol and inhibit the formation of arterial plaque.

Mitchella repens

COMMON NAMES
Partridgeberry, Squaw vine

LATIN NAME
Mitchella repens

FAMILY Rubiaceae

PART USED
Whole herb

DESCRIPTION
An evergreen vine, partridgeberry grows up to a foot
long, with a whitish, trail-
ing stem. A ground-hugger, it
forms "mats" as it grows. Flowers are white and often paired.
Fruits are small, scarlet berries.

HABITAT
Partridgeberry is indigenous to
eastern and central North
America. It can be found from
southwestern Newfoundland
to Minnesota and southward
to Florida and Texas.

**FOLKLORE
AND TRADITIONAL USES**
Partridgeberry is a distinctively
Native American plant. Its
nickname—squaw vine—was
coined by colonists who saw
Native American women
using it. Although primarily
employed in a medicinal capacity, partridgeberry had additional uses among various
tribes, including the following:
as a love potion, as a ceremonial smoke, and as a food. The
fruits were eaten either raw or
dried and in sauces, breads,
and cakes.

MEDICINAL USES
Partridgeberry has a long history of use among Native
American women. Numerous
tribes used it to treat menstrual pains and cramps, to
regulate menstruation and
relieve heavy bleeding, and to
induce childbirth and ease
delivery. Partridgeberry is now
recommended by herbalists for
similar reasons. As a salve, it
is also used to treat nursing
mothers' sore or cracked nipples. Partridgeberry is thought
to contain tannins, glycosides,
and saponins, and it is generally believed to have a tonic
action on the uterus and
ovaries. Partridgeberry
may also be effective as an
abortifacient; for this reason,
it is not recommended for
pregnant women.

Monarda didyma

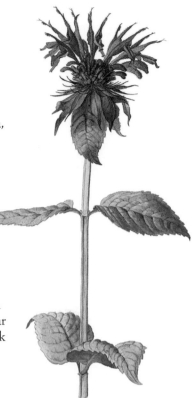

COMMON NAMES
Scarlet bergamot, Oswego tea,
Bee balm

LATIN NAMES
Monarda didyma,
M. fistulosa

FAMILY Labiatae

PART USED
Whole herb

DESCRIPTION
The erect, square, grooved
stems of this perennial, which
grows up to three feet tall, bear
greenish rough leaves and dark
pink, red, or purple flowers
with large, shaggy heads.

HABITAT
Native to eastern North
American, bergamot grows
wild in various habitats. It is
also widely cultivated as a
garden plant.

**FOLKLORE
AND TRADITIONAL USES**
Its aromatic smell, reminiscent
of the bergamot orange (*Citrus
bergamia*), gives bergamot its
name. *Monarda*, its genus, is
named in honor of Spanish
physician Nicholas Monardes,
author of a 1569 herbal of
New World plants. American
settlers, protesting the tax on
East Indian tea after the
Boston Tea Party, drank
Oswego tea prepared from the
leaves and flowers of this herb,
which was introduced to them
by the Oswego tribe. Native
Americans across the United
States used bee balms of various species for a variety of purposes—as perfume, as a
preservative for meats, and as
a food and beverage. A popular
garden plant, bergamot attracts
bumblebees, butterflies, and
hummingbirds.

MEDICINAL USES
Native Americans also had a
variety of medicinal uses for
bergamot and its relatives.
Combating fever and heart disease, increasing urine flow, and
stanching blood were just a
few. Considered an appetite
stimulant and a menstrual reg-
ulator by Native Americans as
well as settlers, bergamot was
traditionally given as a tonic
to young mothers and brides
in 19th-century America.
Herbalists employ the herb to
treat nausea, vomiting, and
upset stomach. Bergamot contains the aromatic antiseptic
thymol, which is widely used
by dentists and modern medical practitioners. Brewed and
ingested, oswego tea treats
flatulence and insomnia.

Nepeta cataria

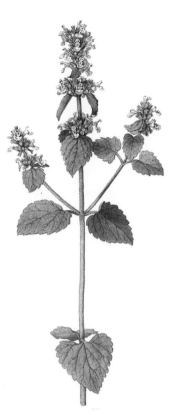

COMMON NAMES
Catnip, Catmint

LATIN NAME
Nepeta cataria

FAMILY Labiatae

PARTS USED
Leaf, flower

DESCRIPTION
A perennial, catnip grows up
to three feet tall and has erect,
angular stems. Leaves are
greenish gray, heart shaped,
and downy. The flowers—
whitish-pink with purple spots
and red anthers—are arranged
in whorls.

HABITAT
Indigenous to Eurasia, catnip
is also cultivated in North
America. This herb grows best
in chalky, gravelly soil.

**FOLKLORE
AND TRADITIONAL USES**
Catnip's aromatic odor acts
as a behavior modifying substance in felines, seeming to
induce a euphoric response. In
ancient Egypt, it was sacred to
Bast, the cat goddess. Today
catnip is used in cat toys and as
a lure for trapping bobcats and
mountain lions. Catnip tea,
once considered highly medicinal, was popular in England
until the introduction of black
tea from China. At that time,
the root was believed to induce
fierceness and hotheadedness.
Hangmen reportedly chewed
the root before executions.
During the 1960s, some people
attempted to use catnip as a
hallucinogen, but its hallucinogenic properties in humans are
not well documented.

MEDICINAL USES
According to 17th century
herbalist Nicholas Culpeper,
catnip was used to treat
bruises, piles, and head scabs.
Its ability to stimulate sweats
without raising body temperature and to induce sleep meant
that catnip tea was also
employed to treat colds, flu,
and fever—as it is today.
Catnip's principal constituent
is nepetalactone, a volatile oil
similar to that found in valerian root. It acts as a mild
sedative to relieve migraines,
menstrual cramps, tension,
and anxiety. Many consider
catnip effective in treating
flatulence and indigestion;
others regard it as a diuretic.
Some people in the American
Ozarks use catnip to treat
aching teeth. A weak catnip
tea is a traditional remedy
to help soothe colicky babies.

Nicotiana rustica

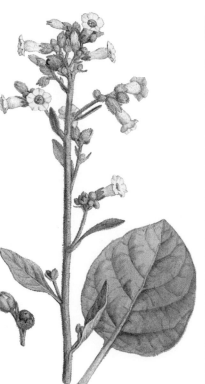

COMMON NAME
Wild tobacco

LATIN NAME
Nicotiana rustica

FAMILY Solanaceae

PART USED
Leaf

DESCRIPTION
Tobacco grows between three and six feet tall, with a thick, upright stem that branches at the top. Leaves are long and pointed. Numerous funnel-shaped flowers, usually pink but sometimes yellow bloom at the top of the plant.

HABITAT
Tobacco originated in the Americas and is now cultivated worldwide.

**FOLKLORE
AND TRADITIONAL USES**
The Maya recorded inhaling tobacco smoke more than 2,000 years ago. When Christopher Columbus came across the Arawak of the Caribbean in 1492, they were smoking loosely rolled cigars. The Karok of California used tobacco as gifts to spirits and to give to guests of lower status. Among the Karok Indians, only men smoked tobacco; the exception was women doctors, who did the work of men and, therefore, were expected to follow the same traditions. Pocahontas's husband, John Rolfe, was the first European settler to grow a crop of tobacco. When tobacco was first introduced in Spain, it was rolled into what we now call "cigars"—cylindrical objects bulging slightly at the middle. These looked like cicadas, thus the Spanish name *cigarro* and, later, the French *cigarette*. Today tobacco is the most widely grown commercial non-food plant in the world.

MEDICINAL USES
Many Native American nations used fresh tobacco leaves as a poultice to kill pain. They also dried the leaves and smoked them as a cure for colds. When tobacco reached Europe, many people there also believed in its medicinal properties. French ambassador to Portugal Jean Nicot, from whose name came the word "nicotine," considered tobacco a cure for headaches and gout. Nicholas Monardes, a Spanish doctor, listed 36 illnesses that tobacco treated. Later, in 1761, John Hill in England proved that snuff causes cancer in the nose. Today tobacco is linked to various forms of cancer.

Oenothera biennis

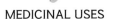

COMMON NAMES
Evening primrose, Fever plant, Scabish

LATIN NAME
Oenothera biennis

FAMILY Onagraceae

PART USED
Seed

DESCRIPTION
This biennial grows up to four feet tall. It has a turniplike root, pointed leaves, and yellow flowers. An oblong capsule holds dark gray to black seeds with sharp edges.

HABITAT
Evening primrose is indigenous to North America, but it can be found throughout much of the world.

**FOLKLORE
AND TRADITIONAL USES**
Evening primrose oil is used in cosmetics, skin lotions, and various toiletries. Many superstitions have arisen about this plant. It is considered unlucky to take primroses into a house in which hens are laying eggs, because it is said that the number of eggs laid will be limited to the number of primroses brought into the house. A primrose blooming during winter was considered to be an omen of death. The expression "primrose path" appears in Hamlet: "Do not as some ungracious Pastors do / Show me the steepe and thorny way to Heaven / Whilst...a...recklesse libertine / Himself the primrose path of dalliance treads."

MEDICINAL USES
Native American women chewed evening primrose seeds to alleviate premenstrual and menstrual discomfort. Both Native Americans and early European settlers of North America treated asthma and gastrointestinal ailments with the seeds. The oil from the seeds is a rich source of gamma-linolenic acid (GLA), an essential fatty acid that supports the production of prostaglandins and thus helps maintain hormonal balance. It is approved in Britain to treat premenstrual syndrome, yet, while available commercially in the United States, this use has not been approved by the FDA. Double-blind research has examined and supported the efficacy of evening primrose oil in treating rheumatoid arthritis and atopic eczema, but more study is needed. The oil has been used for diabetes, dermatitis, and menopause.

Onoclea sensibilis

COMMON NAMES
Sensitive fern, Bead fern

LATIN NAME
Onoclea sensibilis

FAMILIES Polypodiaceae, Onocleaceae

PARTS USED
Frond, rhizome

DESCRIPTION
The sensitive fern can grow up to four feet tall. When fertile, sensitive fern becomes dark green and then turns brown. Firm in texture, it rolls up into beadlike structures. Its coarse, thick rhizome is fibrous and scaled.

HABITAT
Sensitive fern grows in wet, grassy places, open damp woodland, and open hillsides.

FOLKLORE AND TRADITIONAL USES
One of among 12,000 species of ferns, sensitive fern gained its common name from two folk observations—it wilts quickly when picked, and the fronds die with the first autumn frost. The mysterious ability of ferns to regenerate led to an ancient belief that their spores could confer invisibility to a person sprinkled with them. Used in the 1300s to dye wool, ferns have also been employed as bedding for animals and as a mattress stuffing for people, probably because poisons in their dry fronds helped kill fleas. During times of famine, some ferns have been mixed with bread and brewed for beer. Some varieties of young ferns are

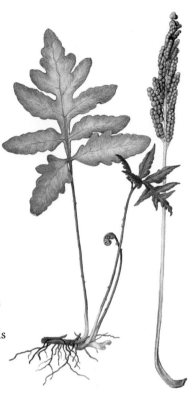

sold as delicacies in Asian markets. In addition, a decoction of sensitive fern has been used to prevent baldness.

MEDICINAL USES
Sensitive fern was employed medicinally by one North American Indian tribe who used it quite widely to treat childbirth pain, female infertility, and cramps. But only a few fern plants have demonstrated true medicinal value. For example, people for centuries have used an oil extracted from the rhizome of the species *Dryopteris filix-mas*, or male fern, to treat tapeworms and liver flukes. Researchers have determined that the chemicals filicin and filmarone found in the male fern's oil are toxic to the worms and that oleoresin paralyzes them and keeps them from attaching to the intestine. Extremely poisonous in high doses, male fern should never be used in self-medication.

Panax ginseng

COMMON NAMES
Ginseng (Asian), Chinese or Korean ginseng

LATIN NAMES
Panax ginseng,
P. trifolium

FAMILY Araliaceae

PART USED
Root

DESCRIPTION
A perennial, ginseng grows up to two and a half feet tall, with a smooth, erect stem. Leaves are thin, finely serrated, grouped in fives, and up to eight inches long. Flowers are greenish yellow or pink and occur in groups of 15 to 30. Fruits are scarlet, smooth, and glossy.

HABITAT
Asian ginseng is indigenous to China and Korea. It is also cultivated in Japan, Russia, and parts of North America. Ginseng thrives in shady locations on rich, moist soil and takes five to seven years to mature from seed.

FOLKLORE AND TRADITIONAL USES
Because of the *Panax ginseng* root's forked shape, which at maturity resembles a man's body, the ancient Chinese named this root *jen shen*, or "man plant." *Panax*, derived from the Greek *panakos* (panacea), refers to the miraculous all-healing virtue ascribed to this plant by the Chinese. Used for centuries in Asia, ginseng was introduced to the West in the 1700s, allegedly

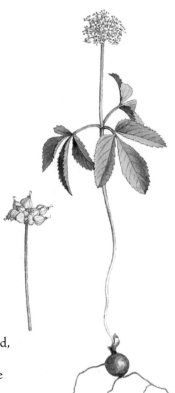

by Jesuit Father Jartoux, who claimed it treated fatigue and pleurisy and aided in convalescence. According to Jartoux, Chinese physicians considered ginseng a necessity in all prescriptions, and only the emperor had the right to collect its roots. The ginseng illustrated here is dwarf ginseng, *Panax trifolium*, which does not have a forked root.

MEDICINAL USES
Ginseng's primary constituents are ginsenosides, which stimulate the cardiovascular and central nervous systems to enhance physical and mental performance; panaxans, which lower blood sugar; and polysaccharides, which strengthen the immune system and help treat diabetes. Ginseng is also thought to have antioxidant, antiaging, and appetite-stimulating properties.

Papaver somniferum

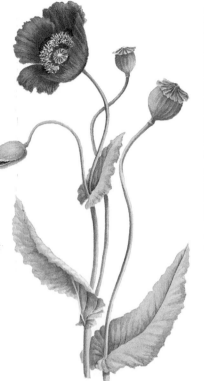

COMMON NAME
Opium poppy

LATIN NAME
Papaver somniferum

FAMILY Papaveraceae

PARTS USED
Capsule, flower

DESCRIPTION
The opium poppy is an erect plant that can measure up to two feet tall. Leaves are toothed and pale green. The large white or red flower is at the top of the stalk. After the petals fall off, a capsule remains.

HABITAT
The poppy is indigenous to Asia Minor but grows anywhere in the temperate regions of the Northern Hemisphere.

FOLKLORE AND TRADITIONAL USES
Humans have cultivated opium poppies since Neolithic times for both medical and spiritual reasons. In Greek legend, the goddess Demeter used poppies to forget the sorrow of losing her daughter Persephone. Greeks at Eleusis took opium to forget the sadness of the death for another year. The Roman god of sleep, Somnus, is often portrayed with poppies. Ceres, the Roman fertility goddess, also used them to reduce pain. The Renaissance doctor Paracelsus claimed that the opium poppy was the source of immortality.

MEDICINAL USES
The Chinese have used the poppy capsules to treat diarrhea, headaches, and asthma. In addition, they have employed the opium latex from the unripe capsules as an antitussive and sedative. Opium poppies contain over 20 alkaloids, including morphine, noscapine, papaverine, and codeine. In 1804 morphine became the first alkaloid to be isolated in the history of chemistry. During the American Civil War, both armies cultivated poppies in the South as a cure for dysentery and as a painkiller. Today, scientists use the poppy's alkaloids primarily as painkillers. Codeine treats minor pains, noscapine counteracts coughing, and papaverine increases blood flow. Scientists have used all of these constituents as the bases for powerful synthetic opiates. Because of their addictive properties, opium products are illegal in many countries.

Passiflora incarnata

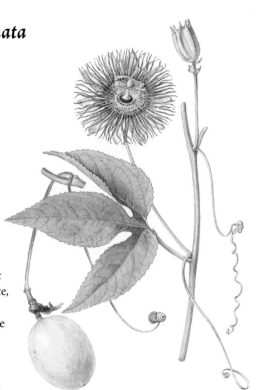

COMMON NAME
Passion flower

LATIN NAME
Passiflora incarnata

FAMILY Passifloraceae

PART USED
Whole herb

DESCRIPTION
A perennial vine, passion flower grows up to 33 feet long. Its leaves are alternate, serrate, and downy. The flowers have pinkish white petals, green-and-white sepals, white-and-purple inner corollas, and thick stigmas. Fruits are orange berries with many seeds and yellow pulp.

HABITAT
Passion flower is indigenous to tropical and subtropical areas of the Americas. It is cultivated throughout the world.

FOLKLORE AND TRADITIONAL USES
The name "passion flower" was given to the plant by Jacomo Bosio, a 17th-century monastic scholar, who considered the appearance of various species as representative of the elements of the Christ's crucifixion. The 72 corona filaments stood for the number of thorns in the crown; the 5 stamens, the 5 wounds; the petals, the 10 true apostles; and the spotted leaf underside, the 30 silver pieces paid to Judas to betray Jesus. Upon discovering the flower, Spanish explorers in Peru saw the flower as a sign of divine approval of their actions. In Peru, New Spain, and the West Indies, descendants of the Spanish explorers still call it the "flower of the five wounds."

MEDICINAL USES
Folk remedies have used passion flower to treat depression, insomnia, and hemorrhoids. An approved sedative in Germany, it is employed today to treat nervous agitation and mild insomnia. Passion flower's mild sedative and spasmolytic properties are attributed to its flavonoids and alkaloids; especially harmalas, which inhibit oxygen consumption by the brain. These compounds are also thought to decrease circulatory and respiratory rates by reducing arterial pressure. Some consider its alkaloids, harmine and harmaline, effective against Parkinson's disease. Other *Passiflora* species contain constituents that act against molds, yeasts, and bacteria.

Paullinia cupana

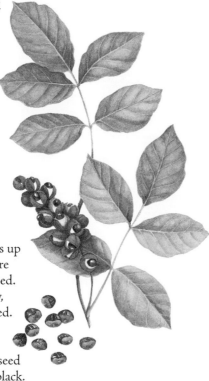

COMMON NAMES
Guarana, Guerana

LATIN NAME
Paullinia cupana

FAMILY Sapindaceae

PART USED
Seed

DESCRIPTION
A perennial shrub with a woody vine, guarana grows up to 30 feet long. Its leaves are compound, large, and ribbed. Flowers are whitish yellow, fragrant, and open clustered. Fruits are reddish orange and berrylike, have three sections, and contain one seed that is purplish brown to black.

HABITAT
Guarana is indigenous to the tropical forests of the Brazilian Amazon. It is also cultivated in other rain forests.

FOLKLORE AND TRADITIONAL USES
Amazonian Indians used guarana as a stimulant and to combat fatigue on long jungle journeys. Carried in baked stick form, it was used as a substitute for food. Today it is employed to help endure periods of fast. Guarana is the key ingredient in many popular South American refreshments, including coffee substitutes, diet beverages, and soft drinks. Guarana seeds are lightly hallucinogenic and are considered to be aphrodisiacs. This herb is also used as a fish-killing drug in Central and South America.

MEDICINAL USES
Guarana has been used by Amazonian tribal peoples for many medicinal purposes, especially to treat diarrhea. The plant's antidiarrheal action is attributed to its high level of tannins, which act as astringents. Guarana also contains a high concentration of caffeine, which, in conjunction with the alkaloids theobromine and theophylline, gives guarana diuretic and stimulant properties. Guarana is used to treat fatigue, mild depression, headache, and migraine, but should not be used long-term. Its potentially serious side-effects include decreased fertility and cardiovascular disease. Guarana is also a vascular muscle relaxant and appetite suppressant, but it is not recommended as part of a weight-loss strategy.

Petroselinum crispum

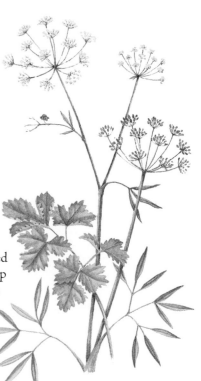

COMMON NAMES
Parsley, Curly parsley

LATIN NAME
Petroselinum crispum

FAMILY Umbelliferae

PARTS USED
Root, seed, leaf

DESCRIPTION
A biennial (although cultivated as an annual), parsley grows up to three feet tall, with an erect stem. Leaves are bright green and crinkled. The small, greenish yellow or white flowers occur in compound umbels. Seeds are tiny, oval, and ribbed.

HABITAT
Parsley is indigenous to the Mediterranean region and to Europe. It is cultivated throughout the world. Parsley grows best in humus-rich, moist, well-drained soil in partial shade.

FOLKLORE AND TRADITIONAL USES
The ancient Greeks regarded parsley as a symbol of death and used it in funeral rites. Because of this association, Greek soldiers feared contact with parsley before battle. The Romans ate parsley sprigs at banquets to absorb wine fumes and to freshen the breath. During the Middle Ages, Europeans considered this herb the signature of the devil, certain to bring about a household's downfall if transplanted. Today it is popular worldwide as a culinary herb and garnish.

MEDICINAL USES
Parsley, used as a medicinal herb for more than 2,000 years, is the source of many volatile oils, mostly concentrated in the seeds. Medieval German herbalist Saint Hildegard of Bingen prescribed parsley wine to improve blood circulation. Parsley's principal constituent, apiol, is effective against chills and fevers. Its secondary constituent, myristicin, in conjunction with apiol gives parsley diuretic properties. It is used to treat cystitis, gout, high blood pressure, and rheumatic conditions. Parsley is rich in the bone strengthener fluorine, the breath freshener chlorophyll, and Vitamins A, C, and E. Parsley root is also a strong uterine stimulant and was once employed to induce abortion.

Phoradendron flavescens

COMMON NAMES
American mistletoe, Mistletoe, Golden bough

LATIN NAMES
Phoradendron flavescens,
Viscum album

FAMILY Loranthaceae

PARTS USED
Leaf, berry, twig

DESCRIPTION
Mistletoe, a semiparasitic plant, clings to the bark of deciduous trees. Its branches are round and knotted at the joints, with leathery evergreen leaves at their ends. Its white, pea-size berries contain single seeds.

HABITAT
Mistletoe grows in temperate areas of Europe and North America, although it can occur as far east as China.

FOLKLORE AND TRADITIONAL USES
According to Norse mythology, the young hero Baldur—killed by an arrow fashioned from mistletoe—was restored to life by Freya, the goddess queen. She then made herself protectress of the plant, proclaiming that those who pass under it must kiss. Believed to be a divine gift from God, it was sacred to the Druids of Europe, the Ainos of Japan, and certain tribes in Africa. Because its strength depends upon its not touching the ground, it is always found hanging. It was hung above doors and used as amulets to ward off evil spirits. Its evergreen leaves symbolized new life and rebirth at the winter solstice. In France and Sweden mistletoe gathered on midsummer's day was believed to possess special healing power.

MEDICINAL USES
The Chinese have used mistletoe as a laxative, a sedative, and a uterine relaxant during pregnancy. Nineteenth-century Eclectic physicians in America also used it to ease menstrual pain, as mistletoe contains tyramine, which stimulates uterine contractions. In folk medicine, the stem was employed for anxiety as a tranquilizer, and the berries were used to treat epilepsy and bleeding in the lungs. In Germany, mistletoe extract is an ingredient in many medications prescribed to regulate blood pressure. Some studies suggest that mistletoe stimulates the immune system; others show that injections of mistletoe extract may decrease the size of tumors.

Phyllanthus niruri

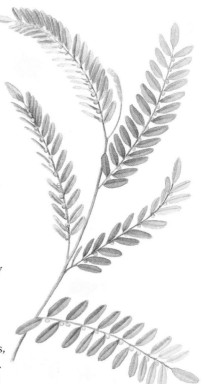

COMMON NAMES
Phyllanthus, Amla

LATIN NAMES
Phyllanthus niruri,
P. amarus

FAMILY Euphorbiaceae

PART USED
Whole herb

DESCRIPTION
A perennial herb with many yellow flowers, phyllanthus grows to about two feet in height. It is a genus of the spurge family and has over 600 different species of trees, shrubs, and low-lying herbs. Some species have flattened stems that resemble leaves; others have deciduous twigs that bear small, alternating leaves.

HABITAT
Phyllanthus is indigenous to central and southern India. It is also cultivated in other countries, including China, the Philippines, Cuba, Nigeria, and Guam.

FOLKLORE AND TRADITIONAL USES
Various species of phyllanthus have a wide variety of purposes. One, *P. acidus*, has light yellow and green fruits that are made into preserves. The leaves and bark of *P. emblica*, called amla or Indian gooseberry, contain tannin and are used in tanning and dyeing. In India people make its dried fruit into ink, hair dye, and detergent. They also use the fresh fruit, which is high in Vitamin C, in drinks and candy. Phyllanthus is not related to what Europeans call gooseberry.

MEDICINAL USES
Many species of phyllanthus have been used in Ayurvedic medicine for more than 2,000 years. It is a traditional remedy for ailments like jaundice, dysentery, diabetes, skin ulcers, and urinary tract infections. Phyllanthus's principal constituents—lignans, alkaloids, and bioflavonoids—have been found to act primarily on the liver, which confirms its traditional use in the treatment of jaundice. *Phyllanthus amarus* attracted the attention of Nobel prize winner Baruch Blumberg. He and others studied its uses in preventing hepatitis B and devised a vaccine. Recently Indian doctors and scientists have also developed a medicine, shown to clear the body of hepatitis in many cases. Phyllanthus inhibits liver cancer, as well, and has potential as a diuretic, hypotensive, and hypoglycemic drug for diabetes.

Physostigma venenosum

COMMON NAMES
Calabar bean, Ordeal bean

LATIN NAME
Physostigma venenosum

FAMILY Leguminosae

PART USED
Seed

DESCRIPTION
A perennial woody climber, calabar bean has a twining vine that can extend more than 50 feet long. The three leaves are large and pinnate. Flowers are purple. Fruits are dark brown pods containing two to three brownish black, kidney-shaped seeds about an inch long.

HABITAT
Calabar bean is indigenous to western Africa in an area around Nigeria once known as Calabar. It is also cultivated in India and parts of South America.

**FOLKLORE
AND TRADITIONAL USES**
Infamous in Africa, the poisonous seeds of the calabar bean were once used as an "ordeal poison" to identify a witch or a person possessed by evil spirits. Made to ingest several beans, the accused was proclaimed innocent only if he or she regurgitated the beans and survived. Western settlers captured by native people and forced to undergo this ordeal soon learned that swallowing the seeds whole prevented the poison's release. Although outlawed in Africa, the calabar-bean ordeal is still practiced in some tribal rituals. Chemicals derived from the bean have been used in agricultural insecticides and chemical warfare nerve gases. A variant was used in the Persian Gulf war.

MEDICINAL USES
Calabar bean's principal constituent is the toxic alkaloid physostigmine, which helps prolong the activity of acetylcholine, a neurotransmitter that stimulates gastric secretion, contracts smooth muscles, and dilates blood vessels. Chiefly employed to treat the eye, physostigmine is used to contract the pupil and drain excess fluid, which helps prevent optic nerve damage and loss of vision symptomatic of glaucoma. It is also used to reverse the central nervous system toxicity of anticholinergic drugs and to stimulate the intestinal tract. Calabar bean is currently being studied for the treatment of Alzheimer's disease.

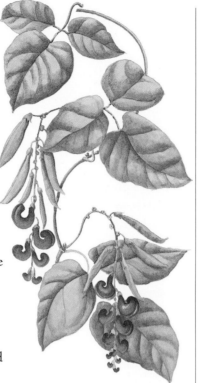

Pilocarpus microphyllus

COMMON NAMES
Jaborandi,
Arruda do mato

LATIN NAMES
Pilocarpus microphyllus,
P. pennatifolius

FAMILY Rutaceae

PARTS USED
Leaf

DESCRIPTION
Jaborandi is a perennial shrub reaching heights of four to five feet. It has large grayish green leaves covered with tiny oil-producing glands; smooth grayish bark; and small, reddish purple flowers.

HABITAT
The jaborandi is native to Brazil.

**FOLKLORE
AND TRADITIONAL USES**
The name "jaborandi" derives from an Amazonian word meaning "slobber weed," as the use of it causes intense salivation. Jaborandi, also known as *alfavaca* in parts of South America, is marketed in the United States and in Latin America as an ingredient in shampoo. In earlier times, Brazilians believed that if they applied it to their heads it would prevent baldness.

MEDICINAL USES
Native Brazilians used jaborandi to treat diabetes and to induce sweating. It was the latter that first attracted the attention of foreign scientists. In the 1870s, Symphronio Continho brought the plant to Europe, where its ability to make people sweat and salivate translated into medicines for dry mouth, a symptom it still combats, especially in people undergoing chemotherapy. Contemporaries of Continho isolated pilocarpine and discovered its use in ophthalmology to contract the pupil and treat glaucoma in early stages. In homeopathic medicine jaborandi was one ingredient in treatments for mumps. Oil from jaborandi leaves contains the alkaloids pilocarpine and jaborine. Pilocarpine mimics or enhances the action of the neurotransmitter acetylcholine—the primary transmitter of nerve impulses of the parasympathetic system. Pilocarpine controls saliva, sweat, and tear glands, as well as contraction of the eye. Pilocarpine can counteract the effects of atropine by stimulating paralyzed nerve endings. Jaborine has qualities similar to atropine.

Piper methysticum

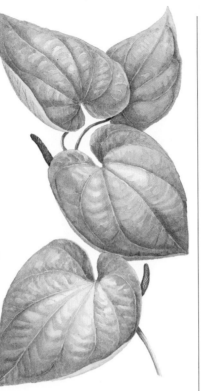

COMMON NAMES
Kava, Kava kava

LATIN NAME
Piper methysticum

FAMILY Piperaceae

PART USED
Rhizome

DESCRIPTION
Kava is a sprawling shrub that can exceed ten feet in height. It has broadly heart-shaped ribbed leaves and numerous small flowers. The rhizome is large and whitish gray, with many roots branching from it.

HABITAT
Kava grows in Polynesia, including Hawaii and other islands in the South Pacific.

FOLKLORE AND TRADITIONAL USES
In the Pacific Islands, kava is used extensively in ceremonies, festivals, and as a sign of good will. The kava-kava beverage is imbibed to foster friendship, to celebrate marriages and births, to mourn deaths, and to placate the gods. It is the beverage of choice to welcome VIPs. For example, Hillary R. Clinton and Lady Bird and President Johnson in Samoa, as well as the pope in Fiji, all drank kava during welcoming ceremonies.

MEDICINAL USES
Because kava numbs any surface it comes into contact with, doctors have used the cut rhizome of kava as a local anesthetic, as well as a treatment for gonorrhea. Kava contains two pain-relieving chemicals, dihydrokawain and dihydromethysticin, which are as strong as aspirin, as well as the lactone, kawain. Kava's main use is as a sedative and as a treatment for nervous anxiety, stress, and restlessness. Scientists are investigating which chemicals produce these effects and have determined that using the whole kava resin works significantly better than kawain alone. Kava also relaxes skeletal muscles and is very effective for treating menstrual cramps. Although it has a sedative effect, kava is not known to be addictive; nor does it dull mental activity. Users report a clear mind while enjoying a relaxed body.

Podophyllum peltatum

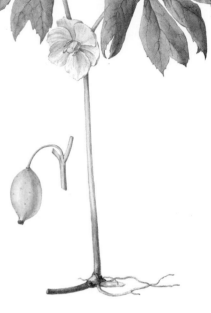

COMMON NAMES
Mayapple, American mandrake, Devil's apple, Duck's foot

LATIN NAME
Podophyllum peltatum

FAMILY Podophyllaceae

PART USED
Rhizome

DESCRIPTION
This perennial grows one to two feet tall. One or two large leaves unfold like umbrellas, and a solitary white blossom forms below them. The mayapple's rhizome is thick and reddish brown. Its fruit is small and yellow.

HABITAT
Indigenous to the eastern United States and southern Canada, American mayapple usually grows in patches.

FOLKLORE AND TRADITIONAL USES
Mayapple gets its Latin name from the Greek words *podos* and *phyllon* (foot-shaped leaves); *peltatum* means "shield-like." While the mayapple's ripe fruit is edible, and jellies and juices are prepared from it, the root, leaves, seeds, and unripe fruit all can be poisonous. To encourage children to stay away from the poisonous mayapple, their elders traditionally taught them that it was tended by the devil. Native Americans used the root, the fruit, or decoctions of the whole plant as insecticides.

MEDICINAL USES
Native North American tribes drank a brew made from the dried, ground rhizome as a treatment for intestinal worms, as an antidote for snakebite, and as a laxative. This herb was formerly used as one of the laxative ingredients in the over-the-counter drug called "Carter's Little Liver Pills." Extracts of mayapple are currently administered externally to treat genital warts and some skin cancers. Podophyllotoxin, a potentially lethal component of mayapple, blocks cell division and has tumor-inhibiting properties. Two drugs derived from it are approved for use in the United States. Etoposide is used to treat testicular and small-cell lung cancer. Teniposide is employed with brain tumors and childhood leukemia. The FDA has warned against mayapple as a laxative because of its potential toxicity.

Polygala senega

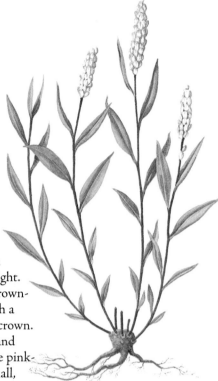

COMMON NAMES
Senega, Senega root,
Seneca snakeroot

LATIN NAME
Polygala senega

FAMILY Polygalaceae

PART USED
Root

DESCRIPTION
A perennial herb, senega
may grow to a foot in height.
Roots are yellowish to brownish gray and twisted, with a
thick, irregular, knotted crown.
Leaves are green, small, and
lance shaped. Flowers are pinkish to greenish white, small,
numerous, and crowded on
a narrow spike up to two
inches long.

HABITAT
Senega is indigenous to central
and western North America. It
is found in the woods and elsewhere on dry, rocky soil.

**FOLKLORE
AND TRADITIONAL USES**
Polygala means "much milk," an
allusion to this herb's profuse
secretions. A related species,
milkwort, is said to increase
milk production in nursing
mothers. *Senega* may be derived
from the Native American
Seneca tribe, who used it as a
remedy for various ailments.
Although other Native American tribes also employed
senega, the Seneca are credited
with revealing it to Scottish
physician John Tennent (1735),
who in turn introduced it to
the Western world of medicine.

MEDICINAL USES
Native Americans have long
used senega for rheumatism,
colds, inflammation, and bleeding wounds. Dr. John Tennent
is credited for learning the
plant's uses from them and
subsequently advancing
senega's use in Europe for
pleurisy and pleuropneumonia.
During the early 19th century,
senega was used as an expectorant cough remedy. Today it
treats bronchitis, tracheitis,
emphysema, and inflammation
of the respiratory tract.
Senega's principal constituents
are saponins, including sene-
gins. These saponins suppress
coughing, while their detergent
activity breaks up phlegm.
Senega is also thought to
stimulate bronchial mucous
gland secretion. Saponins in
senega may hold some potential for treating non-insulin-
dependent diabetes.

Prunella vulgaris

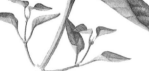

COMMON NAMES
Self-heal, Heal-all,
Heart of the Earth

LATIN NAME
Prunella vulgaris

FAMILY Labiatae

PART USED
Whole herb

DESCRIPTION
Self-heal, a low, creeping
perennial, grows about one
foot tall. With a short rhizome
and freely branching square
stems, this member
of the mint family has bluish
flowers and oblong, pointed
leaves that grow in pairs.

HABITAT
A native Eurasian plant, self-
heal grows wild in temperate
regions throughout the world.

**FOLKLORE
AND TRADITIONAL USES**
Nursemaids would warn their
charges not to pick this plant,
for if they did, the devil would
carry them off. Heal-all and
self-heal, both nicknames of
Prunella vulgaris, are puzzles to
those who study plant lore,
because the medicinal uses are
limited. Some believe the Latin
name was derived from
"brunella," a corruption of the
German word *braüne*, for "a
brown one." Heal-all is an
example of what doctors in
earlier times called the doctrine of signatures: Plants
resembled the part of the body
that they healed.

MEDICINAL USES
This herb was lauded by John
Gerard, 16th-century herbalist
and chief secretary of state to
Queen Elizabeth I. He writes:
"There is not a better wound
herb in the world," and when
mixed with wine and water it
will "make whole and sound all
wounds, inward and outward."
People thought this plant
resembled a mouth and used
it to cure sore throats and
other infections of the mouth.
Self-heal has also been used
to treat diarrhea and boils.
Recently, speculation has it
that extracts from the herb
serve as an HIV inhibitor. In
China it is used as an agent in
lowering blood pressure and as
an antibiotic. A German and
French proverb advises, "He
needs neither physician nor
surgeon that hath Self-Heal
and Sanicle to help himself."

Prunus serotina

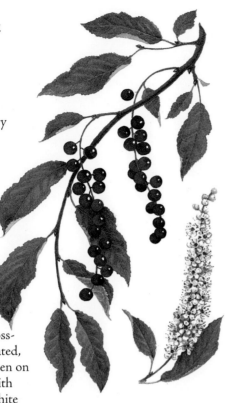

COMMON NAMES
Wild cherry, Black cherry

LATIN NAME
Prunus serotina

FAMILY Rosaceae

PART USED
Bark

DESCRIPTION
A deciduous tree, wild cherry grows up to 90 feet tall. The bark is dark reddish brown (gray in maturity), rough, aromatic, and cross-marked. Leaves are serrated, oval to lance shaped, green on top and pale beneath, with finely toothed edges. White flowers hang in drooping multiple clusters. The fruit is a blackish purple cherry.

HABITAT
Wild cherry is indigenous to North America. It is also cultivated in Europe. This tree grows best in deep, rich, moist, well-drained soil under full sun.

**FOLKLORE
AND TRADITIONAL USES**
Settlers in the Appalachian Mountains used the cherry tree's fruit to brew "rumcherry," a potent liquor. Early New England craftsmen turned to the native tree as a substitute for the more costly and inaccessible Honduras mahogany. Hence, the cherry is sometimes called "the poor man's mahogany." Its finely textured grain has been used for centuries in furniture, musical instruments, and architectural paneling. The slightly bitter-tasting fruit is used to make jelly and wine.

MEDICINAL USES
Wild cherry bark is a popular Native American remedy, long used to treat coughs and colds. Its primary constituent is prunasin, which, when broken down in the body, quells spasms in the smooth muscles that line the bronchioles. Wild cherry syrup is effective in treating coughs, bronchitis, whooping cough, and other lung problems. It is also believed to have a simultaneous mild sedative action. However, wild cherry leaves contain hydrocyanic acid, which is toxic and can cause death if ingested in large amounts.

Pulsatilla vulgaris

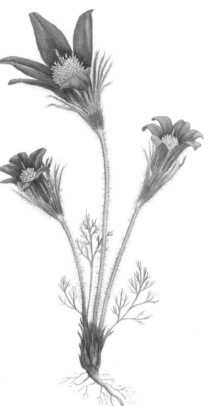

COMMON NAMES
Pulsatilla, Windflower, Anemone, Pasque flower, Easter flower

LATIN NAMES
*Pulsatilla vulgaris,
P. anemone*

FAMILY Ranunculaceae

PART USED
Whole plant

DESCRIPTION
Covered with silky hairs, pulsatilla is a perennial that reaches heights of about 18 inches. It has finely divided leaves and solitary pale violet flowers with yellow stamens, which become feathery seed heads after the blooms fall off.

HABITAT
Pulsatilla is native to northern Europe.

**FOLKLORE
AND TRADITIONAL USES**
In the language of flowers, the windflower speaks of being forsaken. The jealous Greek goddess Flora turned the nymph Anemone into a windflower when she had attracted the attention of her husband, Zephyr. He abandoned Anemone, leaving her blowing in the wind. The flower is also said to have sprung from the blood of Adonis, as Aphrodite, the goddess of love, wept over his slain body. In the 16th century John Gerard, botanist and chief secretary of state to Queen Elizabeth I, claimed to have named it "Pasque flower," Old French for "Easter" (and derived from the Hebrew for "Passover") because it blooms around the time of these holidays. The name, however, could have evolved from its use in coloring Easter eggs.

MEDICINAL USES
Pulsatilla is employed as a homeopathic remedy to treat certain eye and genital diseases, as well as diseases of the gastrointestinal and urinary tracts. Pulsatilla lowers arterial tension, dilates the pupils, and reduces respiration. While there are no known hazards or side effects to the appropriate administration of extremely small therapeutic doses, pulsatilla is poisonous. In improper doses it can cause coma, convulsions, and death by asphyxiation. People should also avoid touching the fresh plant, as it can produce severe reaction on contact. Pregnant women should avoid ingesting it. Experts in Germany who have reviewed the studies and the uses of this herb recommend avoiding it except in homeopathic remedies.

Rauwolfia serpentina

COMMON NAMES
Indian snakeroot, Rauwolfia

LATIN NAME
Rauwolfia serpentina

FAMILY Apocynaceae

PART USED
Root

DESCRIPTION
A climbing evergreen shrub, Indian snakeroot reaches approximately three feet in height, with whorls of elliptical leaves. Its berries are glossy purple to black. The small flowers are white and pink.

HABITAT
Indian snakeroot is indigenous to southern Asia and southeastern Asia. Today the plant is widely cultivated.

FOLKLORE AND TRADITIONAL USES
According to legend, mentioned and discredited by Rudyard Kipling in his story "Rikki Tikki Tavi," mongooses eat Indian snakeroot before engaging in battle with cobras. It is said that natives learned to use the plant as an antidote for snakebites by observing the mongoose. In reality, mongooses can be bitten, but because they fluff out their fur while fighting, a cobra's fangs may not penetrate the skin and, thus, may not harm them.

MEDICINAL USES
Ayurvedic medicine has employed snakeroot to treat bites from poisonous reptiles and insects for thousands of years. The earliest written reference to Indian snakeroot is in the Ayurvedic text *Charaka*

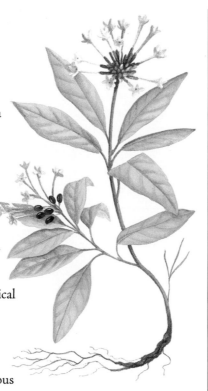

Samhita, a collection of age-old wisdom transmitted orally for thousands of years before being written down in 600 B.C. At that time Indian snakeroot was used to treat snakebite, mental illness, and insomnia. It is said that Mohandas Gandhi chewed on rauwolfia root while meditating. In 1952 Indian snakeroot's integration into Western medicine was fueled by the isolation of its alkaloid reserpine. The term "tranquilizer" was used shortly thereafter when reserpine's effects on the central nervous system were described. Reserpine was the first modern drug developed to effectively treat hypertension, as it acts upon the sympathetic nervous system to reduce vascular resistance and heart rate. The drug is not given to patients with histories of certain mental illnesses, as it can occasionally lead to psychotic depression and suicide.

Rhamnus purshiana

COMMON NAMES
Cascara sagrada (sacred bark), Cascara buckthorn

LATIN NAME
Rhamnus purshiana

FAMILY Rhamnaceae

PART USED
Bark

DESCRIPTION
Bearing greenish flowers and dark purple fruit with glossy black seeds, this deciduous tree usually reaches 20 to 40 feet in height. Ridged bark is brown or red-brown.

HABITAT
Native to western North America, cascara sagrada is cultivated in eastern Africa and on the North American Pacific Coast.

FOLKLORE AND TRADITIONAL USES
The name "cascara sagrada," Spanish for "sacred bark," may have come from its association with the Jesuits who took many plants to Europe from Latin America. Or that name may indicate an appreciation of the plant's ability to heal. Cascara sagrada is a type of buckthorn, a tree whose name means stag's horn. This tree had a variety of uses. Its wood yielded charcoal; its bark and fruits yielded yellow and green dyes. Its bark was an Appalachian folk remedy for cancer and was among the ingredients of the highly controversial Hoxsey Cancer Formula in the first half of the 20th century.

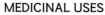

MEDICINAL USES
Originally a Native American remedy for upset stomachs and constipation, cascara sagrada was lauded as a wonder of the New World in Europe when it was brought back by Spanish explorers, who named it cascara sagrada, or sacred bark. Its qualities as a gentle laxative were important in an era where medicine focused on keeping bodily fluids in balance. This herb, which has held a place in the U.S. Pharmacopoeia since 1890, is among the most popular herbal medicines in the world. It is included in many over-the-counter laxatives and is prescribed more than 2.5 million times a year. The bark must be dried for up to one year before it can be used officially as a laxative. Aloe-emodin, found in cascara sagrada, is being researched as a possible treatment for leukemia.

Rosa canina

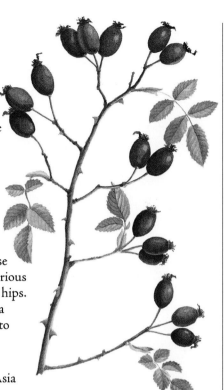

COMMON NAMES
Rose, Rose-hips, Dog rose

LATIN NAME
Rosa canina

FAMILY Rosaceae

PARTS USED
Petal, leaf, rose hip, seed

DESCRIPTION
A perennial shrub, the rose has aromatic flowers in various colors; its fruits are called hips. Plant heights range from a few inches in dwarf form to several feet.

HABITAT
Roses are indigenous to Asia and possibly Iran. They now bloom in temperate and sub-tropical zones everywhere.

FOLKLORE AND TRADITIONAL USES
The Roman naturalist Pliny attributed the name "dog rose" to a belief that the plant's root would prevent the dire consequences of being bitten by a mad dog. Roses are, for many people, the flowers of love and beauty and have been celebrated in song and poems for centuries. In some cultures, the oil of roses was also believed to help an infertile woman conceive. Romans wore rose garlands during their drunken festivals to Bacchus, because they believed it would temper the effects of wine. The rose is linked with almost every religion and is associated with Brahma, Vishnu, Mohammed, Buddha, Confucius, Zoroaster, and Jesus. In Renaissance England, the symbolic meaning of the flower took on a huge importance during the War of the Roses. In addition to their beauty, rose petals are valued for their scent and flavor, and rose hips are sometimes made into jellies, preserves, syrups, tea, and wine.

MEDICINAL USES
In the Middle Ages roses were brought to Europe from Asia and used for a variety of ailments, usually mixed with other ingredients. Herbalists consider rose hips one of the best sources of Vitamin C; they are used with other treatments for colds, flu, and disorders of the urinary tract. They also contain A, K, and many of the B vitamins. Rose oil acts as an astringent and treats inflammation of the mouth and pharynx. The Chinese have used roses, both fruit and petals, for intestinal and uterine disorders.

Salix alba

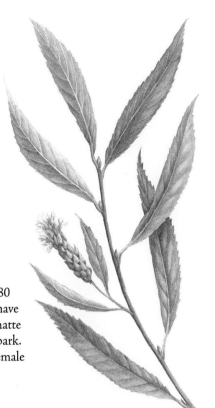

COMMON NAMES
White willow, European willow

LATIN NAME
Salix alba

FAMILY Salicaceae

PART USED
Bark

DESCRIPTION
Willow trees can grow to 80 feet in height. All species have long, narrow, blue-green matte leaves and rough, grayish bark. Male flowers are yellow; female flowers are green.

HABITAT
Indigenous to central and southern Europe, willows are now found in temperate wetlands throughout the world.

FOLKLORE AND TRADITIONAL USES
The words "willow" and "witch" derive from the same word: the Old English *wigle*, or divination. Druids purportedly sacrificed people in wicker—Scandinavian for "willow"—baskets at the full moon. Ancient Egyptians considered the tree a symbol for joy. In Japanese legend the spine of the first human was made from the willow. In ancient Greece it was the emblem of Artemis, representing fertility. It became a symbol of sorrow after the destruction of the first temple in Jerusalem. The Bible thereafter refers to the willow as a source of comforting shade and water. In China it was associated with feminine beauty. Willow wood also is used for making cricket bats and artist's charcoal.

MEDICINAL USES
The cuneiform sign for the willow appears frequently in prescriptions on a 4,000-year-old Sumerian tablet from Nippur. And in recent centuries willow has been used for joint pain and fevers. It has also been recognized as a diuretic, a treatment for eye disease, and an aid in childbirth. The bark and leaves are rich in the glucoside salicin, first isolated in the 1820s. In the 1850s a derivative, acetylsalicylic acid, was synthesized as an active ingredient in aspirin, one of the world's most popular medications. Recently, researchers have learned that aspirin, now totally synthetic, can be taken prophylactically to reduce the likelihood of stroke and heart disease. The drug is thought to work by blocking the synthesis of prostaglandins, hormonelike substances that, among other things, stimulate inflammation and affect clotting of blood.

Sedum telephium

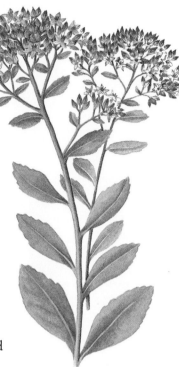

COMMON NAMES
Live-long, Orpine, Stonecrop

LATIN NAMES
Sedum telephium, S. purpureum

FAMILY Crassulaceae

PART USED
Whole herb

DESCRIPTION
Live-long is a perennial that grows up to three feet tall. The rootstock is large and fleshy, with small parsnip-shaped tubers and a whitish gray rind. The broad, flattened leaves are bluish green and up to three inches long. Flowers are whitish pink to reddish purple.

HABITAT
Indigenous to temperate zones, live-long is cultivated in many countries. In the tropics, live-long grows in the mountains; in cooler regions, it thrives in lower locations such as hedge-banks on the shady sides of woods.

FOLKLORE AND TRADITIONAL USES
The name "live-long" derives from this plant's tenacity for life. Because of its fleshy leaves and swollen roots, live-long has a rare ability to stay fresh and alive, long after having been uprooted. The Latin name "telephium" comes from Telephus, son of Hercules, who is said to have used it to cure a battle-wounded leg that had not otherwise healed. Also known as "midsummer men" this herb was once gathered on Midsummer's Eve to determine the future of a love relationship: Two leaves would be placed side-by-side; if they fell toward each other, love was true. In Scandinavia, live-long was planted on the roof to ward off lightning. If the herb suddenly withered, superstition held that someone would die.

MEDICINAL USES
Live-long has been used as a popular folk remedy for diarrhea. The 16th-century German herbalist Hieronymus Tragus states that it was used to treat stomach, lung, liver, and bowel problems, burns, inflammation, and sore throats. Live-long has proven immuno-stimulant and anti-inflammatory properties due to the presence of two major poly-saccharides. These polysaccharides may help inhibit tumors and increase the action of phagocytes, which effectively kill bacteria and viruses.

Serenoa repens

COMMON NAME
Saw palmetto

LATIN NAMES
Serenoa repens, Serrulata, S. serrulata

FAMILY Arecaceae

PART USED
Fruit

DESCRIPTION
Saw palmetto is a palm tree that grows up to ten feet tall. Its crown is made up of yellowish green leaves that are more than two feet long. The saw palmetto's flowers are white and fragrant. Its fruit consists of brownish black, wrinkled berries that contain one brown, hard seed. The panicle holding the seed may weigh up to nine pounds.

HABITAT
Saw palmetto is indigenous to the southern coastal regions of the United States and the West Indies.

FOLKLORE AND TRADITIONAL USES
Palm trees are sources of fruit, oil, and fiber. Throughout history, they have had great economic importance. They also figure prominently in myth. For example, Ulysses blinded Cyclops with the sharpened branch of a green palm tree. And in the Christian religion, the palm is the rod of life. Various palms, including saw palmetto, were thought to have aphrodisiac properties.

MEDICINAL USES
Saw palmetto has been employed as a diuretic, a sperm stimulant, a breast enlarger, and an expectorant. Saw palmetto is chiefly employed to manage prostatic enlargement, or benign prostatic hyperplasia (BPH). A hexane extract inhibits 5-alpha reductase, the enzyme needed for the conversion of testosterone into dihydrotestosterone (DHT). Saw palmetto further antagonizes DHT binding at prostatic receptor sites, which increases the metabolism and excretion of DHT. It is also used to treat BPH-related inflammation. Saw palmetto relieves urinary symptoms and flow measures associated with an enlarged prostate; it does not reduce the enlargement. Saw palmetto preparations have been shown to be effective for treating symptoms of BPH in 18 human clinical trials, with several of them indicating significantly safer effects than the leading pharmaceutical drug.

Silybum marianum

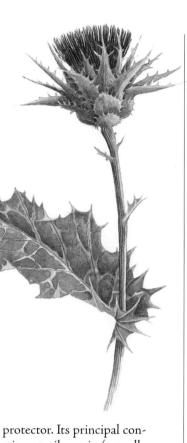

COMMON NAMES
Milk thistle, Marian thistle

LATIN NAME
Silybum marianum

FAMILY Asteraceae

PART USED
Seed

DESCRIPTION
An annual or biennial, milk thistle grows up to six feet tall, with an erect stem. Alternate leaves are grayish green, spiny, and white-veined. When broken, they exude a milky sap. Flowers are reddish purple, ridged, and sharply spined. Fruits are brown, spotted, and glossy, with a white tuft of hair.

HABITAT
Milk thistle is indigenous to Europe. It is also cultivated in North America, South America, and Australia.

**FOLKLORE
AND TRADITIONAL USES**
According to medieval legend, the white markings on milk thistle leaves were caused by a drop of the Virgin Mary's milk. Consequently, the plant became known as our lady's thistle, or *marianum*, from which the common name "milk thistle" is derived. Thistles, briers, and thorns are mentioned many times in the Bible and are often used interchangeably with each other. In the Book of Isaiah "brier" is employed to mean troublesome men.

MEDICINAL USES
Milk thistle has been used medicinally for more than 2,000 years, especially as a liver protector. Its principal constituent, silymarin (actually a combination of three compounds called flavonolignans), helps restructure liver cells to prevent toxins from penetrating that organ. It stimulates the regenerative ability of the liver by helping form new cells. Glutathione compounds, which are potent antioxidants and intermediates in cell metabolism, remove toxins from liver cells. Milk thistle is used to treat jaundice, cirrhosis, hepatitis, toxin-poisoning—such as that induced by alcohol and industrial toxins—and other liver diseases. Milk thistle is also useful as an anti-inflammatory and a bile stimulant. It is employed in Europe to treat amanita mushroom poisoning.

Tanacetum parthenium

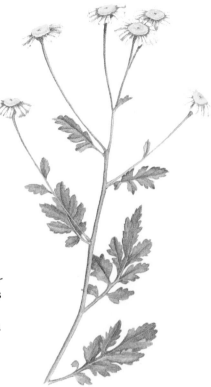

COMMON NAME
Feverfew

LATIN NAME
Tanacetum parthenium

FAMILY Asteraceae

PART USED
Whole herb

DESCRIPTION
A perennial herb, feverfew grows as tall as three feet. Leaves are yellow-green, crenate, and margined. Flowers have white, finely divided feathery petals, centering on a yellow disk.

HABITAT
Feverfew is indigenous to southeast Europe. It is now cultivated all over Europe, Australia, and North America. It requires well-drained soil in full sun.

**FOLKLORE
AND TRADITIONAL USES**
The Latin *parthenium* may refer to this plant's legendary role in saving the life of a man who fell from the Parthenon during its construction (around 400 B.C.). A more plausible explanation is its use for treating menstrual cramps in young women, deriving its name from the Greek *parthenos* (virgin). In the Middle Ages the plant was renamed "featherfoil," which eventually evolved into its present-day common name of "feverfew." Because of its name, feverfew has been mistakenly used as a treatment for fever. Its bitter principle has also been employed in food recipes, liqueurs, and perfumes.

MEDICINAL USES
Recommended over the centuries by the ancient Greeks, the herbalist Nicholas Culpeper (ca 1600), and Canada's Health Protection Branch, feverfew has long been used to treat rheumatism, menstrual discomfort, headache, and hysteria. Parthenolide, a constituent of feverfew, inhibits the release of certain chemicals, including the hormone serotonin, which is produced during a migraine attack, and certain inflammatory mediators, including the hormone prostaglandin, which regulates inflammation. Feverfew is used for prevention of migraines and headaches, despite some evidence against its efficacy, and to relieve arthritis, psoriasis, and dermatitis. Feverfew is also an antihistamine and a preventive against potential strokes and heart attacks. It should not be used by pregnant women.

Taxus brevifolia

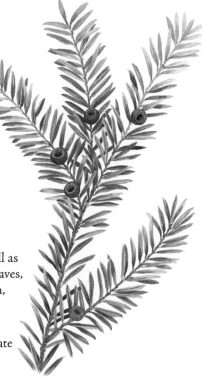

COMMON NAME
Pacific yew

LATIN NAMES
Taxus brevifolia,
T. baccata

FAMILY Taxaceae

PARTS USED
Bark, leaf

DESCRIPTION
Evergreen yews grow as tall as 80 feet. They have spiky leaves, arranged in a spiral pattern, and fleshy red berries.

HABITAT
This tree grows in temperate climates in the Northern Hemisphere.

**FOLKLORE
AND TRADITIONAL USES**
Druids saw the yew as the tree of immortality and held it sacred. Later, Christians planted it in their churchyards. The reason is not clear. Some say it was to keep cattle from eating its poisonous berries; others say it was because a steady supply of the wood was needed for making bows. The Latin name *taxa* comes from the Greek *toxon,* the root word for "poison" and "bow." Legend has it that the famous archer and outlaw Robin Hood was married under a yew tree. Ancient British law protected the yew tree and prescribed penalties for disfiguring yew wood furniture, carvings, or doors. Native Americans also held the yew in high regard. Some tribes saw it as the chief of trees. Although it had a variety of uses, Native Americans, like Europeans, associated it with war and bows.

MEDICINAL USES
The compound paclitaxel, from the bark of this plant, stabilizes microtubules, the part of the cell that maintains shape and aids in cell division. It combats certain cancers, most notably ovarian and breast. In the early 1960s the Pacific yew was part of a widespread search for cancer-fighting plants. More than 20 years later, clinical trials began. In 1994 scientists succeeded in synthesizing paclitaxel from yew needles and bark after concerns that a severe depletion in the numbers of yews could occur. Needles from a related species, *T. baccata,* have been used for many ailments, such as tapeworms, epilepsy, and tonsillitis. Medical experts do not recommend self-prescribing, however, because yew needles and seeds are known to be toxic.

Theobroma cacao

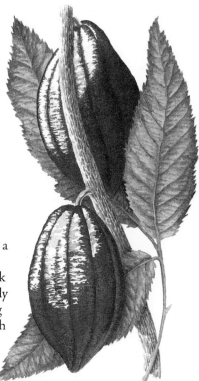

COMMON NAMES
Cocoa, Cacao, Chocolate

LATIN NAME
Theobroma cacao

FAMILY Sterculiaceae

PART USED
Seed

DESCRIPTION
Cocoa, an evergreen tree with a knotty trunk, can grow up to heights exceeding 25 feet. Pink or creamy flowers grow directly on the trunk. Its fruit, ranging in color from yellow to reddish purple to brown, grows in capsules, each containing about 25 seeds.

HABITAT
Native to Mexico and Central America, cocoa grows worldwide in tropical regions.

**FOLKLORE
AND TRADITIONAL USES**
Cocoa's Latin name, *Theobroma,* means "food of the gods." To the Aztec, *xocoatl* (cocoa) was a form of currency and a beverage drunk by nobility from gold goblets. The rest of the world learned about chocolate when Hernando Cortez brought it back from Mexico in 1519. The Spanish succeeded in keeping chocolate a secret for more than a century before its use spread throughout Europe. It was originally consumed solely as a sweet or bitter beverage. Only since about 150 years ago has chocolate been enjoyed as a confection. In the U.S. alone chocolate sales in 1998 amounted to 13 billion dollars.

Cocoa butter is widely used as an ointment base, an emollient, and an ingredient in various topical cosmetic preparations.

MEDICINAL USES
Central Americans have used cocoa for centuries to treat the pains of pregnancy and childbirth, fevers, and coughs. Cocoa's primary alkaloid, theobromine, has an effect similar to that of caffeine—stimulating the muscles, heart, and kidneys—and is closely related to theophylline, which treats asthma. Accordingly, theobromine and caffeine can relieve congestion during colds by opening the bronchial passages in the lungs. Theobromine also relaxes the smooth muscle in the digestive tract. In addition, cocoa contains methylxanthines, which have a diuretic, bronchyolitic, and vasodilatory effect.

Thuja occidentalis

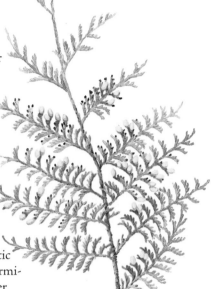

COMMON NAMES
Thuja, Arbor vitae, Swamp cedar, White cedar

LATIN NAME
Thuja occidentalis

FAMILY Coniferae

PARTS USED
Needle, branch

DESCRIPTION
Thuja is a tree reaching 30 to 60 feet tall with horizontal branches and scale-like, green needles. This aromatic evergreen tree has small terminal flowers, which are either dark brown (male) or yellow-green (female).

HABITAT
Thuja grows in Canada and the northern United States. It is cultivated as an ornamental plant in Europe.

FOLKLORE AND TRADITIONAL USES
Ancient peoples burned thuja's aromatic wood along with sacrifices. "Thuja" comes from the Latin form of the Greek word *thero* (to sacrifice). Other species of thuja were used in Egypt for embalming the dead. The botanist Carolus Clusius called the tree *arbor vitae*, Latin for "tree of life," when he saw one that had been imported from Canada to France. Native Americans used the plant for canoes, baskets, and perfumes, and sometimes boiled twigs for broth when other foods were unavailable or scarce. Oriental thuja, or *Platylactus orientalis*, has been popular in China for thousands of years, where it was cultivated for religious and ornamental purposes.

MEDICINAL USES
Native Americans employed thuja for malaria, gout, scurvy, rheumatism, menstrual disorders, and coughs. Thuja's volatile oil acts as a stimulant, a diuretic, and an irritant. Thuja is prepared as an ointment and applied externally to treat joint pain and arthritis. While the parts of the plant usually employed for therapeutic purposes are toxicologically harmless, the compound thujone can be toxic. It can cause vomiting, queasiness, painful diarrhea, and in some cases death. Thuja is used for respiratory tract infections, and in conjunction with antibiotics, in the treatment of bacterial skin infections and *Herpes simplex*. Homeopaths safely treat headache, eye inflammation, colds, and warts with thuja.

Thymus vulgaris

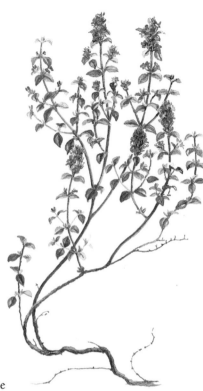

COMMON NAMES
Thyme, Wild thyme

LATIN NAMES
Thymus vulgaris (Garden thyme), *T. serpyllum* (Wild thyme)

FAMILY Labiatae

PARTS USED
Leaf, flower

DESCRIPTION
Wild thyme usually grows close to the ground in dense patches, although it can grow up to a foot tall in sheltered areas. Garden thyme grows only a few inches tall. Both have fine, hairy leaves along the stems and flowers at the tips, which are usually purple.

HABITAT
Both species of thyme grow throughout temperate parts of Europe and Asia. They thrive in well-drained or chalky soil in full sun.

FOLKLORE AND TRADITIONAL USES
Charlemagne ordered thyme grown in his gardens for its culinary and medicinal uses. In the Middle Ages noblewomen embroidered sprigs of thyme on scarves and gave them as symbols of courage to their favorite knights who were leaving for the Crusades. Shakespeare describes thyme as the home of the queen of the fairies.

MEDICINAL USES
Both varieties of thyme have the same properties. The wild thyme is slightly less potent. The aromatic oil extracted from its leaves contains thymol and carvacol, which have preservative, antibacterial, and antifungal properties. Thyme is a bronchial antispasmodic that relaxes muscles in the respiratory tract, an effect that makes it a good treatment for bronchitis and whooping cough. Thyme also relaxes smooth muscles in the gastrointestinal tract and the uterus, making it effective as a digestive aid and as a reliever of menstrual cramps. Externally, its antiseptic properties are good for small cuts. The primary ingredients in a commonly used mouthwash are thymol and eucalyptol.

Trillium erectum

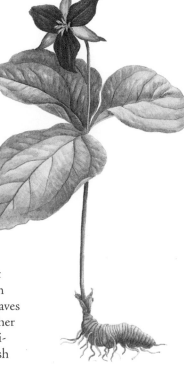

COMMON NAMES
Trillium, Bethroot, Birthroot, Wake robin, Stinking Benjamin

LATIN NAME
Trillium erectum

FAMILY Liliaceae

PARTS USED
Rhizome, root, leaf, flower

DESCRIPTION
Trillium is a perennial that grows to about 16 inches in height, with three broad leaves and one solitary flower, either white, red, or yellow. Its rhizome is yellowish to reddish brown and about the size of a thumb.

HABITAT
Native to North America, trillium grows in shady areas of woodlands.

FOLKLORE AND TRADITIONAL USES
This plant goes by several names. The origins of some, such as "bethroot" and "wake robin," are not well known. The word "trillium" is related to the word for "three" in Latin, Greek, and other languages, corresponding to the plant's three leaves. Perhaps "wake robin" comes from the red color of certain species, or perhaps because the flower blooms in spring when robins abound. The nickname "Stinking Benjamin" derives from the distinctive and unpleasant odor of the flower, which is likened to the smell of rotting meat. Whatever the plant's name, Native Americans from throughout the continent made tea from it or boiled the greens to eat. It was also a charm to foretell love, to detect witchcraft, to protect the teeth, and give general good luck.

MEDICINAL USES
The name "birthroot" signals the most famous use of this plant. Native Americans and European settlers in North America used it to help with the labor of childbirth. Other gynecologically related symptoms this plant was used to relieve included menstrual problems, sore nipples, and discomforts of menopause. Trillium is still employed for many of these same symptoms, as well as for bleeding associated with uterine fibroids. The plant was also used internally for bowel complaints and externally for headaches, sunburn, acne, and boils. Trillium contains the saponin trillin, tannin, and some essential oil.

Urtica gracilis

COMMON NAMES
Nettle, Stinging nettle

LATIN NAMES
Urtica gracilis,
U. dioica

FAMILY Urticaceae

PARTS USED
Leaf, shoot, seed, root

DESCRIPTION
Perennials, nettles grow in clumps and reach heights of about five feet. Their serrated leaves are covered with stinging hairs. The flowers are greenish white.

HABITAT
Native to Eurasia, nettles grow in temperate parts of the Northern Hemisphere.

FOLKLORE AND TRADITIONAL USES
Some believe that the word "nettle" came from "needle" because it has been used by peoples as varied as the Ainu of Japan and the Germans during World War I to make thread and cloth. Archaeologists have discovered nettle-fabric burial shrouds at Bronze Age sites in Denmark. Many Native American groups employed nettles for constructing nets and rope. The Makah rubbed nettles on hunters' bodies to protect them from the weather. They also applied nettles to the body of anyone who had touched a corpse. Many groups also rubbed them on fishing lines to ensure good fishing by removing human odor. Nettles are often cooked as a vegetable and made into soup. Even into the 20th century, England celebrated Oak and Nettle Day, during which, if a person carried an oak leaf, he or she was allowed to pass; if not, the person was stung with a nettle.

MEDICINAL USES
The nettle has been used in medicine for centuries to relieve the pain of gout and rheumatism, to treat mild acne and to eczema, to heal cuts and burns, reduce hemorrhoids, and to augment breast milk production. The nettle is rich in Vitamins A and C and in minerals, particularly iron, potassium, and silica. Modern scientific studies have focused on its diuretic action. It lowers systolic blood pressure by increasing volume, and the root treats symptoms of benign prostatic hyperplasia (BPH) by increasing urine flow and reducing residual urine. Nettle herb is also used for bladder irrigation and to prevent and treat bladder and kidney stones.

Vaccinium macrocarpon

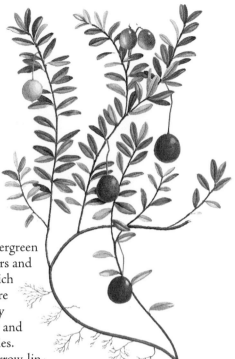

COMMON NAME
Cranberry

LATIN NAME
Vaccinium macrocarpon

FAMILY Ericaceae

PART USED
Berry

DESCRIPTION
The cranberry is an evergreen shrub with long runners and vines. The flowers, which appear in the spring, are light pink to purple. By summer they fall away and leave brilliant red berries. Leaves are tiny and narrow, lining the vines evenly.

HABITAT
The cranberry is native to North America. For best growth it requires boggy soil.

FOLKLORE AND TRADITIONAL USES
The Pilgrims in America supposedly feasted on cranberry dishes at their first Thanksgiving in 1621. Such dishes became a national tradition, however, only after General Ulysses S. Grant ordered them served to Union troops during the Civil War. Native Americans used cranberries as a source of dye. Cranberry juice cocktail is available commercially. Because pure cranberry juice is too acidic and sour to drink, water and sugar are added.

MEDICINAL USES
German researchers in the 1840s discovered that people who have eaten cranberries pass urine with hippuric acid, a bacteria-fighting chemical. Recent studies support the speculation that eating cranberries or drinking their juice can prevent or fight urinary tract infections. Hippuric acid prevents *Escherichia coli (E. coli)* from adhering to the urinary tract. Cranberries also contain arbutin, which fights yeast infections. The berries are also used as a "urinary deodorant." Native Americans are known to have treated wounds with poultices of cranberries. The Pilgrims who used these berries to treat fevers were not misguided; the berries have a high Vitamin C content.

Valeriana officinalis

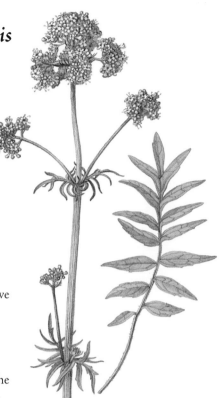

COMMON NAMES
Valerian, Setwell, Phu, All-heal

LATIN NAME
Valeriana officinalis

FAMILY Valerianaceae

PARTS USED
Root, rhizome

DESCRIPTION
Valerian is a perennial that reaches heights of three to five feet, with pairs of fernlike leaves and crowning masses of small, pale pink flowers.

HABITAT
Temperate regions around the globe are home to this plant.

FOLKLORE AND TRADITIONAL USES
Countless legends surround valerian, which was called "phu" for its foul odor in ancient times. Despite its odor, valerian was used as a potent perfume during the Middle Ages. Chaucer's "Miller's Tale" describes a character as "sweet-smelling as the root" of valerian and other herbs. Cats and other small animals are attracted to it. According to early German folklore, the Pied Piper had it squirreled away in his pocket as he lured the rats and eventually the children from Hamelin. Humans have also been attracted to it for centuries. Native Americans used its roots for food and as a flavoring in tobacco.

MEDICINAL USES
Valerian was held in such high esteem in medieval times as a remedy that it received the name "all heal." It has been used as a healing agent for cuts and boils, as an antidote for poison, and in the treatment of epilepsy. It is now primarily employed as an aid for sleep problems, nervousness, headaches, and anxiety. While there is substantial debate over the constituents responsible for valerian's sedative properties, the plant's extract has been proven in experiments with humans and animals to reduce sleeplessness and seems to have no short-term negative effects. In Germany it is the active ingredient in more than a hundred over-the-counter tranquilizers and sleep aids. Recently scientists have learned that the aqueous extract of valerian contains substantial quantities of gamma-aminobutyric acid (GABA)—a neurotransmitter that is thought to inhibit the brain's arousal system.

Vernonia amygdalina

COMMON NAMES
Bitter leaf, *Mujonso*

LATIN NAME
Vernonia amygdalina

FAMILY Asteraceae

PARTS USED
Pith, leaf, root

DESCRIPTION
Bitter leaf is a shrub or small tree that grows up to 23 feet tall. The bark is gray or brown, rough, and flaked. Its branches are brittle. Leaves are green, oblong to lance shaped, veined, and with pale soft hairs beneath. Flowers are white, small, thistly, and clustered. Fruits are small, slightly hairy nutlets.

HABITAT
Bitter leaf is indigenous to Africa, especially sub-Saharan Africa, notably Tanzania. It is usually found on the margins of cultivated fields.

**FOLKLORE
AND TRADITIONAL USES**
Called *mujonso* by the Tanzanians, bitter leaf is eaten in many parts of Africa. The leafy greens are prepared like spinach and used in soups and stews, while "chew sticks" from the root and twigs are enjoyed as an appetizer. In the form of a tonic food called *ndole*, bitter leaf is also believed to restore stamina.

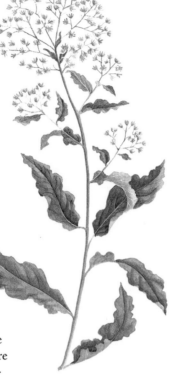

MEDICINAL USES
In the Mahale Mountains National Park in Tanzania, studies have shown that chimpanzees chew the pith of bitter leaf for its antiparasitic and other medicinal properties. African people also use the plant to treat intestinal parasite infestation. Their traditional healers may have studied the behavior of sick animals. Bitter leaf's active constituents are steroid glycosides (type vernonioside B_1), which possess antiparasitic, antitumoral, and antibacterial agents. Used primarily to treat schistosomiasis, a disease caused by parasitic worms, bitter leaf concurrently relieves related problems such as diarrhea and malaise. In sub-Saharan Africa, bitter leaf treats 25 more ailments, including fever, intestinal complaints, and malaria.

Viburnum prunifolium

COMMON NAMES
Black haw, Snowball tree, King's crown, Cramp bark

LATIN NAME
Viburnum prunifolium

FAMILY Caprifoliaceae

PART USED
Bark

DESCRIPTION
This deciduous tree or shrub grows 5 to 15 feet tall, with grooved branches and red-brown bark, flat-topped white flowers, and shiny, blue-black, juicy berries.

HABITAT
Native to the United States, black haw grows as a shrub in northern areas and as a small tree in southern areas.

**FOLKLORE
AND TRADITIONAL USES**
Native Americans made the fruit of black haw into jams and used the stems in baskets. Southern slave owners coercively gave female slaves black haw to increase the production of slave children. This use is mentioned in *King's American Dispensatory*, a 19th-century medical text used by doctors who called their group the Eclectic movement: "It was customary for planters to compel female slaves to drink an infusion of black haw daily whilst pregnant to prevent abortion…."

MEDICINAL USES
Native American women took black haw for medicinal purposes long before the European settlement of North America. They drank decoctions of black haw bark to treat menopause and menstrual cramps, to ease pains following childbirth, and to prevent miscarriage. Related species were used to treat ailments ranging from blood disorders to migraines. Highly valued by the Eclectics, black haw bark soothes irritation in the womb, making this herb a potent aid for women with histories of pregnancy difficulties. Black haw contains scopoletin, a uterine relaxant, perhaps verifying its traditional uses. This bark continues to be popular among modern herbalists.

Vinca rosea

COMMON NAME
Rosy periwinkle

LATIN NAME
Vinca rosea

FAMILY Apocynaceae

PART USED
Whole plant

DESCRIPTION
A perennial subshrub with many branches, rosy periwinkle grows up to two and a half feet tall. Leaves are oval and have a glossy surface. The five-lobed flowers are usually white or light pink. The long seedpods are cylindrical and have a downy texture.

HABITAT
Rosy periwinkle is native to Madagascar, but it has been naturalized worldwide. Other species of the plant are native to the Mediterranean region.

FOLKLORE AND TRADITIONAL USES
Periwinkle was called "sorcerer's violet" by the French, in reference to its use in charms and love potions. Europeans also believed that periwinkle had the power to exorcise evil spirits. Medieval Europeans used it frequently in garlands to protect the bearer. The Italians placed garlands of the plant on the graves of infants, calling it the flower of death. During the Enlightenment in Europe, the French considered periwinkle an emblem of friendship.

MEDICINAL USES
Periwinkle has been used for health problems ranging from memory loss to toothache and from circulatory disorders to intestinal inflammation. Although its effectiveness in treating all these ailments has not been proved, periwinkle has been shown to lower blood sugar and to act as a diuretic. In testing the plant as a drug source for diabetes in the 1950s, an extract was found that proved successful in treating juvenile leukemia, Hodgkin's disease, and other cancers that were previously considered largely incurable. The main alkaloids, vinblastine and vincristine, appear to bind to proteins in some microtubules, facilitating cancer-cell death.

Zingiber officinale

COMMON NAME
Ginger

LATIN NAME
Zingiber officinale

FAMILY Zingiberaceae

PART USED
Root

DESCRIPTION
A perennial herb, ginger extends underground in tuberous joints. In spring it sprouts a green stem up to three feet tall. It has narrow, lance-shaped leaves and yellow and purple flowers.

HABITAT
Ginger is indigenous to Southeast Asia. It is also cultivated in other parts of Asia, Africa, the Caribbean, and other tropical climates. It does best in well-watered soil in partial shade.

FOLKLORE AND TRADITIONAL USES
To facilitate digestion, ancient Greeks wrapped ginger in bread, a practice that evolved into today's gingerbread. Ginger has been associated with red-haired people, who are often labeled hot-tempered. This may be a reflection of the medieval belief that ginger induces liveliness.

MEDICINAL USES
The *Pen Tsao Chung* (3000 B.C.), China's first great herbal, recommended ginger for colds, fever, tetanus, and leprosy. In ancient India, ginger was called *vishwabhesaj,* "the universal medicine." It is commonly used to treat motion sickness and vertigo. Although its specific action is currently unknown, ginger may act directly on the gastrointestinal system, or it may affect the part of the central nervous system that causes nausea. Ginger is also employed to treat indigestion, flu and colds, and arthritis. Its primary constituents, gingerols and shogaol, soothe abdominal cramps and increase intestinal muscle contractions, while the proteolytic enzyme, zingibain, breaks down protein. Gingerols and shogaols also reduce pain and fever, suppress coughs, and have a mild sedative effect. The constituent sesquiterone has a specific action against the most common family of colds, rhinoviruses. Zingibain also displays anti-inflammatory properties, as do ginger's 12 antioxidant compounds.

The terms listed here are defined in reference to plant-based medicine. In some instances they are newly coined words or words whose new meanings reflect a growing understanding of medicinal plants and their importance. To find terms in the book's text, check the Index.

Active agent (compound, element, molecule, substance)
any single, isolatable, bioactive substance that has an identifiable pharmaceutical action.

Alkaloid
an organic compound constructed around a ring of nitrogen atoms; the active agent in many plant-based pharmaceutical drugs. (See also **Secondary metabolite**.)

Allopathy
the name given to mainstream medicine by Samuel Hahnemann, founder of homeopathy.

Alternative medicine
a term applied to medical therapies that lack generally accepted methods of scientific validation. Most treat the body holistically by addressing the interplay of emotional, psychological, and physical factors.

Antioxidant
compound that neutralizes free radicals (oxidants).

Ayurvedic medicine
the ancient Indian system of maintaining health and fighting disease based upon equilibrium with nature; utilizes thousands of plants.

Bioactive
having an effect on living organisms.

Bioavailability
a measure of the degree to which a medically active substance affects the body.

Biochemical farming
chemical-farming techniques that manipulate a plant's chemistry, causing it to produce desired compounds of consistent quality and composition.

Biodiversity
the diversity of living organisms on Earth.

Biopiracy
cultural and commercial exploitation by outsiders of indigenous peoples' knowledge and resources.

Botanical or herbal medicine or remedy
plant-derived substances used for medicinal purposes. Also called botanicals and herbals.

Carcinogens
various agents—including viruses, chemicals, and radiation—that cause cancer.

Cell line
permanently established cell cultures that can be grown indefinitely in a laboratory environment; used to screen plants for bioactive compounds.

Chemical prospecting
the search for bioactive substances in plants and other organic compounds and the subsequent random assessment of their effectiveness on various human diseases.

Combinatorial
describes a pharmaceutical research technique whereby researchers combine known compounds to create new bioactive substances.

Detoxifier
an organic disease-preventing compound that diminishes or removes the poisonous quality of any substance through excretion or chemical transformation.

Doctrine of signatures
a theory upholding that the Creator (or creators) gave plants signs of their medicinal usefulness based on supposed anatomical resemblance to the human body part to be treated.

Ethnobotany
the systematic study of a society's knowledge about locally available plants and their use in medicine, food, agriculture, clothing, and rituals.

Extract
a concentrated preparation of bioactive substances taken from plants.

Flavonoids
water-soluble pigments that serve plants as secondary metabolites and that help maintain the walls of small blood vessels in humans.

Folk/Indigenous/Native/ Traditional medicine/ Remedy
terms used, often interchangeably, to denote household, indigenous, or traditional systems of healing; often these systems date back to antiquity. Most rely on plant-based medicines. (See also **Herbalism**.)

Free radical (oxidant)
the highly reactive molecule that is produced when cells burn oxygen to create energy; can cause clogged arteries, cancer, diabetes, cataracts, and mental decline.

Galenic medicine
a theory that health comes from achieving a balance of humors (fluids) within the human body. Imbalance, or illness, was usually treated with plant-based purgative medicines; dominated Western medical thinking for approximately 2,000 years before falling out of favor after the emergence of modern science. (See also **Humors**.)

Glycoside
an organic substance consisting of a carbohydrate molecule and convertible into sugar. Cardiac glycosides are used to stimulate the heart. Glycosides are secondary metabolites known as terpenoids.

Herb
a seed-producing nonwoody plant—an annual, biennial, or perennial—that dies back at the end of the growing season. The term is often applied generally to any plant of medicinal value.

Herbalism
a therapy that uses plants and plant-derived substances to treat illnesses and maintain health.

Herbal medicine
See **Botanical medicine**.

Heroic medicine
aggressive treatments—such as bleeding, blistering, and inducing vomiting, sweating, and diarrhea—used in premodern Western medicine.

Homeopathy
an approach to medicine founded by Samuel Hahnemann in the 19th century that uses infinitesimal dilutions of medicinal substances, including many from plants, to treat illness.

Humors
the four supposed bodily fluids—blood, phlegm, yellow bile, and black bile—that dominated Galenic medicine. (See also **Galenic medicine.**)

Lead compound
any substance, most often taken from plants and other natural sources, that is known to be bioactive and leads pharmaceutical researchers to devise or discover structurally similar compounds.

Medicine man/Shaman/ Traditional healer
terms used, often interchangeably, to denote a person who is skilled in the use of plants and other natural substances and in the rituals of medicine and healing.

Mineral
an inorganic substance with a distinctive internal crystalline structure.

Modern medicine
a product of an approach to medicine that began with the scientific revolution in Europe in the 15th to 17th centuries and continues into the 21st century. It asserts that medicine should be based on objective, empirical research and experimentation; also called Western medicine.

Molecule
the smallest unit a pure substance can be divided into without losing its defining chemical composition and properties.

Multimodality
the concurrent use of several different treatments, including prescribing more than one medicine to be taken at the same time; often involves combinations of drugs that act in different ways on various parts of the body; often called polypharmacy.

Naturopathy
an approach to medicine that focuses on herbs, nontoxic chemicals, and other natural means such as diet and exercise to stimulate and support the body's inherent power to regain health; draws upon Chinese, Greek, and other approaches to healing.

Nutriceutical
also spelled **nutraceutical**— any substance found in fruits and vegetables that may have minimal or no nutritive value but which helps prevent and treat disease.

Oxidant
See **Free radical.**

Pharmaceutical drug
a medicine based on a single bioactive compound approved by a government agency; dispensed only with a physician's prescription; a product of modern scientific research.

Pharmacopoeia
an officially sanctioned book that lists pharmaceutical compounds and standards for their strength, quality, and preparation. Most countries have their own pharmacopoeia.

Phytoestrogens
plant chemicals that are structurally similar to estrogen and can help lower cholesterol levels, prevent osteoporosis, and provide protection against cancer.

Phytosecretions
chemicals produced by plants.

Placebo
a medicine that lacks any known pharmacological effect but which may provide psychological relief or trigger the patient's own healing mechanisms; usually prescribed to a control group as part of a placebo double-blind experiment.

Polypharmacy
See **Multimodality.**

Prescription drug
See **Pharmaceutical drug.**

Primary metabolite
any compound produced by a plant's metabolism that is essential to cell survival. Functions include giving plants the ability to absorb food and nutrients and reproduce.

Reductionism
the approach that holds that human health, among other things, can be reduced to isolated, mechanical, cause-and-effect operations and principles.

Screening
testing a complex substance such as a chemical derived from a plant to see whether it has any effect on living cells, especially those with a particular disease.

Secondary metabolite
any compound produced by a plant's metabolism that is not essential to cell survival. Functions include defense against predators. The three largest groups of secondary metabolites are alkaloids, phenolics, and terpenoids.

Semisynthetic drug
a drug that is made in the laboratory and is based in part on a chemical formula found in nature.

Single active agent (also compound, molecule, element, or substance)
See **Active agent.**

Synthetic drug
an artificially constructed drug; synthesized versions of natural compounds, e.g. synthetic salicylic acid, are still considered "natural" and not "synthetic" when analyzing the source of drugs.

Tincture
a solution of nonvolatile substances extracted from a plant and put in alcohol or a mixture of water and alcohol.

Traditional healer
See **Medicine man.**

Traditional medicine/ remedy
See **Folk medicine/remedy.**

U.S. Pharmacopoeia
the not-for-profit organization of scientists, physicians, pharmacists, and others interested in health care that produces the *Pharmacopoeia of the United States.* (See also **Pharmacopoeia.**)

Western medicine
See **Modern medicine.**

ADDITIONAL READING

The reader may wish to consult the *National Geographic Index* for related articles, particularly "Nature's Rx" in the April 2000 issue of NATIONAL GEOGRAPHIC. The following sources may also be of interest:

General Reference

Lonnelle Aikman, *Nature's Healing Arts*, 1977; Wade Boyle, *Botanical Substances in the United States Pharmacopoeias 1820-1990*, 1991; Stephen Cummings and Dana Ullman, *Everybody's Guide to Homeopathic Medicines*, 1997; Lawrence Greene, et al., *Adaptation to Malaria*, 1997; Alfred G. Gilman, et al., eds., *Goodman & Gilman's The Pharmacological Basis of Therapeutics*, 1996; Walter H. Lewis, *Medical Botany*, 1971; Robert S. McCaleb, *Encyclopedia of Popular Herbs: An Authoritative Guide to the 40 Most Effective Medicinal Plants*, 1999; Peter Raven, Ray F. Evert, and Susan E. Eichorn, *Biology of Plants*, 1999; J. E. Robbers and Varro E. Tyler, *Tyler's Herbs of Choice: The Therapeutic Use of Phytomedicals*, 1999; Richard Evans Schultes and Siri Von Ries, eds., *Ethnobotany: Evolution of a Discipline*, 1995; Volkmar Schulz, R. Haensel, and Varro E. Tyler, *Rational Phytotherapy: A Physician's Guide to Herbal Medicine*, 1998.

Chinese and Ayurvedic Medicines

Harriet Beinfield and Efrem Korngold, *Between Heaven and Earth: A Guide to Chinese Medicine*, 1991; R. N. Chopra, *Indigenous Drugs of India*, 1994; John D. Keys, *Chinese Herbs: Botany, Chemistry, and Pharmacodynamics*, 1976; Joseph Needham, *Science and Civilization in China* (multi volumes), 1974; Vivek Shanbhag, *A Beginner's Introduction to Ayurvedic Medicine*, 1994; Harmi Sharma and Christopher Clark, *Contemporary Ayurveda*, 1998; K. Chimin Wong and Wu Lien-Teh, *History of Chinese Medicine*, 1973.

History of Medicine and Pharmacology

George A. Bender, *Great Moments in Pharmacy*, 1966; Charles J. Brim, *Medicine in the Bible*, 1936; David Burnie, *Plant*, 1989; Eldon G. Chuinard, *Only One Man Died: The Medical Aspects of the Lewis and Clark Expedition*, 1995; Lawrence I. Conrad, et al., *The Western Medical Tradition: 800 B.C. to A.D. 1800*, 1995; David L. Cowen and William H. Helfland, *Pharmacy: An Illustrated History*, 1990; Jordan Goodman, *Tobacco in History*, 1993; Barbara Griggs, *Green Pharmacy*, 1993; Wolfgang-Hagen Hein, ed., *Botanical Drugs of the Americas in the New and Old World*, 1983; B. Holmstedt and G. Liljestrand, eds., *Readings in Pharmacology*, 1963; Saul Jarcho, *Quinine's Predecessor: Francesco Torti and the Early History of Cinchona*, 1993; Joan Lane, *John Hall and his Patients*, 1996; Albert Lyons and R. Joseph Petrucelli, *Medicine: An Illustrated History*, 1978; Nicholas Monardes, *Joyful Newes Out of the New Founde World*, 1925; A. G. Morton, *History of Botanical Science*, 1981; Roy Porter, *The Greatest Benefit to Mankind: A Medical History of Humanity*, 1997; H. H. Rusby, *Jungle Memories*, 1933; Arthur and Elaine Shapiro, *The Powerful Placebo: From Ancient Priest to Modern Physician*, 1997; Henry E. Sigerist, *A History of Medicine (Vols. 1 & 2)*, 1987; Varro E. Tyler and James E. Robbers, *Pharmacognosy and Pharmacobiotechnology*, 1996; William Withering, *An Account of the Foxglove*, 1785.

Medicines From Traditional Cultures

Wade Davis, *Shadows in the Sun*, 1998; Food and Agricultural Organization of the United Nations, *Medicinal Plants for Forest Conservation and Healthcare*, 1997; Daniel E. Moerman, *Native American Ethnobotany*, 1998; Mark J. Plotkin, *Tales of a Shaman's Apprentice*, 1998.

Herbs and the Healing Power of Fruits and Vegetables

Mark Blumenthal, ed., *The Complete German Commission E Monographs: Therapeutic Guide to Herbal Medicines*, 1998; Lesley Bremness, *Herbs: The Visual Guide to More Than 700 Herb Species From Around the World*, 1994; Jean Carper, *Food—Your Miracle Medicine*, 1998; Andrew Chevallier, *The Encyclopedia of Medicinal Plants*, 1996; James A. Duke, *The Green Pharmacy*, 1997; Facts and Comparisons, *The Review of Natural Products*, 1998; Mitchell Gaynor and Jerry Hickey, *Dr. Gaynor's Cancer Prevention Program*, 1999; Maud Grieve, *A Modern Herbal*, 1931; *Physicians' Desk Reference, PDR for Herbal Medicines*, 1998; World Cancer Research Fund, American Cancer Institute, *Food, Nutrition and the Prevention of Cancer*, 1997; World Health Organization, *Monographs on Selected Medicinal Plants*, 1999.

Drug Regulation and Legal Issues

Harry M. Marks, *The Progress of Experiment*, 1977; Vandana Shiva, *Biopiracy, The Plunder of Nature and Knowledge*, 1997; James Harvey Young, *The Medical Messiahs: A Social History of Health Quackery in Twentieth-Century America*, 1967, and *The Toadstool Millionaires—A Social History of Patent Medicines in America before Federal Regulation*, 1961.

INTERNET RESOURCES

The sites listed below provide useful starting points for additional research of medicinal plants. Some sites may be best for directed research focused on specific topics, while others will probably be more helpful to those seeking general information. Web addresses and website content are subject to change.

Information on Specific Plants and Herbs

American Botanical Council
www.herbalgram.org
Plans to post selections from *The Complete German Commission E Monographs: Therapeutic Guide to Herbal Medicines*, which lists uses, indications, actions, dosage, and side effects for hundreds of approved medicinal herbs.

A Modern Herbal
www.botanical.com
Contains a hyper-text version of Maud Grieve's 1931 work, *A Modern Herbal*, which describes more than 800 medicinal, cosmetic, and culinary herbs. It also provides information on their physical properties, folklore, medicinal uses, and cultivation. This site has links to other plant reference materials.

Herbal Materia Medica
www.healthy.net/clinic/ therapy/herbal/herbic/ herbs/index.html
Offers details on more than 150 medicinal herbs.

Plant Explorer
www.iversonsoftware.com/ business/plant/index.htm
Gives detailed descriptions of more than 800 plants and an overview of the plant kingdom.

Rx List
www.rxlist.com
Provides detailed information about herbal and pharmaceutical drugs, lists of the most frequently prescribed drugs, and answers to frequently asked questions about alternative medicine.

The Complete Herbal (The English Physician)
www.bibliomania.com/ NonFiction/Culpeper/ Herbal or
www.med.yale.edu/library/ historical/culpeper/ culpeper.htm
This classic work, used as a touchstone for herbal practitioners, has been widely reprinted over the past 350 years. In it, 17th-century English physician Nicholas Culpeper attempts to provide remedies through easily available herbs.

Reference Materials and Search Engines

National Library of Medicine
www.nlm.nih.gov
Official website of one of the world's largest medical libraries, located in Bethesda, Maryland, and home to MEDLINE, a searchable database of 11 million abstracts and references from 4,300 biomedical journals. An ideal starting point for directed medical research,

the site also provides a directory of health organizations, an online catalog of journals, books, and audiovisual sources currently in National Library of Medicine collections, and information on biomedical research programs.

Gardenweb
www.gardenweb.com
Provides access to a number of plant-related resources, including a searchable online dictionary of botanical terms.

Plantlink
www.plantamerica.org/ palink.htm
This comprehensive plant search engine automatically searches other major search engines, including AltaVista, Excite, Look-Smart, Lycos, the Mining Co., Thunderstone, and Yahoo! It also allows users to search for websites related to specific plants. Users can search by a plant's scientific, family, or common name. In addition to the search engine, this site provides links to national associations, university departments, government agencies, botanical gardens, and other miscellaneous websites that offer information on plants.

Medicinal Herb FAQ
metalab.unc.edu/ herbmed/mediherb.html
Gives answers to many frequently asked questions on herbal medicine as well as links to mailing lists and other resources.

Botanical Bookmarks
www.graylab.ac.uk/usr/ hodgkiss/botanic.html
Provides links to a number of useful resources on various plant species, botany, biodiversity, and conservation.

Discussion Group

Ethnobotany Café
countrylife.net/ ethnobotany
This site is an online forum for discussion of plants and their uses in different cultures.

Institutions

Royal Botanic Gardens, Kew
www.rbgkew.org.uk

New York Botanical Gardens
www.nybg.org

Missouri Botanical Garden
www.mobot.org

NOTES ON CONTRIBUTORS

Joel L. Swerdlow has written about medical topics for National Geographic since 1991. *Nature's Medicine* builds upon his article "Nature's Rx," which appears in the April 2000 issue of NATIONAL GEOGRAPHIC. Swerdlow is the author of a novel and more than a half-dozen nonfiction books, one of which was made into an NBC movie. He has written for the *Atlantic, Harper's, Rolling Stone,* and numerous other magazines. Before joining the NATIONAL GEOGRAPHIC staff in 1991, he was a visiting professor at Georgetown University and a guest scholar at the Woodrow Wilson International Center in Washington, D.C. His work has been translated into more than three dozen languages.

Lynn Johnson is known for her sensitive documentary photography in both color and black and white. The winner of numerous photography and photojournalism awards, she has produced photo essays for NATIONAL GEOGRAPHIC, *Life, Sports Illustrated, Smithsonian,* and other magazines. Her most recent book is *We Remember: Women Born at the Turn of the Century.* Johnson earned a B.A. in photographic illustration and photojournalism from Rochester Institute of Technology in 1975. Committed to developing

the talent of young photographers, she teaches at the Eddie Adams Workshop and has established a workshop for photography students in coordination with Ithaca College.

Jane Watkins was born in Somerset, England, where she now lives with her two children. She has been selling and exhibiting her botanical paintings for ten years, and has completed assignments for several organizations, including the National Geographic Society. *The Royal Mail* has recently commissioned Watkins to paint roses for the Queen Mother's 100th-birthday commemorative stamp collection.

Mary E. Eaton painted 672 botanical watercolors for the National Geographic Society between 1915 and 1928. Although then NATIONAL GEOGRAPHIC editor Gilbert H. Grosvenor considered Eaton's work "exquisitely beautiful," he was willing to pay only $12.50 per painting. In 1926, the Society agreed to increase her payment to $15 but attempted to make up the difference by offering only $10 for paintings of less colorful specimens. When Eaton complained that "the less colorful subjects take as long to paint—sometimes longer," the Society wisely reconsidered and agreed to meet her price.

AUTHOR'S ACKNOWLEDGMENTS

Nature's Medicine: Plants That Heal reflects the intelligence, imagination, hard work, wisdom, and commitment of many people.

Prime among them is my wife, Marjorie L. Share, who has a habit of asking questions that go beyond accepted wisdom—and a way of being ahead of her time. For years, she's been studying herbs, finding what works, and talking about possibilities that Western science does not yet understand. On her advice, I embarked upon writing this book (and the NATIONAL GEOGRAPHIC article upon which it is built), and her insights and suggestions enhanced every stage of both projects. In this, as in so many other things, she changed the way I see the world.

Bill Allen, Editor of NATIONAL GEOGRAPHIC, is committed to coverage of science and health issues. He and Bob Poole, Associate Editor, gave the support that made this book possible. Also deserving special mention is Michele Callaghan, who assisted in editing the Plant Profiles section, wrote a large number of the profiles, and contributed to this book far beyond the call of official duty. Her insights and persistence, as well as her research, writing, and editing abilities made huge contributions throughout. When the

work had to be done, she got it done to the highest standards. And what's even more important: During our years of working together Michele has provided a living lesson in friendship.

Wisdom, work, and energy also came from many people on the magazine staff (with a sprinkling of people in other divisions of the Society) including (here, and in what follows, everyone is listed in alphabetical order) Kevin Craig, Hugh Grindstaff, Davida Kales, Tom O'Neill, Bob Radzyminski, Heidi Schultz, Heidi Splete, Charlene Valeri, and Susan Welchman; and staff from the National Geographic Library, including Ann Benson, Chuck Brady, Ellie Briscoe, Janet Dombrowski, Elaine Donnelly, Susan Eaton, Barbara Ferry, Nancy Majkowski, Tim Schoepke, Cassandra Shieh, and Mike Terry—without whom many pages of this book would have been blank.

The extraordinary and talented employees of the National Geographic Book Division and freelances who contributed to this book worked hard—with style, a sense of humor, and high standards of excellence. I am especially indebted to Bonnie Lawrence for laying the groundwork for the project; Barbara Payne for her faith in and support of the work; Marty Christian for her brilliance in assembling and refining all the pieces of the book and helping everyone do a better job; Toni Eugene for her patience and talent as the editor of the text and captions; John Agnone for selecting photographs that capture the majesty and complexity of medicinal plants; Lyle Rosbotham for designing a logical and aesthetic layout that encourages people to read the book; Sallie Greenwood, Winfield Swanson, and Marilynh "Minh" Le for their good spirits and capacity to absorb huge amounts of information while ensuring the accuracy of even the most technical details; Alexander Cohn, Dale Herring, and Mary Jennings for researching the art; and Linda Averitt for her fresh eye and editorial skill as a final reader.

Lynn Johnson, an exceptionally talented photographer, gave these pages an amazing and evocative visual grace. She also contributed much of the material used in the photo captions.

Experts (many of whom are affiliated with preeminent research and medical institutions) who contributed their knowledge and wisdom include Patch Adams, Izzy Alter, Clifford Bailey, Doug Beech, Dina Berlin, David Berrisford, Mark Blumenthal, Gerry Bodeker, Robert Bud, Mike Domanski, Jim Duke, Cecelia W. Enns, Nina Etkin, David Friedman, Gerard Geison, Frank Gonzalez, Anita Goodman, Francesca Grifo, Robert Grupp, JoAnn Gutin, Michael Huffman, Martha Kent, Shiyou Li, Harry Marks, Peter Martin, Jim Miller, Brent Mishler, Daniel Nebert, David Newman (who was extraordinarily generous), Anne Niemiec, Nat Quansah, Martin Raff, Ilya Raskin, David Reeve, Harant Semerjian, Monique Simmons, Dennis Stevenson, Kathleen Thomas, Dale Tussing, David Warrell, Merlin Wilcox, and Robert Wright.

Also, representatives from the following institutions provided valuable assistance: American Botanical Council, American Medical Association, Facts and Comparisons (*The Review of Natural Products*), the Food and Drug Administration, GIFTS, Merck, Missouri Botanical Garden, National Cancer Institute, Paracelsian, Pfizer, PhRMA, Smile Herb Shop, United States Pharmacopoeia, and Warner-Lambert/Parke-Davis. All of them may not agree with all of the assertions and analyses in *Nature's Medicine*, but they helped educate me.

Friends who helped included Daniel Callaghan, Dennis Callaghan, Emily Callaghan, Karen Jaffe, Jannie Kinney, Frank Kress, Donna Melville, Joy Midman, Matt Schneider, and Erla Zwingle.

Substantive contributions came from various members of my family including my mother, Professor Gertrude K. Swerdlow; my sister and brother-in-law, Jo Betty Swerdlow, M.D., and Harry Sommer; and my two sons, Paul Z. Swerdlow and Aaron B. Swerdlow. Aaron's contribution is especially worthy of note. At age 16 he wrote first, and very near final, drafts of some of the captions—then worked on rewrites with patience and diligence.

The most exciting group to work with were the young people who provided the energetic heart of this book. Among them were Leah Boonthanom-Perrilloux (who made special contributions to the Plant Profiles and Glossary), Andy Brashear, Ben Brazil, and Samuel Chernawsky, all of whom researched large sections of the book. All are college students or recent college graduates who brought intelligence, humor, and fresh perspectives to every chapter. Most amazing among these extremely impressive young people were Colby University senior Kate Harrington, who worked with me for four months and made me wish she would come work at the Society full-time; and Ari Johnson, who was a 14-year-old high school freshman when we began to work together and is graduating as this book goes to press. In my opinion Ari's skills as a researcher, writer, and editor already approach—and in many cases have achieved—professional levels. With such young people, the future is in good hands.

For the many friendships that have developed, thank you. I am enriched and look forward to more adventures together. I hope that I have overlooked no one, and for any oversight I apologize. All the errors and shortcomings in this book are my own.

BOOK DIVISION ACKNOWLEDGMENTS

The Book Division acknowledges the invaluable assistance of contributing editor Bonnie S. Lawrence at the project's inception and the editorial skills of consulting editor Carolinda E. Averitt near the book's completion. We also recognize the major contribution, particularly on the Plant Profiles, of our general consultant Mark Blumenthal, director of the American Botanical Council. In addition, we extend thanks to our many colleagues at the Society who, through their cooperation and assistance, helped make this book a reality. Most particularly, we acknowledge the NATIONAL GEOGRAPHIC magazine, the Library, the Indexing division under manager Anne Marie Houppert's steady hand, and the document reproduction center.

NATURE'S MEDICINE
Plants That Heal

By Joel L. Swerdlow
Photographs by Lynn Johnson

Published by the National Geographic Society

John M. Fahey, Jr., *President and Chief Executive Officer*
Gilbert M. Grosvenor, *Chairman of the Board*
Nina D. Hoffman, *Senior Vice President*

Prepared by the Book Division

William R. Gray, *Vice President and Director*
Charles Kogod, *Assistant Director*
Barbara A. Payne, *Editorial Director and Managing Editor*
David Griffin, *Design Director*

Staff for This Book

Martha Crawford Christian, *Editor*
Toni Eugene, *Text Editor*
John Agnone, *Illustrations Editor*
Lyle Rosbotham, *Art Director*
Sallie M. Greenwood, *Senior Researcher*
Winfield Swanson, *Researcher*

Staff for Plant Profiles

Michele Tussing Callaghan, *Assistant Editor,
Contributing Writer, and Researcher*
Marilynh "Minh" Le, *Researcher*
Leah Boonthanom-Perrilloux, Katherine L. Harrington,
and Ari Johnson, *Research Assistants and Contributing Writers*
Alexander L. Cohn, Dale-Marie Herring,
and Mary Jennings, *Art Research Assistants*

R. Gary Colbert, *Production Director*
Lewis R. Bassford, *Production Project Manager*
Janet Dustin, *Illustrations Assistant*
Peggy Candore, *Assistant to the Director*
Kathleen Barber, *Indexer*

Manufacturing and Quality Control

George V. White, *Director*
John T. Dunn, *Associate Director*
Vincent P. Ryan, *Manager*
Phillip L. Schlosser, *Financial Analyst*

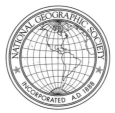

The world's largest nonprofit scientific and educational organization, the National Geographic Society was founded in 1888 "for the increase and diffusion of geographic knowledge." Since then it has supported scientific exploration and spread information to its more than nine million members worldwide.

The National Geographic Society educates and inspires millions every day through magazines, books, television programs, videos, maps and atlases, research grants, the National Geography Bee, teacher workshops, and innovative classroom materials.

The Society is supported through membership dues and income from the sale of its educational products. Members receive NATIONAL GEOGRAPHIC magazine—the Society's official journal—discounts on Society products, and other benefits.

For more information about the National Geographic Society and its educational programs and publications, please call 1-800-NGS-LINE (647-5463), or write to the following address:

National Geographic Society
1145 17th Street N.W.
Washington, D.C. 20036-4688 U.S.A.

Visit the Society's website at www.nationalgeographic.com.

Composition for this book by the National Geographic Society Book Division. Printed and bound by Quad/Graphics, West Allis, Wisconsin. Color separations by Digital Color Image, Pennsauken, New Jersey. Dust jacket printed by the Miken Co., Cheektowaga, New York.

Portions of this book appeared in a different form in the April 2000 NATIONAL GEOGRAPHIC magazine.

Lines reprinted on pages 314-315 are from *You're Only Old Once!* by Dr. Seuss. Copyright © 1986 by Dr. Seuss Enterprises, L.P. Reprinted by permission of Random House Children's Books, a division of Random House, Inc.

Library of Congress Cataloging-in-Publication Data
Swerdlow, Joel L.
    Nature's medicine : a chronicle of mankind's search for healing plants through the ages / Joel L. Swerdlow ; photographs by Lynn Johnson.
        p. cm.
    Includes bibliographical references and index.
    ISBN 0-7922-7586-1(reg.)—ISBN 0-7922-7587-X (dlx.)
        1. Materia medica, Vegetable. 2. Medicinal plants. 3. Pharmacognosy.
    I. Title

RS164 .S947 2000
615'.32—dc21   99-089037
                                                                    CIP